Immunoassays

The Practical Approach Series

Related **Practical Approach** Series Titles

Flow Cytometry 3e*

Monoclonal Antibodies

Spectrophotometry and
Spectrofluorimetry

Immunodiagnostics

Lymphocytes 2e

Immobilized Biomolecules in
Analysis

Gel Electrophoresis of
Proteins 3e

Complement

MHC 1

MHC 2

Affinity Separations

Immunochemistry I

Immunochemistry II

Protein Function 2e

Protein Structure 2e

Antibody Engineering

Platelets

HIV Volume I

HIV Volume II

Non-isotopic Methods
in Molecular Biology

Enzyme Assays

* indicates a forthcoming title

Please see the **Practical Approach** series website at
http://www.oup.co.uk/pas
for full contents lists of all Practical Approach titles.

Immunoassays

A Practical Approach

Edited by

James P. Gosling

Department of Biochemistry and National
Diagnostic Centre, National University of
Ireland Gallway

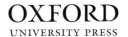

OXFORD
UNIVERSITY PRESS

OXFORD
UNIVERSITY PRESS

Great Clarendon Street, Oxford OX2 6DP

Oxford University Press is a department of the University of Oxford.
It furthers the University's objective of excellence in research,
scholarship, and education by publishing worldwide in

Oxford New York

Athens Auckland Bangkok Bogotá Buenos Aires Calcutta Cape Town
Chennai Dar es Salaam Delhi Florence Hong Kong Istanbul Karachi
Kuala Lumpur Madrid Melbourne Mexico City Mumbai Nairobi Paris
São Paulo Singapore Taipei Tokyo Toronto Warsaw

with associated companies in Berlin Ibadan

Oxford is a registered trade mark of Oxford University Press in the UK
and in certain other countries

Published in the United States by Oxford University Press Inc., New York

British Library Cataloguing in Publication Data
Data available

Library of Congress Cataloguing in Publication Data

1 3 5 7 9 10 8 6 4 2

ISBN 0-19-963711-3 (Hbk.)
ISBN 0-19-963710-5 (Pbk.)

Typeset in Swift by Footnote Graphics, Warminster, Wilts
Printed in Great Britain on acid-free paper
by The Bath Press, Bath, Avon

Preface

It is in the last 30 years that measurement methods based on the specific recognition of analytes by binding proteins and oligonucleotides have become so important that such binding may be regarded as a fundamental analytical principle, equivalent in importance to those underlying spectrophotometry and chromatography. Measurement procedures that use antibodies as specific binding reagents are termed immunoassays, as are assays that use antigens for the measurement of specific antibodies.

Immunoassays were first applied to proteins and other natural antigens but, since antibodies can be raised against all molecules with immunologically distinctive characteristics, they are now used to measure an enormous range of steroids, drugs, peptides, sugars, vitamins, molecular complexes, viral particles and cells. Immunoassays are essential to routine measurements in all areas of pure and applied biology and chemistry. Without immunoassays (and their efficient exploitation of the tight and specific binding of antibodies and antigens) these measurements would be much more complex, or even impracticable.

Many books on immunoassay have been published but this may be the first comprehensive immunoassay manual designed to help those in any of the biological and chemical sciences develop any type of immunoassay for any suitable analyte. The 10 chapters progress from considerations of assay design, to the preparation of components, to the development of assays and, finally to their proper operation.

Chapter 1 is a general introduction that describes immunoglobulins, explains antigen–antibody binding and surveys the wide choice of immunoassay designs and formats. Chapters 2-6 discuss assay components, their preparation, characterization, storage and commercial availability. All are comprehensive and attempt to meet the needs of most if not all assay developers, whatever the intended assay design (label-free, sandwich or competitive), label type or application (hapten, protein or specific antibody).

Chapters 7-9 are concerned with assembling the components to give a valid assay and using that assay to generate true results. Optimization is defined broadly so as to include the elimination of interference and the improvement of accuracy, as well as the minimization of imprecision and detection limits.

Comprehensive and thorough validation procedures are described for both quantitative and qualitative assays. Chapter 9 may be the first ever explanation of immunoassay data processing that meets the needs of both occasional and regular users of immunoassays.

An assay is only as good as its results and Chapter 10 provides all the information and procedures needed to assess and control any quantitative immunoassay whatever its analytical goals. It may be particularly suited to developers of assays for *new* analytes since it also explains, in simple terms, how comparability of results may be monitored as an assay is distributed to other laboratories (external quality assessment).

The average user of this book will not be a specialist developer of immunoassays but rather a biological scientist or chemist who needs to measure a drug, hormone, peptide, specific protein, antibody or pathogen. They will be a user or modifier of immunoassay kits, or a developer of immunoassays with commercial reagents who may also need to raise an antibody or prepare a label or conjugate. In summary, they want comprehensive practical knowledge of immunoassays in one affordable book. This may be the only specialist immunoassay book on their shelf. Specialist developers or users of immunoassays in clinical or research laboratories, or in commercial companies, will also want this book as part of their core collection of books on immunoassay methodology.

This book also complements and is complemented by other books in the *Practical Approach Series*, in particular *Peptide Antigens* (ed. G. B. Wisdom), *Immunochemistry I* and *II* (eds A. P. Johnstone and M. W. Turner) and *Antibody Engineering* (eds J, McCafferty, H. R. Hoogenboom and D. J. Chiswell).

I wish to thank the contributors for all their efforts and patience, and for the benefit of their expertise. Hopefully, their combined contributions will help analysts all over the world to develop better immunoassays more quickly and more cheaply. I also thank my wife Elizabeth and family, Marcus and Daniel, for their support. The material help of the Department of Biochemistry, NUI, Galway is also greatly appreciated.

J.P.G
March 2000

Contents

CONTENTS

Protocol list

Solid-phase formats

Conjugation of haptens and carriers

Sensitivity

Accuracy

Specificity

Abbreviations

4-MU-Gal	4-methylumbelliferyl-β-D-galactopyranoside
4-MUP	4-methylumbelliferyl-phosphate
4PL	four parameter logistic
Ab	antibody
ABTS	2,2'-azino-bis[3-ethylbenzthiazloline-6-sulfonic acid
Ag	antigen
AMPPD	3-(2'-spiroadamantane)-4-methoxy-4-(3″-phosphoryloxy)phenyl-1,2-dioxetane
AP	alkaline phosphatase
APG	p-azidophenylglyoxal monohydrate
BAPA	5-(biotinamido)-pentylamine
BCIG	5-bromo-4-chloro-3-indolyl-β-D-galactopyranoside
BCIP/NBT	bromochloroindolyl phosphate/nitro blue tetrazolium
BSA	bovine serum albumin
CBSA	cationized BSA
CDI	carbonyldiimidazole
CDR	complementarity determining region
CEDIA	combined enzyme donor immunoassay
CMO	carboxymethyloxime
CRM	Certified reference materials
CUSUM	cumulative sum (chart)
CV	coefficient of variation
DAB	3,3'-diaminobenzidine [3,3',4,4'-tertraaminobiphenyl]
DCCD	dicyclohexylcarbodiimide
DEA	diethanolamine
DELFIA®	dissociation enhanced lanthanide flourescence immunoassay
DMA	dimethyl adipimidate
DMF	N,N-dimethylformamide
DMP	dimethyl pimelimidate
DMS	dimethyl subetimidate
DMSO	dimethyl sulfoxide
DNA	deoxyribonucleic acid
DTBP	dimethyl 3,3'-dithiobispropionimidate

DTT	dithiolthreitol
EDAC	1-ethyl-3-(3- dimethylaminopropyl)carbodiimide
EDTA	ethylenediamine-tetra acetic acid
EGTA	ethyleneglycol-bis(aminoethyl)-N,N,N',N'-tetraacetic acid
EIA	enzyme immunoassay
ELISA	enzyme-linked immunosorbent assay
EMIT®	enztme modulated immunotest
EQA	external quality assessment
Fab	antigen-binding fragment
Fc	crystalizable (constant) fragment
FCS	fetal calf serum
FITC	fluorescein isothiocyanate
FPLC®	fast protein liquid chromatography
FSH	follicle stimulating hormone
Fv	variable fragment
GCMS	gas chromatography–mass spectrometry
Gly	glycine
H chain	heavy chain (of immunoglobulin)
Ha	hapten
HAMA	human anti-mouse antibodies
HAS	human serum albumin
HAT	hypoxanthine, aminopterin and thymidine (growth medium)
HAZA	hypoxanthine, azaserine and aminopterin (growth medium)
hCG	human chorionic gonadotrophin
HES	hybriboma-enhancing supplement
HIV	human immunodeficiency virus
HLA	human leucocyte antigen
HPAA	p-hydroxyphenylacetic acid
HPLC	high-performance liquid chromatography
HPPA	3-[p-hydroxyphenyl] propionic acid
HRP	horseradish peroxidase
HS	hemisuccinate
ID GCMS	Isotope dilution GCMS
IEMA	immunoenzymometric assay
IFMA	immunofluorimetric assay
Ig	immunogloulin
IQC	Internal quality control
IRMA	immunoradiometric assay
IS	International Standards
IVD	*in vitro* diagnostic (industry)
L chain	light chain (of immunoglobulin)
LC-ESI	liquid chromatography–electrospray ionization
LH	luteinizing hormone
LLD	lower limit of detection
MALDI	matrix-assisted laser desorption ionisation
MAP	multiple antigenic peptides

MES	2-[*N*-morpholino] ethane sulphonic acid
MHC	major histocompatability complex
NBCS	newborn calf serum
NHS	*N*-hydroxysuccinimide ester
NIBSC	National Institute for Biological Standards and Control (UK)
NSB	nonspecific binding
OD	optical density (absorbance)
ONPG	*o*-nitrophenyl-β-D-galactopyranoside
OPD	*o*-phenylenediamine dihydrochloride
PABC	protein–avidin–biotin-capture
PAGE	polyacrylamide gel electrophoresis
PBS	phosphate buffered saline
PBSTA	PBS with Tween and azide
PEG	polyethylene glycol
PNPP	*p*-nitrophenyl phosphate
PVDF	polyvinylidine dichloride
QA	quality assurance
QC	quality control
RAC	repeat analytical controls
RIA	radioimmunoassay
RMV	Reference method value
RU	resonance units
SAMSA	*S*-acetylmercaptosuccinic anhydride
SATA	succinimidyl acetylthioacetate
SATP	succinimidyl acetylthiopropionate
SD	standard deviation
SDS-PAGE	sodium dodecyl sulphate PAGE
Ser	serine
SFv	single chain Fv
SIAB	*N*-succinimidyl (4-iodoacetyl) aminobenzoate
SMCC	4-[*N*-maleimidomethyl)-cyclohexane-1-carboxylate
SPDP	*N*-Succinimidyl-3-(2-pyridyldithio) propionate
SPDP	succinimidyl 3-(2-pyridyldithio)propionate
SPR	surface plasmon resonance
sulfo-HSAB	*N*-hydroxysulphosuccinimidyl-4-azidobenzoate
TBS	Tris buffered saline
TCEP	Tris-(2-carboxyethyl)phosphine
TMB	3,3′,5,5′–tetramethylbenzidine
TNBS	Epinitrobenzenesulphonic acid
TSH	thyroid stimulating hormone
UK NEQAS	United Kingdom National External Quality Assessment Schemes
WHO	World Health Organization

Chapter 1
Analysis by specific binding

James P. Gosling

Department of Biochemistry and National Diagnostic Centre, National University of Ireland Galway, Galway, Ireland

1 Introduction

In the last 30 years analytical methods that depend on the recognition of analytes by high-affinity, specific binding proteins and oligonucleotides have found so many applications in diverse areas of biochemical analysis that they now represent a standard analytical principle, such as colorimetry or chromatography.

While there are many kinds of high-affinity, specific binding proteins in nature (hormone receptors, for example), the special properties of antibodies have made them the most popular choice for protein binding assays (*Table 1*). Measurement procedures that use antibodies as specific binding reagents are called immunoassays, as are assays that use antigens for the detection or quantification of specific antibodies. It is because of the extraordinary affinity, specificity and variety of antibody–antigen binding reactions, that immunoassays are used for routine analyses and for research purposes throughout the biological and medical sciences.

Often, an immunoassay is chosen to measure a particular analyte because no other type of assay is technically feasible, which is true for specific antibodies, most proteins and for many other complex biomolecules. However, an immunoassay is also frequently chosen because it matches the analytical and practical requirements *and* is more cost effective than any alternative method.

Immunoanalysis is a highly developed science that is supported by continuous, world-wide research and an extensive range of books (references 1–54 represent

Table 1. The advantages of antibodies compared with other binding proteins

---

Stable, soluble and abundant

Standard procedures for preparation, selection, isolation, coupling and immobilization

Suitable for antigens, weak antigens and non-antigenic small molecules ($M_r > 150$)

Available as a mixture with related specificities (polyclonal), or with a single binding specificity (monoclonal)

Bivalent (IgG) or polyvalent (IgM), but smaller monovalent fragments easily prepared

Available with a range of different constant regions (Ig class or species)

Amenable to modification and systematic improvement with recombinant DNA methods

---

a reasonably complete selection). There are few books with a clear emphasis on practical advice. Exceptions include the widely used, but now at least partly out of date, manuals on radioimmunoassay by Chard (24) and on enzyme immunoassay by Tijssen (34). Related volumes in the Practical Approach Series with chapters that are directly relevant to immunoassay include those on peptide antigens (55), antibody engineering (56) and immunochemistry (two volumes) (57). Journal reviews on immunoassay are mainly concerned with specialized aspects, with some exceptions (58–62).

2 Requirements for high-affinity specific binding

2.1 Immunoglobulins

2.1.1 Immunoglobulin G (IgG)

IgG, the class of antibody used predominantly in immunoassays, is a 150 000 Da glycoprotein containing two identical heavy (H, $\approx$ 420 residues) and two identical light (L, $\approx$ 215 residues) polypeptide chains (*Figure 1*). H chains in immunoglobulins are named with the equivalent lower-case Greek letter (IgG$_1$ has γ_1 heavy chains). L chains in any Ig class can be either λ or κ, each having a characteristic, constant sequence towards the *C*-terminal. Most of the areas this section are covered in more detail in basic texts on immunology and immunochemistry (63, 64)

The sequences of the $\approx$ 110 residues at the *N*-termini of both the H and L chains vary enormously to give rise to the multiplicity of specific IgG antibodies. The remainders of the H chains towards the *C*-terminals are constant within an Ig subclass or class and animal species, except for allotypic variation which is equivalent to the normal genetic variation that affects all proteins. The effector functions of each Ig in the humoral immune system are determined by the structure of the H chain constant region.

The entire H and L chains consist of homologous segments of about 110 amino acid residues that form structural domains with a characteristic antiparallel, β-barrel configuration (the immunoglobulin fold). This structural motif occurs in pairs in the immunoglobulins, each pair constituting a double domain, with six such 'domains' in IgG (*Figure 1*).

Immunoglobulins are flexible molecules because this facilitates their binding simultaneously to adjacent identical antigens on the surface of a pathogen and enables the aggregation of soluble antigens. While all inter-domain regions can flex and bend, the greatest flexibility (particularly in certain classes and subclasses) is associated with the 'hinge regions' of the H chains, near the *C*-termini of the L chains.

The two identical antigen-binding sites (also called paratopes) of IgG are composed from about 50 amino acid residues found in groups (the hypervariable regions) scattered along the variable segments of the H and L chains. In the three-dimensional structures of all immunoglobulins the hypervariable regions occur as loops that constitute the complementarity-determining regions (CDR). The six CDRs in any paratope are named CDR-L1 to CDR-L3 and CDR-H1 to CDR-H3, and

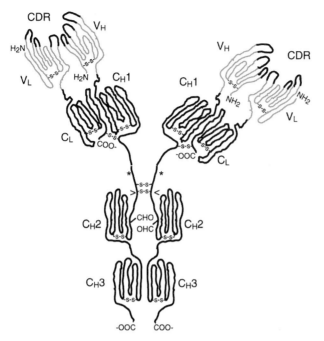

Figure 1. This diagrammatic representation of an IgG molecule is designed to emphasize its six structurally analogous globular double-domains, with the 'base' and the 'arms' connected by the long 'tethers' of the hinge region.

The six double-domains are $2 \times V_L/V_H$, $2 \times C_L/C_H1$, C_H2/C_H2 and C_H3/C_H3, where V indicates variable, C constant, H heavy chain and L light chain. The V_L/V_H domains constitute the variable regions and contain the two identical binding sites. They are shown by thin line except for the hypervariable segments making up the complementarity determining regions (CDR) of the binding sites. The constant domains C_L/C_H1, C_H2/C_H2 and C_H3/C_H3 constitute the rest of the structure. The intradomain and interchain disulfhydryl bonds are shown as '-s-s-'.

The approximate locations of the sites in the hinge region susceptible to cleavage by papain (*), which is used to prepare Fab and Fc fragments, and to cleavage by pepsin ($<$, $>$), which is used to prepare $F(ab')_2$ and Fab' fragments, are indicated (see *Figure 1.2*). IgG, like the other immunoglobulins, is a glycoprotein and has carbohydrate (CHO) chains attached via serine residues to the heavy chains in the C_H2/C_H2 domain. The base of the IgG molecule, consisting of the C_H2/C_H2 and C_H3/C_H3 domains, has a range of essential biological functions including binding sites for complement and macrophage receptors.

IgG is inherently highly flexible. Because of the extended peptide segments of the hinge region, the Fab arms can move quite freely and over a wide range relative to each other and to the Fc base. In addition, there is also some flexibility between each domain pair, particularly at the elbow of the Fab arms where angles differing by up to 40° are observed. However, there are differences in flexibility between immunoglobulin classes and subclasses. IgG3 has a greatly extended hinge region with multiple disulphide bonds between the H chains, human IgA2 has an abbreviated hinge region, and IgM and IgE have reduced hinge regions but with an extra pair of flexible domains.

they vary not only in sequence but in length. The CDR-H3 loop can adopt the greatest variety of conformations, largely because it can be up to 25 residues long. It is CDR variability that accounts for almost all of the immense range of antibody specificity.

3

The ranges of IgG subclasses differ in humans (IgG1, IgG2, IgG3, IgG4), from those in mice (IgG1, IgG2a, IgG2b, IgG3), and in rats (IgG1, IgG2a, IgG2b, IgG2c).

2.1.2 IgM

Of the other immunoglobulin classes (IgA, IgD, IgE and IgM), only IgM antibodies are used to any significant extent as immunoassay reagents. However, the appeal of IgM is limited by its often lower affinity for mono-epitopic antigens compared with IgG, and by a greater inherent tendency to bind nonspecifically. IgM has a total of seven immunoglobulin double domains because of longer H chains, and soluble IgM is pentameric (M_r 950 000), giving very high-avidity binding to poly-epitopic entities.

2.1.3 Affinity maturation

During a primary immune response the first specific antibodies are IgM but 'class-switching' ensures that the same (or similar, see below) heavy chain variable regions (and light chains) are later associated with IgG, IgA or other antibodies classes. In serum, IgG is usually the dominant class during the late primary response, and during subsequent responses. In addition, early IgG antibodies generally bind to antigen with higher affinity than the earlier IgM antibodies, and later IgG antibodies have, on average, even greater affinity. This process is termed affinity maturation and comes about because somatic mutations in the DNA segments corresponding to the variable regions of L and H chains occur frequently in B lymphocytes, and lymphocytes displaying higher affinity antibodies are preferentially selected as the immune response develops.

2.1.4 Antibody fragments

The exposed hinge or 'tether' region of IgG is highly susceptible to proteolytic cleavage by suitable enzymes, a fact that has been exploited in investigations and applications of antibodies since the beginnings of molecular immunology. It was Rodney Porter who showed that limited digestion with papain gave what are termed Fab ($M_r \approx 50\ 000$) and Fc fragments ($M_r \approx 50\ 000$) and Alfred Nisonoff who found that pepsin cut slightly nearer the C-termini and below the inter-H chain disulfhydryl links to give F(ab')$_2$ fragments ($M_r \approx 100\ 000$). Such studies led to the first proposals of accurate, general structures for antibodies. F(ab')$_2$ dimers are easily reduced to give Fab'. Fab' and Fab fragments (*Figure 2*) have found many application in immunoassays because of their relatively small size, reduced tendency to bind 'non-specifically' and lower reactivity to various factors commonly found in serum samples.

Later, occasional antibodies were found to be susceptible to proteolytic cleavage at the junctions between the variable and constant domains on both the H and L chains and the first Fv fragments were isolated. Fv ($M_r \approx 25\,000$) represents a minimal antibody and recombinant DNA methods have now made feasible the preparation of stable, single-chain Fv (sFv) fragments of any monoclonal antibody, and of chimeric proteins incorporating antibody-binding sites (*Figure 2*). The affinities of Fab, Fab' and Fv fragments are generally identical to the corresponding intact antibodies.

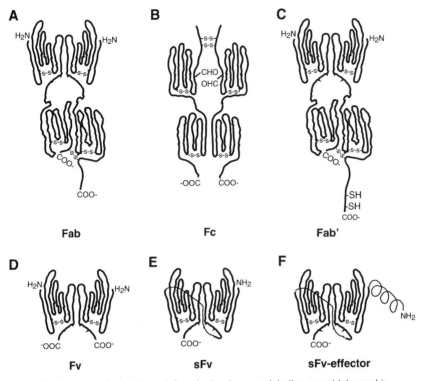

Figure 2. Fragments derived from IgG and other immunoglobulins are widely used in immunoassays and in other applications of antibodies. Fab (A) and Fc (B) are generated from IgG by limited proteolysis of IgG with papain. Careful treatment with pepsin cleaves the arms from the base a little nearer the C-termini of the H chains giving what is termed F(ab')$_2$, but the C_H2/C_H2 and C_H3/C_H3 domains are also cut at a number of other sites, giving a variety of peptides. F(ab')$_2$ are used directly for some applications but, more often, they are reduced to give Fab' fragments (C) which have the important advantage of having free sulfhydryl groups (two in human IgG1 and three in the commonly used IgG1 and IgG2a subclasses from BALB/c mice) that can be used to conjugate Fab' to give labels or immobilized reagents. Fv fragments (D) can be prepared by recombinant DNA methods but are prone to dissociate, so single-chain sFv binding proteins (E), which are coded for by genes assembled from segments for the H and L chain variable regions joined by a synthetic oligonucleotide coding for a linker peptide (e.g. the 15-residue segment [Gyl$_4$Ser$_3$]$_3$), are often used. However, once a protein is to be produced by recombinant means other possibilities for innovation immediately present themselves, including the preparation of chimeric proteins with the incorporation of an effector peptide to give a sFv-effector construct (F). For immunoassays the effector could act directly (enzyme, fluorescent protein) or indirectly (peptide hapten) as a label.

2.2 Antigen–antibody binding

2.2.1 Paratopes

Haptens are molecules of limited molecular weight (≥ 150 g/mol), which are not naturally antigenic but when conjugated to protein (bovine serum albumin, for example, with 20–30 hapten molecules per molecule of BSA) give an immunogen that can be used to generate antibodies that specifically bind free hapten with high affinity.

When an antibody-binding site, or paratope, is complexed with its specific hapten, the hapten is generally found to be located in a pocket, cavity or groove surrounded by functional groups of the peptide residues and backbone that are structurally complementary to adjacent portions of the hapten molecule. CDR loops commonly flex and move to accommodate binding, and high-affinity paratopes frequently give complexes in which the hapten is buried to the extent of 80–90% or greater.

When a paratope is complexed with the antigenic determinant region (epitope) of its specific protein antigen, the apparent area of close contact is usually relatively large, being about 700–900 Å^2, with about 20 amino acid residues on each reactant apparently participating. Within this area of contact there may be clefts to accommodate projecting side-chains on the antigen and vice versa. In all antibody–hapten or antibody–antigen complexes various structural adjustments of the epitope as well as of the paratope can occur. This is termed induced fit. The resultant contact is often close, but frequently there is room between the two interacting molecules to accommodate water molecules or ions. However, many of the residues and individual atoms in a protein epitope that are apparently in close contact with a paratope may actually contribute little to binding.

2.2.2 Epitopes

Each large antigen has a theoretically unlimited number of epitopes, a number that is limited in practice by immune tolerance in the immunized animal towards surface regions that share structural features with self proteins, and by the difficulty of differentiating between overlapping epitopes. Structurally, protein epitopes are similar to paratopes and are made up of a number of amino acid residues that are scattered, singly or in small groups, along the amino acid sequence but are close together on the surface of the intact antigen. Thus, epitopes are said to be generally discontinuous. However, a single short peptide may represent a large fraction of an epitope and may, in isolation, be specifically bound by an antibody against the protein that it represents. Correspondingly, antibodies raised against such a peptide may bind to the region of the cognate protein containing the same sequence (55). Epitopes containing such sequences may be referred to as continuous epitopes. Not unusually continuous epitopes correspond to exposed termini.

2.2.3 The binding reaction

Antigen–antibody interactions are reversible and high-affinity binding requires a combination of easy association and reluctant dissociation. Association can be regarded as occurring in two phases, with the first requiring the overcoming of repulsive forces and the second involving the establishment of multiple hydrogen, ionic and van der Waals attractive interactions between atoms on the paratope and epitope. (See Section 1.4 of Chapter 3 for a more formal treatment of binding affinity.)

Any interaction must be preceded by a 'coming together', i.e. a collision. The rate at which collisions occur is dependent on rates of diffusion, which, in turn, is influenced by molecular mass and shape, temperature and on whether both reactants are mobile. Therefore, haptens tend to associate more readily with their specific antibodies than large antigens, and hapten analytes more readily than hapten–enzyme conjugates. In addition, antigen–antibody interactions reach equilibrium less quickly when the antibody or antigen is immobilized to a solid phase as opposed to when both are free to diffuse. This effect is maximal when the solid phase surface is of limited area and is localized, as is the case with antibody- or antigen-coated tubes or microtitre wells. Therefore, many automated immunoassays, which require short incubation times, involve the use of microparticulate solid-phase media or are designed such that the binding reaction occurs in liquid phase and separation is effected later.

Apart from temperature, other physiochemical conditions of the surrounding aqueous environment are influential, particularly pH, ionic strength and, occasionally, the presence of particular ions species that may participate in the binding reaction. An appropriate pH, which is usually near pH 7, ensures that acidic and basic groups on both species are suitably dissociated or associated, and in more dilute salt solution electrostatic forces operate at longer ranges. Furthermore, the addition of various species (such as ammonium sulphate and polyethylene glycol) which reduce the shield of water molecules that exists around all molecules in aqueous solution, may act to promote association. However, adjustment of any of the above parameters may influence not just specific binding but also nonspecific binding (which is fundamentally similar but must always be made negligible or kept to a minimum) and the exact conformations of antibody and antigen. Therefore, optimal reaction conditions can only be estimated experimentally.

3 The variety of immunoassays

3.1 Representing assay complexes in text

Most of the reagents used and the complexes of antibodies, antigens and other components that form during the operation of immunoassays can readily be represented by text rather than only in diagrams or figures, provided that a standard notation system is followed. The rules that are used here are very simple. The analyte is shown in bold type, e.g **A′**, **Ha** or **Ab** for the general analytes antigen, hapten and antibody, respectively. Where any one of a number of labelling substance could be used, it is represented by L. The hyphen (-) sign indicates associations established before commencement of the assay such as an antibody enzyme conjugate (Ab-enz) or an antibody immobilized on a solid phase (sp-Ab). In contrast, the en dash (–) represents associations formed during the course of the assay procedure. For example, the final complex of a solid phase ELISA for an antigen is described as: sp-Ab–**Ag**–Ab-enzyme. Unusual components are accommodated by spelling out their names, and standard abbreviations are used when the class (IgG, IgM) or type of antibody (mono-

Table 2. Classification of immunoassays into four groups

1. Label free	Agglutination	Haemagglutination
		Latex agglutination
	Precipitation	Ouchterlony gel diffusion
		Rocket immunoelectrophoresis
		Immunoturbidimetry/nephelometry
	Immunosensors	Resonant mirror waveguide (IAsys™)
		Surface plasmon resonance (BIAcore™)
2. Reagent excess	One site	Immunostaining
		Western blotting
	Two site	Immunoenzymometric assay, ELISA,
		Immunofluorimetric assay,
		Immunoradiometric assay
3. Reagent limited	Labelled antigen *or* antibody	Radioimmunoassay,
		Enzyme immunoassay,
		Fluoroimmunoassay
	Separation free	EMIT, CEDIA
4. Ambient analyte	Microarray/microchip	Microspot®

clonal, mAb) or antibody fragment (Fab′, F[ab′]2) or its origin (goat, G; human, H; mouse, M; rabbit, R; sheep, S) is relevant.

3.2 Classification

Table 2 represents a system whereby most, if not all, immunoassays can be classified into four Groups, examples of some of which are illustrated in *Figure 3*. In this context, it should also be borne in mind that binding proteins other than antibodies can be used as specific binding reagents in assays that are the exact equivalents to those mentioned below. For example, intrinsic factor and β-lactoglobin are used as specific binding reagents in Group 2-type assays for vitamin B_{12} and folate, respectively (65). A combination of an antibody and a particular lectin may also be used specifically to measure glycoproteins with specified carbohydrate residues (66).

Most quantitative immunoassays developed for research purposes or for applications of limited scale (which are the major concern of this book) are simple immunoprecipitation assays (Group 1), reagent excess, sandwich assays with either direct or indirect labels (Group 2) or reagent limited, competitive assays with a separation step (Group 3).

3.2.1 Label-free assays

Provided that the concentrations are sufficient, the molecular complexes (*Figure 3A*) ([Ab–**Ag**]$_n$) generated by antibody–antigen interaction are visible to the naked eye, but in laboratory situations smaller amounts may be detected and measured owing to their ability to scatter a beam of light. Complex formation indicates that both reactants are present, so that a constant concentration of a reagent antibody can used to measure specific antigen, and reagent antigen can be used to detect specific antibody. If the reagent species is previously coated onto cells or very small particles, binding at much lower concentrations causes detectable precipitation or agglutination of the coated particles.

A variety of assays based on these elementary principles are in common use, including Ouchterlony immunodiffusion assay, rocket immunoelectrophoresis, haemagglutination testing, latex agglutination assay (*Figure 3B*), and immuno-turbidometric and nephelometric assays (67). The main limitations of such assays are restricted sensitivity (lower detection limits) and, in some cases, the fact that very high concentrations of analyte can inhibit complex formation, necessitating safeguards that make the procedures more complex. Some of these Group 1 assays date back to the discovery of antibodies and none have a true 'label' (e.g. antigen conjugated to enzyme).

Other types of immunoassays that are label-free depend on immunosensors, and a variety of instruments that can directly detect antibody–antigen inter-actions are now commercially available (68). Most depend on generating an evanescent wave on a sensor surface with immobilized ligand, which allows continuous monitoring of binding to the ligand. Immunosensors allow the easy investigation of kinetic interactions and, with the advent of lower-cost special-ized instruments, may in the future find wide application in immunoanalysis. (The use of immunosensor instruments in the characterization of antibodies is further discussed in Section 4.2.4 of Chapter 3.)

3.2.2 Reagent-excess assays

Group 2 of *Table 2* contains assays that are typified by the use of an excess concentration of labelled antibody or antigen for the detection specific antigen or antibody.

'One-site' reagent excess assays include Western blotting, whereby proteins absorbed to nitrocellulose filters are located by 'probing' with labelled specific antibodies (nitrocellulose–**Ag**–Ab-L) and immunostaining, such as immuno-fluoresence assay whereby antigen in a tissue section is visualized with specific antibodies conjugated to fluorescein (cell matrix-**Ag**-Ab-fluorescein) (*Figure 3C*).

However, separate binding reactions specific for two different sites on the analyte may be involved, giving rise to a trimolecular, or larger, complex with the analyte in the middle, hence the terms 'two-site assay' and 'sandwich assay' (*Figure 3D–F*). For example, two monoclonal antibodies against different, non-overlapping epitopes on the analyte may be used to detect a protein hormone such as human chorionic gonadotropin (hCG) with high specificity (sp-mAb$_1$-**hCG**-mAb$_2$-L). Similarly, two-site assays can be used to detect specific antibodies of a particular immunoglobulin class or subclass (*Figure 3G*). For example, a purified allergen and an antibody against human IgE may be used to detect specific antibodies of the IgE class that bind to the allergen in question (sp-allergen–**IgE**–Ab-L).

Assays for specific antibodies that employ immobilized antigen to capture the target antibody and labelled antigen of the same kind to titrate the bound antibody via its free antigen-binding site (IgG) or sites (IgM or IgA) are, strictly speaking, two-site assays (*Figure 3H*) (sp-Ag–**Ab**–Ag-L). However, since both sites

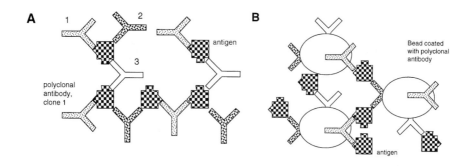

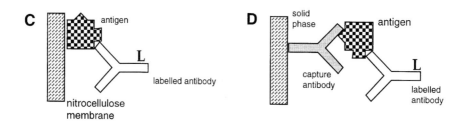

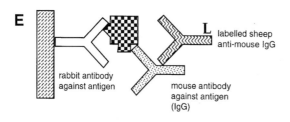

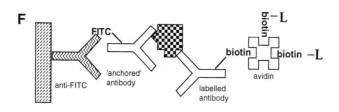

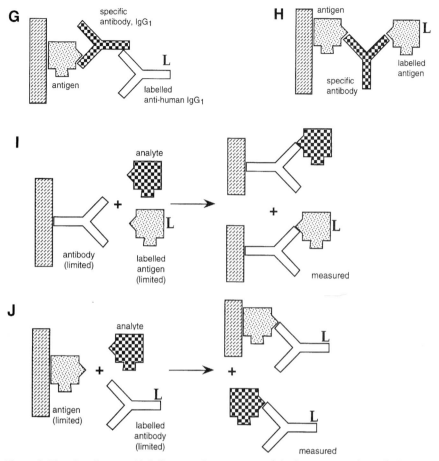

Figure 3. The nine diagrams (A–I) illustrate the structures of the immune complexes that are measured in a range of immunoassays of different design. They may be related to *Table 2* as follows: A and B, Group 1 label-free assays; C to H, Group 2 reagent-excess assays; and I and J, Group 3 reagent-limited, competitive assays.

A. Precipitated complexes equivalent to that illustrated here result when a polyclonal antibody is mixed with its large molecular weight antigen. They may be visible (Ouchterlony immunodiffusion assay, immunoelectrophoresis) or may be measured by their ability to scatter light (immunoturbidimetric and immunonephelometric assays). If the concentration of a specific antibody is constant, increasing the concentration of its antigen causes increased precipitation over a certain range of antigen concentration and vice versa. In liquid solution, precipitation may be hastened and maximized by the addition of reagents that promote precipitation, such as polyethylene glycol, or by attaching the reagent antibody or antigen to microbeads.

B. Agglutinated complexes (as shown here) results when antibody-coated latex beads are mixed with antigen. While a suspension of antibody-coated latex beads has a milky appearance, when strong agglutination occurs the solution clears but with tiny, diffuse clumps distributed throughout. In a latex agglutination assay for a specific antigen (as here) agglutination is caused by the addition of sample with antigen, otherwise the solution remains unchanged. Many variants of agglutination assays have been devised, such as those with antigen-coated particles and soluble antibody (agglutination inhibition assay of antigen) for the detection of specific antibody, or with alternative particles (haemagglutination assay).

Caption continued on page 12

11

C. This simple complex of labelled antibody with immobilized antigen is intended to represent the final complexes obtained after any of a number of varied immunoassay procedures. For example, the Western blotting of a two-dimensional electrophoretogram of a complex protein mixture to identify a specific protein, or (imagining the solid phase to be part of a subcellular complex) the immunostaining of a tissue section to investigate the location and distribution of a specific antigen. In either case, the labelling substance, L, could be a fluorescent compound, an enzyme or a radioisotopic atom (probably ^{125}I), and for electron microscopic studies it could be the electron-dense protein, ferritin. For all such assays, excess, high specific activity labelled antibody is applied, which, ideally, have no tendency to bind nonspecifically. Endpoint determination or visualization would depend on the type of label used.

D. Solid-phase, two-site assay for antigen with direct immobilization of one antibody to the solid phase and direct labelling of the other antibody. This is the traditional arrangement for a reagent-excess, sandwich immunoassay, but a large variety of solid phase materials, labelling substances and label measurement procedures are used. Analyte may be added to both antibody reagents together (one-step procedure), or the complex may be built up stepwise with thorough washing of the solid-phase after each step.

E. As D, but with indirect measurement of the 'sandwich' by means of labelled sheep anti-mouse IgG. Here, the Fc of the mouse antibody acts as a 'tag' on the primary label and is titrated with the secondary label. Obviously, other combinations of species may be used as the origins of the antibodies, but the two antibodies of the sandwich must be from different species.

F. This assay involves indirect measurement with biotinylated antibody as primary label, and indirect immobilization with FITC acting as a specific 'anchor'. Biotinylation of both the antibody to be labelled and the secondary labelling substance (L) (e.g. an enzyme) and the use of an avidin bridge allows for the binding of up to three labels per complex. Conjugating FITC to the antibody to be immobilized and the use of immobilized anti-FITC antibodies enables procedures in which the antibody–analyte–label complex is allowed to form in solution and then immobilized by the late addition of solid-phase (e.g. beads) with anti-FITC attached. This may allow very short incubation times for high-performance assays.

G. Solid-phase, reagent-excess, 'antibody-capture' assay for specific antibodies of a particular class or subclass. Most assays to measure antibodies against a particular pathogen, allergen or autoantigen are of this type, and the use of a variety of solid-phase materials, reagent types and formulations gives rise to a wide range of assays suitable for different applications. Depending on the specificity of the labelled antibody, this design allows a narrow or broad range of antibody subclasses (only IgG1 or all IgG subclasses) or classes (only IgG, only IgM, or IgG and IgM) to be included. Sometimes, when specific antibodies of a specific minor class (e.g. IgE) or subclass (e.g. IgG4) are to be measured, an 'antigen capture' design is used, whereby the anti-class antibody is immobilized and antigen is labelled, directly (sp-Ab–**Ab**–Ag-L) or indirectly (e.g sp-Ab–**Ab**–Ag-biotin–avidin-L).

H. 'Double-antigen' assays for specific antibody are becoming increasingly popular for screening assays because they detect all antibodies that bind a particular antigen, irrespective of class. In particular, pentameric antibodies of the IgM class, which occur soonest after a primary infection, may be detected with enhanced sensitivity because multiple copies of the labelled antigen can bind (not shown).

I. Labelled-antigen, reagent-limited assay for hapten analytes is the most common type of competitive assay. Antibody is used at a constant, limited concentration and, usually, so also is the labelled antigen. After incubation the unbound label is removed and the amount of label bound to antibody is measured. The amount of label bound is inversely related to analyte concentration. Most immunoassays for smaller analytes such as steroids and many drugs are of this design. If the reagents can be prepared such that the binding of the labelled antigen activates or inhibits the activity of the labelling substance, a separation-free assay is possible and no solid phase is needed.

J. Labelled-antibody reagent-limited assay for an antigen. Both immobilized antigen and labelled antibody are normally used in constant, limited concentrations. After incubation, unbound components (including labelled antibody bound to analyte) are removed and the amount of label bound to immobilized antigen is measured.

are identical, such 'antibody bridge' assays may be regarded as resembling one-site assays with respect to their specificity.

3.2.3 Reagent-limited assays

Group 3 contains reagent-limited assays which are typified by classical RIA. These are also commonly referred to as competitive assays and may have labelled antigen (*Figure 3I*) or labelled antibody (*Figure 3J*). They are used to measure the concentrations of large antigens and, more commonly, of smaller analytes such as steroids or drugs. In contrast to almost all other immunoassays, the immune complexes measured or detected (sp-Ab–Ag-L or sp-Ag–Ab-L) do not contain the analyte and, therefore, all such assays give inverse (i.e. falling as opposed to rising) standard curves when the concentration of bound label is plotted against analyte concentration. Competitive assays are inherently less sensitive than reagent excess assays (69).

Importantly, competitive assays can be designed to obviate the need for a separation step to isolate the bound and free fractions before label measurement, when they are referred to as 'separation-free' or homogeneous assays. To avoid the need for a separation step, the binding reaction must influence the ability of the label to generate the endpoint signal. Ideally, such modulation should be 100% efficient and the limited lower detection limits generally achievable testify to the fact that this is often not realized. Separation-free assays include the commercial systems EMIT® (Syva), and CEDIA®, which are widely employed in the manual and automated measurement of therapeutic, toxic and illegal drugs. Such assays are difficult to develop and optimize, and are not often developed for small-scale laboratory applications.

3.2.4 Ambient analyte assays

Ambient analyte immunoassays (Group 4) are performed under conditions where the concentration of capture antibodies (or antigen molecules) is so low that their presence does not affect the concentration of free analyte in the reaction medium. As with many receptors in endocrine systems, fractional binding site occupancy is independent both of the amount of capture agent and reaction volume. To make possible such a system very high specific activity, fluorescent labels are used, and the small amount of capture ligand is coated at very high density within a 'microspot'. This principle was invented by Roger Ekins and is being exploited in the development of an ultrasensitive microarray-based multi-analyte assay system by Boehringer Mannheim GmbH (70).

3.3 Nomenclature

The names of immunoassays are confusing and make it difficult for readers to understand similarities and differences, as well as the diversity of immunoassay designs. In general, most assay names contain 'immuno', the combining form of the adjective 'immune', and another combining word indicating the type of label employed, e.g. radioimmunoassay (RIA) or enzyme immunoassay (EIA). If receptor is employed rather than antibody the corresponding name is radio-receptor assay.

The use of the terms RIA and EIA is usually restricted to reagent-limited, competitive assays, and reagent-excess assays are commonly distinguished by reversing the order of the combining forms, as in IRMA, IFMA, or IEMA. The term immunometric assay is used to refer to reagent excess assays in general. However, similar names are sometimes used for competitive assays with labelled antibody. The acronym ELISA is generally used for all kinds of microtitre plate assays with enzymatic labels and, when encountered, cannot be relied upon to indicate a particular assay mechanism. In general, EIA is to be preferred for assays equivalent to RIA and IEMA for assays equivalent to IRMA.

3.4 The variety of formats

The versatility of immunoassays is made possible by the wide variety of formats that can be implemented for assays of similar basic design. For example the basic reagent-excess sandwich assay (*Figure 3D*) may be used for high-performance, high-throughput, laboratory-based applications or for simple, test devices to be used by untrained persons and sold over the counter in normal retail outlets. Much of the variety in format is dependent on the different solid phase materials and their 'shapes' (e.g. microtitre wells, microparticles or membranes) and on the different labels/endpoints (e.g. radioactive, fluorescent, enzymatic or coloured particles) that are used.

4 The limitations of binding assays

Absolute specificity that depends on a binding reaction alone is unattainable. Whether the binding protein is an antibody, a hormone receptor or a lectin, the existence of crossreacting molecules in (unrefined) samples to be analysed is a continuous possibility. After all, the science of pharmacology depends largely on finding or devising substances that strongly crossreact with 'specific' binding sites.

With hapten analytes, a structurally similar crossreactant may be able to bind to the specific paratope in a slightly different orientation (71), or a mol-ecule with a single different functional group may bind because of the existence of a sufficiently large 'pocket' in the binding site. There is also the well-accepted fact that changes at or near the site through which the hapten was conjugated to the immunogen carrier molecule often have little effect on affinity. Dissimilar crossreactants, which may be defined as such by crude comparisons of chemical formulae or two-dimensional representations, are also always possible.

Large protein, glycoprotein or complex carbohydrate antigens interact with a large area of the paratope, thereby making effective epitope uniqueness more feasible. Nevertheless, crossreacting molecules do occur and, in addition, the achievement of adequate specificity may be exacerbated by analyte hetero-geneity. Two-site assays require the recognition of two spatially distinct epitopes and can be exploited to improve specificity when analytes are large, but then there are two interactions that are susceptible to general interference instead of one. In addition, protein analytes are subject to genetic variation, so that subpopulations may exist that express a variant epitope that is not recognized by a reagent antibody (72)

When the analytes are specific antibodies, the required specificity may be quite different from one application to another. The purity and suitability of the antigen reagent is critical and, when class (or subclass) specificity is also required, a two-site design is normally used, so that the specificity of the class-specific antibody used is also vital. Epitope (as opposed to antigen) specificity may be required in some applications. This can be achieved by using a peptide to represent the epitope, or a (labelled) monoclonal antibody binding to the 'same' epitope can be used in a one-site competitive assay (73). In all these designs antibodies against other 'similar' antigens or polyspecific antibodies may be detected, and may even give rise to false positive diagnoses.

However, no analytical method is absolutely specific in practice and the best perform as well as they do because they involve at least two stages: one to separate the analyte from the general constituents of its sample matrix and one to measure it. For example, analyte is normally presented to a mass spectrometer only after it has been extensively purified by means of a high-resolution chromatographic method. In contrast, most immunoassay methods are expected to be accurate and precise when presented with untreated samples. The only preliminary treatment that is generally acceptable is dilution.

Nevertheless, any really effective answer to interference and crossreactivity as they affect immunoassays must also involve the use of preliminary purification steps. Otherwise the accuracy of any immunoassay is completely dependent on the careful selection and purity of antibodies (and/or antigens) and other reagents, careful optimization, thorough analytical and biological validation, thorough quality control procedures, and a good track record when used by operators who are alert to problems (and luck).

References

1. Diczfalusy, E. and Diczfalusy, A. (eds) (1969). *Acta Endocrinol.* Suppl. **142**.
2. Diczfalusy, E. and Diczfalusy, A. (eds) (1970). *Acta Endocrinol.* Suppl. **147**.
3. Kirkham, K. E. and Hunter, W. M. (eds) (1971). *Radioimmunoassay Methods.* Churchill Livingstone, Edinburgh.
4. Odell, W. and Daughaday, W. H. (eds) (1971). *Principles of competitive protein-binding assays.* Lippincott, Philadelphia.
5. Websterman, J. G. (ed.) (1971). *Radioimmunoassay.* Hospital Medicine Publications, London.
6. International Atomic Energy Agency (1974). *Radioimmunoassay and related procedures in medicine.* IAEA, Vienna, Austria.
7. Pasternak, C. A. (ed.) (1975). *Radioimmunoassay in clinical biochemistry.* Heyden, London.
8. Cameron, E. H. D., Hillier, S. G., and Griffiths, K. (eds) (1975). *Steroid immunoassay.* Alpha Omega, Cardiff.
9. Lorraine, J. A. and Bell, E. T. (eds) (1976). *Hormone assays and their clinical application.* Churchill Livingstone, Edinburgh.

10. International Atomic Energy Agency (1978). *Radioimmunoassay and related procedures in medicine, second symposium.* IAEA, Vienna.
11. Pal, S. B. (ed.) (1978). *Enzyme labelled immunoassay of hormones and drugs.* Walter de Gruyter, Berlin.
12. Richie, R. F. (ed.) (1978). *Automated imunoanalysis, parts 1 and 2.* Marcel Dekker, New York.
13. Jaffe, B. M and Behrman, H. R. (eds) (1979). *Method of hormone radioimmunoassay.* Academic Press, New York.
14. Nakamura, W. R., Dito, W. R., and Tucker, E. S. (eds) (1979). *Immunoassays in the clinical laboratory.* Alan R. Liss, New York.
15. Langone, J. J. and van Vunakis, H. V. (eds) (1980). *Methods Enzymol.* **70.**
16. Maggio, E.T. (ed.) (1980) *Enzyme-immunoassay.* CRC Press Inc., Boca Raton.
17. Malvano, R. (ed.) (1980). *Immunoenzymatic assay techniques.* Martinus Nijhoff, The Hague.
18. Albertini, A. and Ekins, R. (eds) (1981). *Monoclonal antibodies and developments in immunoassay.* Elsevier/North Holland, Amsterdam.
19. Clausen, J. (1981). *Immunochemical techniques for the identification and estimation of macromolecules.* Elsevier North Holland, Amsterdam.
20. Langone, J. J. and van Vunakis, H. V. (eds) (1981). *Methods Enzymol.* **73**.
21. Langone, J. J. and van Vunakis, H. V. (eds) (1981). *Methods Enzymol.* **74**.
22. Ishikawa, E., Kawai, T., and Miyai, K. (eds) (1981). *Enzyme immunoassay.* Igaku-Shoin, Tokyo.
23. Voller, A., Bartlett, A., and Bidwell, D. (eds) (1981) *Immunoassays for the 80s.* MTP Press Ltd, Lancaster.
24. Chard, T. (1982). *An introduction to radioimmunoassay and related techniques*, 2nd edn. Elsevier North Holland, Amsterdam.
25. International Atomic Energy Agency (1982). *Radioimmunoassay and related procedures in medicine, third symposium.* IAEA, Vienna.
26. Langone, J. J. and van Vunakis, H. (eds) (1982). *Methods Enzymol.* **84.**
27. Avrameas, S. P., Dreut, P., Masseyeff, R., and Feldman, G. (eds) (1983). *Immunoenzymatic techniques.* Elsevier, Amsterdam.
28. Hunter, W. M. and Corrie, J. E. T. (eds) (1983). *Immunoassays for clinical chemistry.* Churchill Livingstone, Edinburgh.
29. Langone, J. J. and van Vunakis, H. (eds) (1983). *Methods Enzymol.* **92.**
30. Butt, W. R. (ed.) (1984) *Practical immunoassay. The state of the art.* Marcel Dekker Inc., New York.
31. Read, G. F. *et al.* (eds) (1984). *Immunoassays of steroids in saliva.* Alpha Omega, Cardiff.
32. Collins, W. P. (ed.) (1985). *Alternative immunoassays.* John Wiley & Sons, Chicester.
33. Ngo, T. T. and Lenhoff, H. M. (eds) (1985). *Enzyme-mediated immunoassay.* Plenum Press, New York.
34. Tijssen, P. (1985). *Practice and theory of enzyme immunoassays.* Elsevier, Amsterdam.
35. Pal, S. B. (ed.) (1986). *Immunoassay technology*, Vol 2. Walter de Gruyter, Berlin.
36. Chan, D. W. and Perlstein, M. T. (eds) (1987). *Immunoassay. A practical guide.* Academic Press, San Diego.
37. Morris, B. A., Clifford, M. N., and Jackman, R. (eds) (1987). *Immunoassays for veterinary and food analysis–1.* Elsevier, London.
38. Ngo, T. T. (ed.) (1987). *Electrochemical sensors in immunological analysis.* Plenum Press, New York.
39. Albertson, B. D. and Haseltine, F. P. (eds) (1988). *Non-radiometric assays. Technology and application in polypeptide and steroid hormone detection.* Alan R Liss, New York.
40. Collins, W. P. (ed.) (1988). *Complementary immunoassays.* John Wiley & Sons, Chichester.
41. Kemeny, D. M. and Challcombe, S. J. (eds) (1988) *ELISA and other solid phase immunoassays. Theoretical and practical aspects.* John Wiley & Sons, Chichester.

42. Butler, J. E. (ed.) (1991). *Immunochemistry of solid-phase immunoassay.* CRC Press, Boca Raton.

43. Hemmila, I. A. (1991). *Applications of fluorescence in immunoassays.* Wiley, New York.

44. Chan, D. W. (ed.) (1992) *Immunoassay automation.* Academic Press, San Diego.

45. Nakamura R. M., Kasahara, Y., and Rechnitz, G. A. (eds) (1992). *Immunochemical assays and biosensor technology for the 1990s.* American Society for Microbiology, Washington D.C.

46. Wyatt, G. M., Lee, H. A., and Morgon M. R. A. (1992). *Immunoassays for food poisoning bacteria and bacterial toxins.* Chapman & Hall, London.

47. Masseyeff, R. F., Albert, W. H., and Staines, N. A. (eds) (1993). *Methods of Immunological Analysis, vol. 1 Fundamentals.* VCH, Weinheim

48. Masseyeff, R. F., Albert, W. H., and Staines, N. A. (eds) (1993). *Methods of Immunological Analysis, Vol. 2 Samples and reagents.* VCH, Weinheim

49. Gosling, J. P. and Reen, D. J. (eds) (1993) *Immunotechnology.* Portland Press, London.

50. Wild, D. (ed.) (1994). *The Immunoassay Handbook.* Stockton Press, New York,

51. Gosling, J. P. and Basso, L. V. (eds) (1994) *Immunoasay: Laboratory Analysis and Clinical Applications.* Butterworth Heineman, Boston.

52. Kurz, D. A., Skerrit, J. H., and Stanker, L. H. (eds) (1995). *New frontiers in agrochemical immunoassay.* AOAC International, Arlington.

53. Diamandes, E. P. and Chrisopoulos, T. K. (eds) (1996) *Textbook of Immunological Assays.* Academic Press, New York.

54. Price, C. P. and Newman, D. J. (eds) (1997). *Principles and Practice of Immunoassay*, 2nd edn. Macmillan, London.

55. Wisdom, G. B. (1994) *Peptide antigens, a practical approach.* IRL Press, Oxford.

56. McCafferty, J., Hoogenboom, H. R., and Chiswell, D. J. (eds) (1996). *Antibody engineering. A practical approach.* IRL Press, Oxford.

57. Johnstone, A. P. and Turner, M. W. (eds) (1997). *Immunochemistry, a practical approach,* Vols 1 and 2. IRL Press, Oxford.

58. Gosling, J. P. (1990). *Clin. Chem.* **36**, 1408.

59. Kricka, L. J. (1993). *J. Clin. Immunoassay* **16**, 267.

60. Gosling, J. P. (1994). *Biochem. Ed.* **22**, 176.

61. Kricka, L.J. (1994). *Clin. Chem.* **40**, 347.

62. Morgan, C. L., Newman, D. J., and Price, C. P. (1996). *Clin. Chem.* **42**, 193.

63. Day, E. D. (1990). *Advanced immunochemistry.* Wiley–Liss, New York.

64. van Oss, C. J. and van Regenmortel, M. H. V. (eds) (1994). *Immunochemistry.* Marcel Dekker, New York.

65. Dacie, J. V. and Lewis, S. M. (1991). *Practical haematology*, 7th edn. Churchill Livingstone, Edinburgh.

66. Kinoshita, N., Suzuki, S., Matsuda, Y., and Taniguchi, N. (1989). *Clin. Chim. Acta* **179**, 143.

67. Price, C. P. and Newman, D. J. (1997). In *Principles and Practice of Immunoassay* (eds C. P. Price and D. J. Newman)*, 2nd edn., pp. 443–480. Macmillan Press, London.

68. Purvis, D. R., Pollard-Knight, D., and Lowe, C.R. (1997). *Principles and Practice of Immunoassay* (eds C. P. Price and D. J. Newman)*, 2nd edn., p. 511. Macmillan Press, London.

69. Jackson, T. M. and Ekins, P.P. (1986) *Clin. Chem.,* **87**, 13.

70. Finckh, P., Berger, H., Karl, J., Eichenlaub, U., Weindel, K., Hornauer, H., Lenz, H., Sluka, P., Ehrleich Weinreich, G., Chu, F., and Ekins, R. (1998). *Proceedings of the UK NEQAS Endocrinology Meeting, 1998,* No. 4, p. 155. Association of Clinical Biochemists, London

71. Arevalo, J. H., Taussig, M. J., and Wilson, I. A. (1993). *Nature,* **365**, 859.

72. Pettersson, K., Ding, Y.Q., and Huhtaniemi, I. (1991). *J. Clin. Endocrinol. Metab.* **74**, 164.

73. Kemeny, D.M. (1992) *J. Immunol. Methods* **150**, 57.

Chapter 2
Raising antibodies

M. M. Kane* and J. N. Banks†

*Immunodiagnostics Group, National Diagnostics Centre, National University of Ireland Galway, Galway, Ireland and †Central Science Laboratory, Sand Hutton, York YO4 ILZ, UK

1 Introduction

1.1 Monoclonal and polyclonal antibodies

Antibodies are essential components of immunoassays, and the versatility of immunoassays results from the unique features of these proteins. Antibodies can recognize and bind to their antigen with high affinity and specificity, even when they are part of a complex mixture, enabling sensitive measurements of antigens or antibodies in a variety of matrices.

Early immunoassay developers relied entirely on polyclonal antibodies prepared from the sera of animals, and developed many very successful assays. However, because of increasingly exacting requirements for high specificity and for continuity of supply, monoclonal antibodies are now often used, where possible. Each polyclonal 'antibody' is a heterogeneous mixture of antibody molecules arising from a variety of constantly evolving B-lymphocytes, so that even successive bleeds from one animal are unique. In contrast, ever since Kohler and Milstein (1) first described immortalizing individual B lymphocytes by cell–cell fusions, it has been possible to produce hybridoma cell lines that secrete only one particular type of antibody. Therefore, all monoclonal antibodies are homogeneous and can be produced in unlimited quantities, thus providing reproducible reagents for the long-term manufacture of assay kits and other applications.

Methods based on the manipulation of antibody genes now allow the generation of antibodies, a variety of antibody fragments and chimeric proteins containing antibody-derived binding sites (2). These methods are complex and strange to those who raise 'normal' antibodies and, to date, have been primarily directed at the development of human antibodies and fragments that are intended for *in vivo* diagnostic or therapeutic applications. One exception is the development of recombinant human antibodies for blood group and HLA typing (3). Therefore, the generation of monoclonal antibodies for immunoassay development still relies very heavily on traditional hybridoma technology applied to mice and, to a smaller extent, to rats.

However, polyclonal antibodies are still widely used as primary antibodies, particularly in competitive immunoassays, and the great majority of antibodies used as secondary reagents are polyclonal. Their great advantage is the relative simplicity and low cost of the procedures used for raising them. They are often sufficiently specific for the purposes of their users and long-term continuity of supply may not be seen as a problem, particularly when larger animals are immunized.

1.2 Antibodies and immunoassays

Choosing antibodies for immunoassay development involves the consideration of many factors, some of which may not be scientific.

Double-antibody sandwich immunoassays can be set up with two monoclonal antibodies or, as quite often happens, with a polyclonal and a monoclonal antibody combination. The latter is particularly common among commercial assays because of patent restrictions on the use of two monoclonal antibodies in such assays. With monoclonals, matched pairs that react with different epitopes on the analyte, and can therefore bind the analyte simultaneously, are selected.

Analysis of small molecules (< 5000 Da) by immunoassay is still largely limited to competitive (i.e. reagent-limited) formats. The use of monoclonal antibodies for competitive assays has trailed behind their use in sandwich assays, largely because of the poor yield of high-affinity monoclonal antibodies and the important inverse relationship between antibody affinity and detection limit in competitive assays (4). It is important to remember, however, that good, high-affinity polyclonal antisera are also difficult to raise. In general, the range of affinities of the antibodies arising from a fusion reflects the polyclonal response generated by immunization. Thus, high-affinity antibodies can be produced and the prospect of a continuous supply of a consistent product also makes them the antibody of choice for commercial assays.

Polyclonal antisera can show good specificity because the different antibody populations react with the variety of epitopes that characterize the antigen. The specificity of a polyclonal antiserum can also be 'improved' by removal of antibodies giving rise to an unwanted crossreaction by cross-absorption (5). Conversely, a monoclonal antibody may be 'too specific' if it reacts with an epitope that is polymorphic within the population of molecules to be measured (6). Broadly specific monoclonal antibodies also occur when they react with an epitope that is not unique to an analyte. However, such antibodies may be exploited for the development of broad-spectrum assays, e.g. for the detection of fungi (7) or for low molecular weight generic haptens that have a common structural feature, such as organophosphate pesticides (8). Multispecific mono-clonal antibody molecules have also been described which can bind a number of apparently dissimilar compounds (9).

The multiple interactions with antigen that are characteristic of polyclonal antibodies have long been exploited in immunoassays with agglutination-dependent end-points, e.g. particle-enhanced immunoassays. Only when their specific epitope is present in multiple copies on the antigen can individual monoclonal antibodies be used in direct agglutination assays (10). Cocktails or combinations of selected monoclonal antibodies (i.e. synthetic and definable 'polyclonal' antibodies) can be used in agglutination assays but there are very few examples in the literature. Monoclonal antibodies, however, have often been used in agglutination inhibition assays (11).

2 Animals and cell lines

Increasingly strict and detailed licences are required in an increasing number of countries for all uses of live animals in laboratory procedures and, therefore, for their use in the production of both polyclonal and monoclonal antibodies. The relevant regulations concerning their use should be consulted long before obtaining the necessary animals, because additional training and capital investment in facilities may be needed. In the UK, the Home Office requires that such work be performed in a 'Designated Establishment' that meets all the requirements of animal welfare. The procedures associated with antibody production must have a 'Personal Licence'.

2.1 Raising monoclonal antibodies

Monoclonal antibodies are usually produced (*Figure 1*) in animal species and strains from which myeloma cell lines have been derived that are suitable for fusing with their B lymphocytes (spleen cells). Thus, hybridoma cell generation and monoclonal antibody production are generally confined to certain strains of mice and rats. When B lymphocytes and myeloma cells from different species are fused, the resulting hybrid, and frequently highly unstable, cells are called hetero-hybridoma cells (12). Myeloma cell lines are available in Europe from the European Collection of Animal Cell Cultures and Imperial Laboratories and in the USA from the American Type Culture Collection.

For mice, many useful myeloma cell lines have been derived from BALB/c mice (1, 13). The two lines, NS1 (P3-NS1/1.Ag4.1) and SP2 (SP2/0-Ag14), are used in both of our laboratories and are perhaps the most widely used. These cell lines are commonly fused to B lymphocytes from immunized BALB/c mice, although cells of both these lines can be fused with B lymphocytes from other mouse strains. 'Within-strain' fusions may often provide more stable hybridoma cells, but the main reason for their popularity in the past was that the resulting hybridoma cells could be grown as antibody-secreting tumours (ascites) in mice of the same strain (see Section 5.5).

For rats, three myeloma cell lines, Y3 (210-RCY3-Ag1,2,3), 983 (IR983F) and YB2 (YB2–0), have been derived from the LOU rat which was bred at the Cancer Institute of the Louvain Medical School in Brussels, Belgium (14, 15). Of these three lines, the Y3 is generally not recommended as it secretes κ light chain and, after fusion, this property is retained by its hybridomas (16). However, in

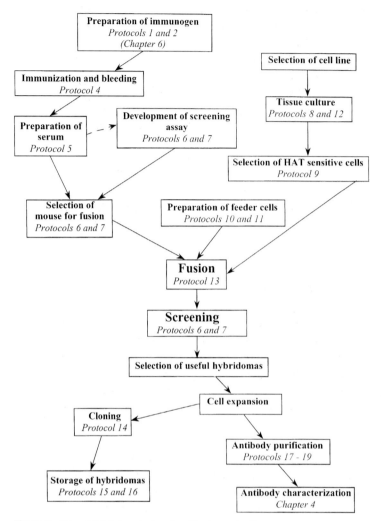

Figure 1. Flow-chart for monoclonal antibody production.

one of our laboratories (Central Science Laboratory, CSL), because of unrelated problems with other cell lines, we have resorted to using Y3 and have obtained useful antibodies, such as antibodies against plant pathogenic viruses (e.g. 17).

The properties of rat monoclonal antibodies are comparable to those from mice in our hands, and others (15). Therefore, rats offer a viable alternative to mice for the production of monoclonal antibodies. Mice are probably much more frequently used because, being smaller, they are easier to handle, require smaller cages, and require less antigen for immunization (see Section 3.1). In addition, general reagents (e.g. anti-species Ig, enzyme conjugates, isotyping reagents) are more readily available.

However, rats, being larger, offer a significant number of practical advantages that may be decisive in some situations. A mouse spleen contains roughly 1×10^8 cells whereas a rat spleen contains in excess of 3×10^8 cells. Since 1×10^8 cells are used for fusion, two aliquots of 1×10^8 rat cells can be saved (frozen in liquid nitrogen) for later fusion with different screening or selection protocols, or kept in reserve in case of contamination problems. In one of our laboratories (CSL), we regularly freeze half or two-thirds of the rat spleen (see Section 5 for relevant protocols) without any adverse effects. This has also been tried with mouse spleens, but without the same success. Most workers check the immune response after the immunization period by testing a blood sample. While it is possible to obtain 100–200 µl of serum from a mouse, more than 1 ml can be obtained from a rat (depending on the regulations in individual countries). The greater the amount of serum, the more antigens can be screened, aiding selection of the animal most likely to yield an antibody with the desired attributes. In addition, the extra serum may be used as positive control material for the optimization of screening procedures.

2.2 Raising polyclonal antibodies

Rabbits, hamsters, guinea pigs and chickens are the most commonly used animals for polyclonal antibody production in the laboratory (*Figure 2*). Rabbits are favoured, probably because the antibodies they produce are well characterized and easily purified. Rabbits are also easy and economical to keep and can be safely repeatedly bled over fairly long periods (up to several years), thereby producing up to several-hundred millilitres of serum. In the UK, the maximum amount of blood that can be taken from a rabbit over a 4-week rolling period is 7.5 ml/kg body weight, up to a maximum of 25 ml (depending on welfare regulations).

When rabbits are used for polyclonal production and the response is considered to be sufficient, a selected animal can be boosted at regular intervals (>4 weeks) and fairly large bleeds taken 7–10 days after each boost. Alternatively, if large volumes are not required, a complete bleed can be taken when the required response is obtained. In this way up to 100 ml of blood can be obtained from a mature rabbit. If the former option is taken, it must be remembered that each bleed will be unique because antibody populations change with time and, therefore, there may be detectable differences in titre and specificity between the batches of antisera collected.

The other laboratory animals mentioned are generally only used either when the amount of antigen available is limiting or when only small volumes of sera are required and, in these cases, mice or rats can be used instead. Typically a single bleed from a rat, hamster, guinea pig (they are hard to bleed) or chicken will yield 1–2 ml of serum. The maximum volume of blood that can be obtained in a single bleed from a mouse is about 200 µl. Most laboratory rabbits, hamsters, guinea pigs and chickens are outbred and they have a wider range of immune response to proteins than the inbred animals (mice and rats) used in the production of monoclonals. Thus, there might be a greater possibility of

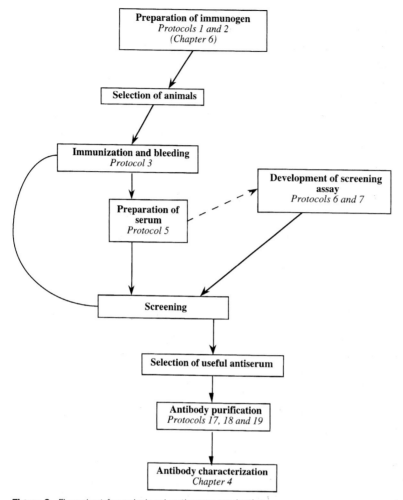

Figure 2. Flow chart for polyclonal antiserum production.

producing good antibodies, both in terms of affinity and specificity, with these animals.

Chickens should be considered for highly conserved mammalian antigens because the phylogenetic distance between these animal groups should provide an enhanced response, as recently reviewed by Jensenius and Koch (18). In terms of the amount of antigen needed and route of administration, the immunization of chickens and rabbits are comparable. The yield of antibody can, however, be much greater with chickens as the egg yolk is a ready source of antibodies. Each yolk can provide approximately the same amount of antibody (1–10 mg of specific IgY out of total of up to about 100 mg) as a 25-ml bleed from a rabbit. Chicken antibodies also have the advantage that they do not react with mammalian rheumatoid factor or activate mammalian complement. However, methods for the purification of IgY from egg yolks can involve difficult and time-consuming steps, which probably explains why chickens are not used as much as other animals. Kits for the purification of IgY are now available (e.g. from Promega) which aim to simplify the task.

Sheep, pigs, donkeys and horses are generally only used when large volumes of serum are required and the choice of species is usually dictated by the availability of suitable facilities and by cost. Larger amounts of antigen will be needed with these species, commensurate with their larger body volume (see Section 3.1). As with all species, there is considerable individual variation in immune response so that the immunization of at least two animals, and more if possible, is recommended.

3 Immunization

The aim of immunization is to elicit a specific and strong immune response to the antigen of interest. When a polyclonal antiserum is to be produced, the quality of the resulting antibody is entirely dependent on the success of the immunization. Even for monoclonal antibody production, immunization is the most important step as it must ensure that activated B cells secreting useful antibodies will be available for fusion with the myeloma cells.

There are a wide variety of standard immunization protocols and many are designed to maximize the response of the immune system to a particular type of antigen or to influence the properties of the antibodies generated. It is often also necessary to devise customized schedules for particular antigens. Factors that must be considered include the species and strain of animal to be immunized (see Section 2), the form and dose of the immunogen, the choice of adjuvant (if any), and the route, number and timing of the initial and 'booster' immunizations.

3.1 The immunogen

The immunogen used can vary from a highly purified soluble or insoluble protein, polysaccharide, lipid, or nucleic acid, or a conjugate of small molecules and protein, to complex mixtures, or even whole microorganisms or mammalian cells. It is always wise to consider carefully what is required with respect to the antibody and what is feasible with respect to the immunogen before proceeding further with an immunization programme.

The specificity of a polyclonal antiserum is usually limited by the purity and physiochemical uniqueness of the antigen used to raise it. A high degree of purity may be essential, especially if the same contaminants will be present in the matrix of the samples to be assayed. Although not as critical for monoclonal production with its inherent selection stages, the use of pure antigen increases the chances of obtaining a large repertoire of B lymphocytes secreting antibodies against the antigen, and not against contaminants that may have 'strong' epitopes.

A useful approach to immunizing small animals, when only impure antigen is available, is to separate the mixture by PAGE or SDS-PAGE and use the 'band' from the gel that contains the antigen (after lyophilization and/or grinding) as the immunogen (19) (See also Section 2 of Chapter 6). Alternatively, it may be possible to immunize with plasmid DNA expression vectors that encode the protein of interest (20). Suitable vectors can apparently give rise to short-term expression of the encoded proteins, leading to specific immune responses in the immunized animals.

Lower molecular weight antigens (generally < 5000 kDa) are conjugated to carrier proteins in order to make them immunogenic or to improve their immunogenicity. Conjugation may also be useful in improving the immune response to highly conserved antigens, which might otherwise be poor immunogens. The preparation of immunogens and conjugation procedures are covered in more detail in Chapter 6.

Antibodies are generally considered difficult to raise against lipids, probably because of their hydrophobicity and consequent inaccessibility to the immune system. However, it is important to remember that many very good antibodies have been raised against steroids when conjugated to proteins (21) and anti-phospholipid antibodies have also been described (22). Nucleic acids are also generally considered to be poor antigens, although antibodies against nucleic acids arise in a number of autoimmune diseases (23). Monoclonal anti-nucleic antibodies have been produced from autoimmune animals with some sequence specificity (24) and anti-nucleic acid antibodies that can distinguish between single and double stranded DNA have been described (25).

The optimal dose of immunogen needed to generate a strong immune response varies from antigen to antigen, and even from animal to animal of the species and strain to be immunized. A balance has to reached between using too much or too little antigen, which lead to either tolerance or an absence of response. The appropriate dose for each antigen has, in many cases, to be determined empirically, although following general guidelines will often result in success. Suggested doses are: mice 50 µg, rats 100 µg, rabbits 200 µg, chickens 100 µg and goats 1000 µg, although much lower doses have been used successfully with each species. Generally, lower amounts of antigen (50% initial dose) are administered in the secondary immunizations or 'boosts', as low antigen levels at the time when the immune response is maturing are thought to promote the production of high-affinity antibodies. This 'affinity maturation' seems to continue in some cases as long as the immunization schedule is continued. We have raised our highest-affinity monoclonal antibodies to progesterone when a mouse in which the initial immunization had been given approximately 15 months previously was used in the fusion (21)

3.2 Adjuvants

Adjuvants are generally essential components in immunization protocols and they are particularly necessary when immunizing with soluble proteins. Adjuvants promote a sustained immune response, most frequently by facilitating the formation of a depot of antigen that is released slowly over time, thus increasing the exposure of the immune system to the antigen. Some adjuvants also contain components that act as nonspecific stimulators of the immune system. Oil-in-water adjuvant emulsions are easily ingested by macrophages, which direct the antigen to the spleen or lymph nodes where the immune response takes place. The most common adjuvant remains Freund's adjuvant, a mixture of mineral oil and surfactant, which in its complete form also contains killed mycobacteria (*Mycobacterium tuberculosis* or *Mycobacterium butyricum*) as an immune stimulant (*Protocol 1*). An alternative is to adsorb the antigen onto aluminium salts, which has fewer side-effects than Freund's adjuvant and is widely used for human immunizations (*Protocol 2*).

A common immunization protocol for both rabbits and mice involves a primary immunization with complete Freund's adjuvant, followed by a number of boosts with Freund's incomplete adjuvant given at intervals of 2–4 weeks until the response is optimum. A number of animals should be immunized with each immunogen as there may be considerable individual variation in the responses obtained.

Tip

It should be remembered that many of the strains of animals used for immunization are inbred and may be incapable of responding to a particular immunogen. Also, depending on the nature of the antigen, a particular adjuvant may be more or less effective. Therefore if resources permit, it is recommended to immunize at least two animal strains with immunogen prepared with at least two different types of adjuvant.

Protocol 1
Preparation of immunogen using Freund's adjuvant

Materials

- Antigen
- PBS
- Freund's complete or incomplete adjuvant
- 16 × 100 mm test-tube
- 1 ml or 2 ml Ventura syringe
- 18- and 21-gauge needles

Procedure

1. Dissolve/suspend antigen in PBS, so that the desired dose is contained in 0.5 times the final injection volume.
2. If using complete adjuvant, mix well ensuring that the mycobacteria are fully suspended in the oil.
3. A number of alternative methods can be used to generate the emulsion:
    (a) With a syringe or a positive displacement pipette, add adjuvant into the test-tube.

Protocol 1 continued

   (b) While vortexing the adjuvant vigorously, add drop-wise an equal volume of the antigen solution/suspension. A white emulsion will form very quickly. It is important that the antigen solution is not added in excess. If in any doubt about the calibration of pipettes, etc. it is better to err on the side of excess adjuvant.

   (c) Continue mixing for 2–3 min until the emulsion visibly thickens and no longer rises up the side of the tube.

or

   (a) To the antigen solution, add an equal volume of the adjuvant (either complete or incomplete adjuvant).

   (b) Mix with a 10-ml syringe and a large-gauge needle by rapidly drawing up and dispelling the mixture several times.

or

   (a) Using two syringes which can be attached by means of a Luer lock mechanism, take up antigen into one syringe and adjuvant into a second, expel the air from each syringe and then attach the connecting mechanism.

   (b) Starting by adding the antigen solution into the adjuvant, rapidly pass the mixture back and forth between the syringes until the mixture thickens. Care should be taken that the attaching device is tightly in position as considerable force will have to be exerted as the mixture thickens (otherwise the emulsion may end up on an adjacent wall!).

4. The resulting emulsion should be thick and creamy. To check that a stable emulsion has been formed, take up a small drop with a Pasteur pipette and place it on the surface of a beaker of water. It should fail to disperse.

5. Draw the emulsion up into the syringe using an 18-gauge needle. Leave to stand on end to allow the emulsion to settle in the syringe.

6. Change to a 21-gauge needle and expel air from the syringe before injection.

Footnote: Because the emulsion will stick to the walls of the tube, syringes, etc., some of the mixture will be lost during preparation. It is therefore advisable to make more than is required. Most antigen/adjuvant emulsions can be stored at 4°C for 1–2 months, so it is possible to make up enough for the complete immunization schedule and so minimize the loss.

Protocol 2

Preparation of immunogen using alum as adjuvant

Materials

- Antigen
- PBS
- Alumina Cγ gel (Sigma 8628)
- 16 × 100 mm test-tube
- 1 ml or 2 ml Ventura syringe
- 21-gauge needles

Protocol 2 continued

Procedure

1. Dissolve/suspend antigen in PBS, so that the desired dose is contained in 0.9 times the final injection volume.

2. Mix Alumina Cγ gel well.

3. Add Alumina Cγ gel into antigen (10 μL Alumina C per 100 μL antigen) and vortex well.

4. Draw up into the syringe using a 21 gauge needle. Leave to stand for at least 5 min before injection.

3.3 Injection route and timing

Subcutaneous and intramuscular routes are commonly used in the rabbit, with the immunogen in a total volume of approximately 1 ml distributed over three to four sites (*Protocol 3*). We have found intradermal immunization at multiple sites to give a slow but prolonged response, and this is especially useful if the antigen is in short supply. The rabbit is bled from the ear vein at the start to check for native antibodies which may react with the antigen and again 7–10 days after each boost to check whether a specific immune response has taken place. Subcutaneous and intramuscular routes are also common for larger animals, although the total volume injected may be larger.

For mice and rats both peritoneal and subcutaneous routes of immunization are common and 300 to 500 μl can be injected at a time (*Protocol 4*). It is usual to bleed these animals at the start and again only once after one to three boosts to confirm that immune responses have been generated and to measure the response (titre, specificity) in each animal (*Protocol 5*). When the antigen is in very low supply, intrasplenic immunization can be used (26), although it is more complex than the usual routes and is not recommended. After selection of the animal that is to supply cells for fusion, it is subjected to a final boosting regime. This may be a single, intravenous injection of a small quantity (e.g. 10 μg) of antigen in 100 μl PBS given 4 days prior to the fusion (day –4). Alternatively, it may involve an intravenous boost of 10 μg on day –4 followed by two intra-peritoneal boosts of 10 μg each on days – 3 and – 2 (21).

For some applications, there is a requirement for a specific antibody class or subclass because of their different effector functions. Shortly after a single immunization, most activated B-lymphocytes will secrete IgM antibodies and bleeds at this time will be rich in antigen-specific IgM; monoclonals generated will be predominantly IgM. Boosting is necessary to promote class-switching to IgG. The IgG isotype generated can be influenced by the adjuvant used, with aluminium adjuvants tending to favour production of IgG1 and IgE antibodies, and IgG2a production being enhanced by complete Freund's adjuvant (27, 28). IgA producers have been selected following immunization by gastric intubation (29) or following fusion with gut-associated lymphoid tissue (30).

Protocol 3

Immunization of rabbits

Materials

- Immunogen prepared as described in Protocol 1 (or Protocol 2)
- Rabbits (2–2.5 kg)
- Rabbit restraining box

Procedure

1. Prepare antigen in Freund's complete adjuvant as described in Protocol 1 with the required dose of antigen per animal in a maximum volume of 1 ml.
2. Place rabbit in the restrainer.
3. Take a small bleed from the animal by shaving the hair over a small section of the vein on the outer edge of the ear. Rub the ear between the fingers to stimulate blood flow through it. Using a sterile scalpel, nick the vein and allow the blood to drip into a clean serum tube. Three to five millilitres of blood is sufficient. Stop the bleeding; if necessary, apply pressure over an antiseptic swab.
4. For immunization, pinch up the skin over one of the shoulders and inject approximately one-quarter of the total dose for each animal. Ensure that the needle only pierces the skin once and does not come through the other side of the skin fold.
5. Repeat step 3 at three other sites along the back, e.g. over the second shoulder and over the two hips.
6. Boosts are given at 4, 8 and 12 weeks and whenever necessary, thereafter. For boosts, prepare the immunogen in the same way as previously. In general, use only half the dose of antigen per boost compared with that given in the initial immunization. If using Freund's adjuvant, use the incomplete form for all boosts.
7. Take small bleeds (as described in step 3 above) 7–10 days after each boost to check that the animal is responding.
8. Take a large bleed (up to 25 ml) when the response is considered adequate in the same manner as described in step 3 above, but, in addition, stimulate blood flow to the ear by rubbing a tissue soaked in xylene briefly over the ear prior to piercing the vein.

Footnote: Remember, all animal experimentation requires a licence and proper training in animal handling techniques.

Protocol 4

Immunization of mice for monoclonal antibody production

Materials

- Immunogen prepared as described in Protocol 1 (or Protocol 2)
- Balb/C mice (6–8 weeks old)
- Mouse restrainer

Procedure

1. Prepare antigen in complete Freund's adjuvant as described in *Protocol 1* with the required dose of antigen per animal in a maximum volume of 300 μl.

2. If necessary, warm mice by placing mouse box close to an infrared lamp.

3. Remove mouse and place in the restrainer.

4. Take a small bleed from the animal by cutting off a small section of the tail using a sterile scalpel and allowing the blood to drip into a clean Eppendorf tube. Approximately 150–200 μl of blood is sufficient. Stop the bleeding; if necessary, apply pressure over an antiseptic swab.

5. For subcutaneous immunization, remove the animal from the restrainer and place on top of cage grid. Pinch up the skin at the scruff of neck and inject the required amount for each animal. Ensure that the needle only pierces the skin once and does not come through the other side of the skin fold. This is the usual route of injection when Freund's complete adjuvant is being used.

6. For intraperitoneal immunization, remove the animal from the restrainer and place on top of cage grid. Hold the animal in the palm of the hand by pinching up the skin at the scruff of neck with the thumb and forefinger and restraining the tail with the little finger. The animal should not be free to move and the skin should be stretched over the abdominal cavity. Piercing the skin and peritoneum halfway between the mid-line and the top of the leg, inject the required amount of immunogen. This is the most commonly used route of injection for mice.

7. Administer booster doses, usually two or three times, at 2-weekly or 4-weekly intervals. For boosts, prepare the immunogen in the same way as previously. The antigen dose per boost is usually only half that given in the initial immunization. If using Freund's adjuvant, use the incomplete form for all boosts.

8. Bleed again (as described in step 4 above) 7–10 days after the second or third boost to check that the animal is responding and to allow selection of the most suitable animal for the fusion.

9. Give an intravenous boost 4 days prior to the fusion. Prepare the immunogen by dissolving the antigen in sterile PBS (10 μg/100 μl) and taking it up into a 1-ml syringe fitted with a 27-gauge needle. Place the warmed mouse in the restrainer. Starting low down in the tail, insert the needle into the tail vein and inject the 100 μl of immunogen. The tail vein is seen to clear when the immunogen passes into the vein. If the vein is missed, try a different vein (there are four veins in the tail) or again further up the same vein. If this is not successful, inject the remainder intraperitoneally.

Footnote: Remember all that animal experimentation requires a licence and proper training in animal handling techniques.

Protocol 5

Preparation of serum

Materials

- Blood
- Serum tubes
- Bench centrifuge

Procedure

1. After collection, leave blood at room temperature for approximately 1 h to clot.
2. For maximum yield of serum, transfer to 4°C for a further hour to cause clot to contract.
3. Centrifuge blood at 3000 **g** for 15 min.
4. Pour serum into a clean tube.
5. Store at 4°C. For long-term storage, store in aliquots at −20°C. Do not repeatedly freeze and thaw.

4 Monitoring immunizations

4.1 General and when raising polyclonal antisera

To monitor the progress of immunizations, a screening procedure is necessary that will provide information on the effectiveness and characteristics of the antibodies being produced. This enables decisions to be made on continuation of boosting, selection of the best responding animal, etc. A fuller characterization of selected antibodies comes later (see Chapter 3), but much time and effort can be saved if the initial screening procedure gives information on those aspects of the desired antibodies which are most important for the intended application. For example, if antibodies of both the IgG and IgM classes are of interest, or if an isotype that fixes complement is desired, then the screening procedure should be designed to include only the required antibody (sub)class(es).

If possible, the screening procedure should be developed and validated in advance with the aid of antibodies with similar properties to the desired antibody. Otherwise, as in the case of a novel antigen, the procedure should be based on a simple well-tried format, with reagents of confirmed quality, and used to search for increases in titre between the bleeds taken before and after the immunization is commenced. Once bleeds with reasonable titres have been obtained they can be used to check the screening procedure itself to determine if it could benefit from further optimization. However, if no increase in titre is found in any animal, one is faced with a classical conundrum. Either all the immunizations were ineffective, which can happen with an antigen of possibly poor immunogenicity, or the screening procedure is defective. Neither should be trusted completely and both should be reviewed with the use of extra controls and, if necessary, with similar reagents or antigens that are known to be effective.

The primary role of screening is to identify the animals giving the most appropriate response to the immunization protocol. If the procedure used detects only antibodies having the desired characteristics, strength of titre (defined as the dilution of antiserum giving a specified response in a screening assay) may be the sole criterion. However, the basic screening procedure may be supplemented with variants so that the specificity, affinity or other properties of at least the most promising bleeds can be assessed.

4.2 When raising monoclonal antibodies

In the production of monoclonal antibodies, the screening procedure has an extra function as it is also used to select the hybridomas secreting the desired antibody. The most interesting hybridomas should be selected as soon as possible after the fusion so that the maximum attention can be given to a smaller number of cell lines.

Fresh and used tissue culture supernatant should be checked in the screening procedure to ensure that they do not interfere. Although not all of the wells in the 96-well culture plates will contain living cells, it is more efficient to simply transfer aliquots of media directly to corresponding wells in the 96-well assay plate. Cell densities should be as high as possible before screening to ensure there is sufficient antibody for detection, but it is also important to screen early so that the cells in positive wells can be cloned as soon as possible and over-growth by non-producing clones is avoided. When coming to a compromise, it should be remembered that (while still ensuring cells are kept alive) the media in the wells should not have been changed for at least 3–4 days so that the antibody concentration in the medium is as high as possible. Screening is usually carried out between 10 and 14 days following the fusion.

4.3 Screening procedures

For most purposes, a colorimetric, microtitre plate, antibody capture ELISA with anti-species antibody coupled to enzyme (well wall-Ag-**Ab**-Ab-Enzyme) is the basic method used for the screening of both sera and culture supernatants. The principles of such tests are long established and well documented (31–33), and they are particularly suitable for soluble protein and glycoprotein antigens (*Protocol 6*).

For each antigen the optimal coating concentration should be checked by serial dilution to maximize sensitivity and to minimize background and negative control readings. Too much antigen coated on the plate will result in a build up of layers that are unstable during washing steps and too little will result in poor sensitivity. However, reduced sensitivity may sometimes be worthwhile since limiting concentrations of antigen favour the detection of higher-affinity antibodies. A concentration of about 1–10 μg antigen/ml coating buffer has been found to be a suitable starting point. Particulate antigens such as cells, micro-organisms, spores, etc., may need to be covalently coupled to the plate surface and a suitable method using glutaraldehyde and poly-L-lysine has been developed (34). (See also Chapter 5.)

For the detection of antibodies to haptens, the plate wells are usually coated with a hapten–carrier protein conjugate equivalent to that used as immunogen. This is because it is often difficult to immobilize haptens directly onto poly-styrene and, even if they can be immobilized, they may be inaccessible to the antibody because they are bound too close to the plastic surface. If the same carrier protein is used for immunization and screening, difficulties will arise owing to detection of antibodies to the carrier protein as well as anti-hapten antibodies. Therefore, a conjugate prepared with a different carrier protein is generally used for screening. There may still be significant crossreactions, which may be attributed to the presence of similarly-modified amino acid residues in both carrier proteins, arising from the conjugation procedure (35). Controls are, therefore, very necessary in these assays and should include testing of binding activity against carrier proteins both unmodified and following a blank (i.e. hapten omitted) conjugation procedure.

However, we have found that the best option for detection of anti-hapten antibodies is to use an antigen capture assay format (*Protocol 7*). This procedure can be quite simple, although it is somewhat insensitive. The antibodies to be detected (if any) (and serum or culture medium proteins) are directly coated onto microtitre plate wells followed by identification of the wells containing anti-hapten antibodies by addition of labelled hapten molecules, e.g. a hapten–enzyme conjugate (well wall-**Ab**–Ag-enzyme). Alternatively, and more sensitively, the wells are precoated with an anti-species antibody, e.g. rabbit anti-species total immunoglobulin antibody or rabbit anti-species IgG Fc region antibody (well wall-Ab–**Ab**–Ag-enzyme).

It is not always possible to identify the most suitable antibodies based on their performance in one type of screening assay. In the production of specific monoclonal antibodies to *Fusarium* species of 'field fungi' (36), each bleed was tested against several different *Fusarium* species plus some other taxonomically more distinct fungi. Mice whose sera showed the greatest reactivity with the homologous rather than the heterologous fungi were considered to be the most likely candidates for specific monoclonal production and were therefore selected for fusion.

After a fusion, it may be necessary to carry out a primary screen on all wells for immunoglobulin production with anti-species/(sub)class antibodies (wall-**Ig**-Ab-enzyme or wall-Ab-**IgG**-Ab-enzyme) and then to screen only positive wells for specific antibodies to the antigen of interest. This is useful if purified antigen is scarce, or if the antigen has not yet been purified. In that case, the secondary screen may involve preliminary fractionation of the antigen preparation by PAGE and Western blotting, which is not suitable for large numbers of samples.

In the production of highly specific antibodies to progesterone in the labora-tory of one of us (National Diagnostics Centre) a multistaged screening procedure was found to be beneficial. Clones secreting antibodies binding to progesterone conjugate were first identified, the supernatants titered to estimate limiting antibody concentrations, and the affinities roughly estimated by looking at displacement of conjugate by a very limited range of progesterone concentrations. The crossreactivities with a small number of 'analytically important', related steroids were then tested before clones were selected for further culture and characterization.

To obtain sufficient culture supernatant for complex screening procedures, either of two approaches may be taken. A single sample, of say 100 μl, of supernatant may be taken for the initial screening procedure and then, when antibody concentration has built up again in the supernatant (within about 2 days), further aliquots taken from the positive wells for subsequent screening. This procedure was used during the development of the anti-progesterone antibodies above. Alternatively, if there is reason to believe that the screening assays are sufficiently sensitive, a single aliquot per well may be taken, diluted (up to fivefold) and used to carry out a range (up to 10 assays at 50 μl per singlicate assay) of screening assays simultaneously. This method was used during the development of the broad-spectrum anti-fungal antibodies mentioned above.

Protocol 6

A typical screening procedure: antibody capture

Materials

- Microtitre plate
- Glass universal containers
- Antigen
- Coating buffer: 50 mM Na_2CO_3, 0.1 g/l thimerosal, pH 9.6
- Wash solution: 0.5 ml Tween 20/l in 150 mM NaCl

- Blocking solution: 0.1% BSA in PBS
- 0.01% BSA in PBS
- Anti-species antibody–horseradish peroxidase conjugate
- TMB solution (Sigma T8540; see Section 2.1.1 of Chapter 4)
- 1 M H_2SO_4

Procedure

1. Dilute antigen in coating buffer (10 μg/ml) in a glass universal container.

2. To coat plates add 100 μl antigen solution per well and incubate at 37°C for 90 min.

3. Empty wells by flicking plate sharply over a sink. Then wash wells three times as follows: fill wells with wash solution, leave for approximately 10 s then empty as before.

4. To block wells add 250 μl blocking solution, incubate at 37°C for 30 min, empty and wash as step 3.

5. Add 100 μl diluted serum (in PBS/0.01% BSA) or tissue culture supernatant to duplicate wells, incubate at 37°C for 60 min, empty and wash as step 3.

Protocol 6 continued

6. Add 100 μl diluted conjugate (in PBS/0.01% BSA) to each well, incubate at 37°C for 60 min, empty and wash as step 3.

7. Develop colour by adding 100 μl TMB solution to each well. Leave plate at room temperature in the dark for 15 min.

8. Add 50 μl H_2SO_4 solution, mix gently and read absorbance at 450 nm.

Footnote: This procedure is merely a guideline. There are many possible variations on each step. It cannot be over-emphasized that the screening assays must be thoroughly optimized and validated prior to carrying out the fusion.

Protocol 7

A typical screening procedure: antigen capture

Materials

- Microtitre plate
- Glass universal containers
- Anti-species antibody
- Coating buffer: 50 mM Na_2CO_3, 0.1 g/l thimerosal, pH 9.6
- 0.01% BSA in PBS

- Wash solution: 0.5 ml/l Tween 20 in 150 mM NaCl
- Antigen horseradish peroxidase conjugate
- TMB solution (Sigma T8540; see Section 2.1.1 of Chapter 4)
- 1 M H_2SO_4

Procedure

1. Dilute anti-species antibody (1 in 1000 approximately, or as recommended) in coating buffer in a glass universal container.

2. Coat plates by adding 100 μl anti-species antibody solution into wells and incubating at 37°C for 90 min.

3. Empty wells by flicking sharply over a sink. Then wash wells three times as follows: fill wells with wash solution, leave for approximately 10 s then empty as before.

4. Add 100 μl diluted serum (in PBS/0.01% BSA) or tissue culture supernatant to duplicate wells, incubate at 37°C for 60 min, empty and wash as step 3.

5. Add 100 μl diluted conjugate (in PBS/0.01% BSA) to each well, incubate at 37°C for 60 min, empty and wash as step 3.

6. Develop colour by adding 100 μl TMB solution to each well. Leave plate at room temperature in the dark for 15 min

7. Add 50 μl H_2SO_4 solution. Mix gently and read absorbance at 450 nm.

Footnote: See comments at end of *Protocol 6*.

5 Making and manipulating hybridoma cells

5.1 Facilities and media

For the production of monoclonal antibodies, the main requirement is a cell culture room, a laminar flow hood, a CO_2 incubator, an inverted microscope, a centrifuge, a liquid nitrogen cell storage unit, access to an autoclave and dedicated variable and multichannel pipettes. This room should be located away from general laboratory activities to potential sources of contamination. It is now common practice to use sterile disposable pipettes, flasks, etc., and ready-to-use, sterile media preparations as much as possible. This, while increasing costs, reduces the time involved in washing, sterilizing, etc., but, more importantly, also eliminates many potential problems, including those arising from improper washing, ineffective sterilization and poor water quality. Expertise in basic cell culture techniques is also required and it would be wise to invest in some general cell culture handbooks (e.g. 37).

A wide variety of media and media supplements can be used for culture of myeloma and hybridoma cells (*Table 1*). Media such as RPMI-1640 or DMEM are commonly used with the addition of a number of supplements (*Protocol 8*). The most important of these is FCS, which is often added at concentrations up to 20%. A number of serum replacement supplements are available but FCS is still commonly used during, and immediately before and after fusions. Importantly, the efficiency of fusions can be dependent on the FCS batch used and, therefore, prior testing of a number of different batches for ability to support myeloma growth and for fusion efficiency is recommended before purchasing a large quantity. The addition of glutamine (≈ 2 mM) is essential unless the medium already contains a stable form of this nutrient. Hypoxanthine, aminopterin and thymidine are added to the culture medium (HAT medium) used immediately following the fusion, to select for growth of hybrids. Myeloma cells should be periodically checked for HAT sensitivity by the addition of 8-azaguanine to the growth medium for a few days (*Protocol 9*). Some workers favour selection by HAZA medium, which contains azaserine, as this is thought to also block the growth of mycoplasma. However, azaserine is a carcinogen and a teratogen, so appropriate safety

Table 1. Media recipes: volume of supplements per 100 ml complete medium

Medium	FCS (ml)	Glutamine (200 mM) (ml)	Penicillin (5000 U/ml), streptomycin (5 mg/ml) (ml)	HAT (50×) (ml)	HT (50×) (ml)	Amphotericin B (ml)	Hybridoma-enhancing medium (ml)	DMSO (ml)
Serum-free		1	2			2		
Growth	10	1	2					
HAT	10	1		2				
HT	10	1	2		2			
Cloning	10	1	2				10	
Freezing	90							10

measures need to be taken if it is used. Before reverting to regular growth medium, hybridoma cells are grown in HT medium (no aminopterin) for a few days.

Protocol 8

Preparation of regular culture medium

Materials

- Sterile medium, RPMI-1640 or DMEM
- Sterile FCS
- Sterile 200 mM glutamine
- Sterile 5000 units/ml penicillin, 5 mg/ml streptomycin

- Sterile flask, pipettes
- Pipette aid

Procedure

1. Use aseptic procedures throughout.
2. In a sterile hood, transfer approximately 80 ml of RPMI-1640 (or DMEM) into a sterile flask.
3. Add 10 ml FCS, 1 ml glutamine and 2 ml penicillin/streptomycin.
4. Make up to 100 ml with RPMI or DMEM. Mix gently.
5. After preparation, leave an aliquot overnight at 37°C to confirm sterility. Any colour change or turbidity indicates contamination and the batch should be discarded. Store the clear medium at 4°C for a maximum of 1 week.

Protocol 9

Selection of HAT sensitive cells

Materials

- 8-Azaguanine
- Double distilled water
- 10 M NaOH

- 0.2 μm filter
- Complete culture medium

Procedure

1. To 6 mg azaguanine, add 9 ml of double-distilled water. Add 10 M NaOH drop-wise until dissolved (3–6 drops). Make up to 10 ml with water.
2. Sterilize by passing through a 0.2-μm filter.
3. To 100 ml complete culture medium, add 0.5 ml azaguanine solution.
4. Grow myeloma cells in this medium for 4–5 days to ensure they are HAT-sensitive. Only cells that are HAT-sensitive will grow in the presence of azaguanine.

Antibiotic supplementation (e.g. penicillin 100 units/ml; streptomycin 100 μg/ml) is desirable during a fusion to reduce the risk of contamination resulting from the large number of manipulations involved. Anti-fungal agents such as amphotericin B should be used with caution as they have been reported to reduce overall fusion efficiency and hence the number of hybridomas resulting from a fusion. Concentrated solutions of glutamine, antibiotics, anti-fungal agents, HAT and HT are commercially available from a variety of suppliers (e.g. Gibco, Sigma, etc.) and should be stored frozen in aliquots as they lose activity at 4°C.

Following a fusion or during cloning, viable cells will be at a very low density in the growth chamber. Because lone cells or cells at low densities do not grow well, it is necessary to have additional growth factors in the medium. These can be supplied by 'feeder cells' (Protocol 10), or by the use of media supplements, such as hybridoma enhancing supplement (HES, Sigma) or a 'home-produced' spleen lymphokine preparation (Protocol 11). The supplements have the advantage that changes are more apparent when the progress of growth is checked microscopically.

Protocol 10

Preparation of splenocyte feeder cells.

Materials

- Mice
- Three 10 cm diameter sterile Petri dishes
- Sterile forceps and scissors, disposable pipettes, centrifuge tubes
- Pipette aid
- Tissue sieve with 50 or 60 mesh screen
- Bench centrifuge
- Bunsen burner
- 70% alcohol
- Serum-free medium
- HAT medium or cloning medium

Procedure

1. One spleen is needed per four 96-well plates.
2. Add 5 ml of serum-free medium to Petri dishes 1 and 2 and 10 ml to a third Petri dish.
3. Swab bench-top where dissection is to take place with 70% alcohol.
4. Turn on Bunsen burner when it is safe to do so.
5. Lay out sterile dissection instruments and dissection board.
6. In the animal house, kill the number of mice required by cervical dislocation and immerse in a beaker of 70% alcohol.
7. On returning to the tissue culture room, change your laboratory coat and wash your hands.
8. Using forceps and scissors, lift up the skin and make a small cut in the skin over

Protocol 10 continued

the spleen. Using two forceps, hold the skin at either side of the cut and tear the skin by pulling. The spleen should be visible under the peritoneum.

9. Using fresh sterile forceps and scissors, lift and cut the peritoneum over the spleen. Cut back the peritoneum until the spleen is fully exposed.

10. Holding the spleen in a fresh sterile forceps, cut it free and remove it placing it quickly into one of the Petri dishes. Discard the mouse remains.

11. Repeat steps 8–10 with each mouse, placing all spleens into the same Petri dish.

12. Turn off the Bunsen burner, swab each Petri dish with 70% alcohol, change gloves and move Petri dish into the laminar flow cabinet.

13. Trim each spleen in turn using another sterile forceps and scissors. Transfer spleens to the second Petri dish and rinse well with serum-free medium.

14. Remove tissue sieve from sterilization bag and put standing in the third Petri dish.

15. Remove plunger from a sterile 10 ml syringe aseptically.

16. Transfer spleens into sieve and using the syringe plunger mash the spleen tissue until the cell contents are seen to run freely into the medium. The spleen capsule(s) should remain on the sieve.

17. With a pipette, transfer the medium with cells to a sterile centrifuge tube.

18. Spin at 1500 **g** for 10 min in the bench centrifuge.

19. Remove the supernatant, tap the tube gently against a solid surface to dislodge the cells from the wall of the tube.

20. Resuspend the cells in 10 ml of serum-free medium and repeat steps 18 and 19.

21. Resuspend the feeder cells in the required volume of HAT medium if they are to be used for a fusion, or of cloning medium if they are to be used for cloning.

Protocol 11

Spleen lymphokine preparation

Materials

- Mice
- Three 10 cm diameter sterile Petri dishes
- Sterile forceps and scissors, disposable pipettes, centrifuge tubes
- Pipette aid
- Tissue sieve with 50 or 60 mesh screen
- Bench centrifuge
- 70% alcohol
- Hepes-buffered saline solution (HBSS)
- Heparin
- Regular growth medium

Procedure

1. Kill a normal mouse by cervical dislocation under anaesthesia.

2. Swab mouse with 70% alcohol and open peritoneal cavity.

Protocol 11 continued

3. Remove spleen aseptically into a sterile Petri dish containing 10 ml HBSS with heparin at 5 IU, warmed to 37°C.

4. Tease out spleen as for a fusion using 'bent needles' or by 'sieve and syringe plunger'.

5. Transfer cell suspension to a plastic universal and centrifuge at 1500 **g** for 3 min at room temperature.

6. Decant HBSS and heparin and resuspend pellet in 30 ml growth medium.

7. Transfer into 80 ml tissue culture flask and incubate for 3 days at 37°C with 5% CO_2.

8. After 3–5 days, centrifuge down cells at 1500 **g** for 5 min at room temperature and collect supernatant.

9. Filter (0.2 μm filter) supernatant and store at −20°C in aliquots of 1 ml.

10. Dilute 1:20 in growth medium for use in replacement of feeder cells.

5.2 Fusions and selection of hybridomas

Although a fusion procedure is complete within 5 min, considerable time must be expended in preparation to ensure a successful outcome. The animal to be used in the fusion must have been selected and the final boost(s) administered. There should be several flasks of myeloma cells available in their log phase of growth (1–5×10^5 cells/ml), with viability greater than 93% (*Protocol 12*). The cells should also have been tested recently for HAT sensitivity (*Protocol 9*). Finally, the animal is killed, the spleen removed and the cells prepared for fusion with the myeloma cells.

There are a small number of important points to be kept in mind when carrying out the fusion procedure with PEG as the fusing agent (*Protocol 13*). The most critical step is exposure of the cells to PEG. Any traces of serum, which would have a protective effect on the myeloma cells and reduce the efficiency of the fusion, should have been removed by washing well with serum-free medium prior to the addition of PEG. Careful attention must be paid to the timing of exposure to PEG and the subsequent dilution steps, as prolonged exposure is lethal. The cells should have minimum and very gently handling for several hours after the fusion while plasma and organelle membranes reassume their normal states.

Following fusion, the cells are generally resuspended in medium containing either HAT or HAZA within a few hours to enable the selection of hybridoma cells and the exclusion of myeloma cells. Some groups prefer to use normal medium for 24 h to give the cells a chance to recover before switching to the selective medium. The selective medium is also supplemented at this stage with either 'feeder cells' (*Protocol 10*), the spleen lymphokine preparation (*Protocol 11*) or HES (see previous section) to support growth of the hybridoma cells. The resuspended cells are then aliquotted into the wells of 96-well tissue culture plates. The density at which the cells are plated out after fusion also varies. Most often the cells are resuspended in 100 ml of medium and are plated out over five 96-well plates (200 μl per well), but this volume may be increased and as many as 20 plates have been used. Such greater dilution may reduce competition between multiple clones of hybridoma cells growing in the same wells but it makes the screening procedure onerous. The procedure followed for feeding cells also varies. Some groups leave the cells alone for approximately 10 days, at which time the supernatants are screened while others feed the cells after 5–6 days (i.e. at least 4 days before screening).

After about 10 days, there is generally good growth of hybridomas and the wells are screened for the presence of the desired antibody (see Section 4.3). Following identification of the wells containing hybridomas secreting the desired antibody, the cells from each such well are expanded (i.e. diluted, aliquoted and cultured) into 24-well plates in preparation for cloning. At each cell expansion stage, it is strongly recommended to continue to maintain the cells remaining in the original well (in this case the master well of the fusion plates) as a back-up, in case the cells fail to thrive when expanded or in case of contamination. Freezing of the hybridoma cells in liquid nitrogen as soon as possible is also recommended as such back-up cells can prove very useful if the hybridomas later lose their antibody-producing genes.

A very successful fusion (i.e. one generating a high number of potentially useful hybridomas) will require considerable work input as the cell numbers expand and it is wise to plan for this eventuality if you do not want to risk losing some useful hybridomas. We put an upper limit of twelve on the number of hybridomas cloned following a fusion. Any further potentially useful clones are simply expanded until there are sufficient cells for freezing down (Protocol 15).

Protocol 12

Determination of cell viability

Materials

- Cell suspension
- Trypan blue solution (0.4 g/25 ml PBS)
- Sterile pipettes
- Pipette aid
- Neubauer haemocytometer and cover-slip
- Microscope

Procedure

1. Prepare the haemocytometer by rubbing with alcohol and drying with a lint-free cloth.

2. Apply a cover-slip over the counting chambers and press onto the haemocytometer along the edges only. The cover-slip is properly attached when an optical interference pattern can be seen along the edges.

Protocol 12 continued

3. Ensure that the cell suspension is thoroughly mixed before aseptically transferring an aliquot to a small vial.

4. Prepare a 1 in 2 dilution of the cell suspension in Trypan blue solution. Mix well.

5. Take up approximately 20 µl of the diluted cell suspension with a pipette and, touching the tip of the pipette against the edge of the cover-slip, allow the counting chamber to fill by capillary action. Do not let the chamber overflow.

6. Count all viable cells (the clear bright cells with 'halos') in the centre and four large corner squares of the counting grid. Cells touching the lower and left-hand perimeter lines should be ignored to avoid double counting. For accuracy, between 20 and 100 cells should be counted. If less than 20 cells are counted in five squares, more squares should be counted; if more than 100, the process should be repeated with an increased initial dilution factor.

7. Count all the cells (viable and nonviable) present in the same squares. Calculate the viable cells as a percentage of the total cells present.

8. The viable cell density in cells/ml of the original suspension is the number of viable cells counted divided by 5 (5 large squares counted), multiplied by 2 (the dilution factor used above) and multiplied by 10^4.

Protocol 13

Fusion procedure

Materials

- Sterile scissors, forceps, pipette tips, troughs, 96-well tissue culture plates, 50 ml centrifuge tubes, 1, 2 and 10 ml pipettes and syringes, 21-gauge needles, Petri dishes, 25 cm^2 tissue culture flask

- Pipette aid

- 70% alcohol

- PEG 1500 (tissue culture grade, Boehringer Mannheim.

- Serum-free medium (approximately 100 ml)

- HAT medium (120 ml) containing feeder cells if used: this amount is sufficient for five plates and controls. If more or less plates are going to be used, the quantity should be adjusted accordingly

- HT medium (50 ml)

- Spleen lymphokine preparation (*Protocol 10*) or HES

- SP2 myeloma cell (section 2.1)

Procedure

Day before fusion:

1. In the morning, split the SP2/O cells to 2×10^5/ml in three tissue culture flasks and to 10^5/ml in two flasks to ensure there will be a sufficient number of actively dividing cells for the fusion (in case of any error in counting or transferring to new flasks).

2. Prepare splenocyte feeder cells (*Protocol 9*) if they are being used.

Protocol 13 continued

Day of fusion:

1. Take samples of all myeloma cultures for total and viable cell counts.

2. Selecting from the flask with highest viability (the viability should be $> 95\%$), transfer a volume of cell suspension containing 10^7 cells to a 50-ml tube. Place the cells in the incubator until needed.

3. Remove PEG from the fridge and leave at room temperature until needed.

4. When everything is ready, kill the immunized mouse and collect the spleen cells as described for preparation of feeder cells (*Protocol 10*, steps 1 to 19).

5. Resuspend the cells in 10 ml of serum-free medium and centrifuge at 1500 **g** for 10 min. At the same time, spin down the myeloma cells which will be used in the fusion.

6. Decant supernatant from each tube, tap tubes gently to dislodge cells and separately wash both cell populations with 10 ml of serum-free medium. Spin down and decant the supernatants as before.

7. Resuspend each pellet in 10.5 ml of serum-free medium. Retain 0.5 ml of each cell type in separate test-tubes as controls.

8. Combine the remaining 10 ml of spleen cells and 10 ml of myeloma cells and spin down as before. Remove the supernatant completely with a pipette. Do not decant. Flick the tube vigorously to break up any clumps of cells and to distribute the cells around the end of the tube.

9. Add 1 ml of PEG very gently over 1 min. Allow to slowly run down the side of the tube while rotating the tube slowly. Wait 1 min.

10. Slowly dilute the PEG using HT medium. Holding the tube almost horizontal and the pipette within 2.5 cm of the PEG/cell suspension and rotating the tube slowly, gradually add 3 ml HT medium over the next 3 min. To ensure slow dilution, it is best to use a 1 or 2 ml pipette at this stage. Wait 2 min, then, add 4 ml over 1 min, wait 4 min and finally add 8 ml over 1 min. Increase the speed of tube rotation as you progress to the final addition.

11. Centrifuge at 1500 **g** for 10 min. Decant the supernatant and flick the tube gently to resuspend the cells. (Note: the cells are very fragile at this time.) Resuspend the cells in 5 ml of HT medium. Pipette very gently to break up clumps and transfer the cell suspension to a 25-cm^2 flask.

12. Place in the incubator for 1–2 h.

13. Control spleen cells and myeloma cells should be diluted in 10 ml of the HAT medium prepared previously and also placed in the incubator.

14. After 1–2 h, carefully transfer the hybridoma cells into a 50-ml centrifuge tube. Rinse the flask two or three times with more medium to harvest all cells from the flask. Do not shake the flask until the last rinse to avoid damaging the cells. Check the flask under the microscope to confirm all cells are removed.

15. Centrifuge at 1500 **g** for 10 min. Remove the supernatant.

Protocol 13 continued

16. Resuspend the cells in the HAT medium. Plate out the cells onto 96-well plates at 200 μl per well. Leave wells A1 and B1 empty on all plates to enable controls to be included with each plate during the screening assay; also plate out the control spleen cells and the control myeloma cells.

17. Place all plates in the CO_2 incubator.

Days after fusion:

1. Check all plates microscopically on the first or second day after the fusion to ensure no contamination is present

2. By day 5 or 6 after the fusion, colonies should be visible microscopically in some wells. Control wells should also be checked to ensure that no growth has taken place (i.e. to check that HAT medium is working).

3. Feed cells on day 5 or 6. With sterile glass Pasteur pipettes and a gentle vacuum pump, aspirate approximately half of well contents and replace with fresh HAT medium. This should be done gently as cells may still be quite delicate after the fusion.

4. Supernatants should be ready for screening by day 10–12 following the fusion. At least 4 days should have elapsed since the cells were last fed when screening is carried out.

5. After selection of useful hybridomas, feed and expand cells as necessary. Keep feeding cells with HAT medium until the myeloma control cells are dead (approximately 14 days). Cells should then be switched to HT medium for two to three feeds before reverting to regular culture medium. Cells should be fed at least once every 5 days. If colonies remain small, they may be boosted by using feeder cells, lymphokine preparation or HES again.

5.3 Cloning and further selections

Two methods of cloning have been described: cloning by limiting dilution and cloning on soft agar. The former is most widely used and, in our laboratories, we find this method to be the most convenient (*Protocol 14*). For the limiting dilution method, the aim is to get growth of positive clones, i.e. antibody-producing clones, from the lowest dilution of cells possible. This will give the highest chance that the clones were derived from a single parent cell, i.e. that they are monoclonal. Antibody-secreting cells, usually from the well of a 24-well plate, are harvested, counted and then serially diluted to a range of low densities, such as 50, 5 and 0.5 cells/ml. Feeder cells, spleen lymphokine preparation or HES will be needed as growth supplements, as before (Section 5.1). When 200 μl volumes of each of these dilutions are pipetted into the wells of a 96-well plate, this will correspond to about 10, 1 and '0.1' cells/well, respectively.

After 5–7 days, examine the wells under the microscope. Differences between the different dilutions should be apparent. In addition, provided the wells have not been agitated too much, individual clones will appear as tight clusters of cells, and wells with single clones can be identified. After about 7–9 days, all wells with clones should be screened and those secreting the desired antibody selected, giving preference to those from wells with single clones. Give particular preference to those from the lowest density plate where clusters are more likely to be monoclonal.

Select a maximum of six positive clones from each original master well to expand up to 30 ml cultures for freezing and further cloning. It should always be borne in mind that antibodies showing similar properties in the screening assays are likely to have originated from the same parent cell and, therefore, saving all of them will not usually be worthwhile. However, it is always worth saving at least two or three clones, as hybridoma cell lines can die or stop producing antibody due to genetic instability. Because they 'shed' some of their surplus complement of genetic material by a random process, not all clones from cells that initially secreted antibody will necessarily lose the ability to secrete antibody as they stabilize.

Thereafter, the selected clones should be cloned for a second time and screened as before to ensure that the cell lines are truly monoclonal and stable. After the second cloning stage, some of the cells should again be frozen and large quantities of antibody-containing culture supernatants should be produced (100–200 ml) for antibody characterization, purification and assay development.

Some workers, however, prefer cloning on soft agar, by which the cells are diluted and then grown on an appropriate agar surface (1, 38, 39). When growth has occurred, individual colonies ('clones') are clearly visible on the surface of the agar. However, it is not possible to screen quickly at this stage, except by haemolytic overlay (1) or immunoprecipitation (40), because the antibodies being produced by each of the colonies diffuse into the medium. Instead, cells from each clone are picked off, expanded in liquid culture and the culture medium screened.

We find the limiting dilution method more convenient because (a) there is no need to transfer clones from agar to tissue culture medium, thereby reducing the chances of contamination, and (b) the cloning plates can be easily screened by the direct transfer of supernatants to the assay plates.

Protocol 14

Cloning by limiting dilution

Materials

- Cloning medium (50 ml per clone) containing feeder cells if used
- Sterile centrifuge tubes (50 ml), serum tubes (5 ml), 10 ml pipettes, automatic pipette tips, 96-well tissue culture plates
- Pipette aid
- Automatic pipettes
- Multichannel pipette
- Haemocytometer and cover slip

Protocol 14 continued

Procedure

1. With a sterile plastic Pasteur pipette, resuspend cells in the selected well and transfer some of the cells and medium to a labelled sterile tube. Mix and remove a few drops of the cell suspension for counting. Place the remainder of the cells in the incubator. Do not work with more than four clones at any one time.

2. Count the cells (see *Protocol 12*).

3. Dilute the cells in cloning medium to densities of 1.5 and 0.5 cells/ml. At least 20 ml of each density is required. It is important to ensure that the cell suspensions are mixed thoroughly by flicking the tube before removing the appropriate aliquot for dilution. It is important also not to use too small an aliquot of the denser suspension, but rather to make dilutions in stages. This reduces the potential error.

4. Using a sterile trough and the multichannel pipette, dispense each cell suspension into the wells of a 96-well culture plate at 200 μl per well and one plate per cell density. (Note: ensure that cell suspensions are mixed thoroughly before each manipulation and always fill multichannel pipette from the bottom of the trough, otherwise the cloning procedure may fail because cells have not been transferred to the wells.)

5. Place plates in the CO_2 incubator.

6. Clones should be visible after 5–7 days. Count the number of wells with cell growth in each plate. Statistically, if there are less than nine wells with growth on an entire plate, then there is a high probability ($> 95\%$) that growth in each well is monoclonal. Note the wells with only one visible clone (cluster) of cells.

7. Screen the supernatants from all wells with growth for production of antibody of interest after about 7–9 days. Clones showing high levels of antibody production should be selected from the lowest density plate and, if possible, from wells that appeared to contain a single clone for further expansion.

5.4 Maintenance and storage

At each stage of the procedures for raising monoclonal antibodies through to second cloning, cells from the previous stages (i.e. after fusion and first cloning) should be saved by keeping the cells growing and/or by freezing. After selection at the second cloning and expansion to produce sufficient antibody for testing, purification, etc., cells should also be saved by storing in liquid nitrogen in case of accidents and instability. However, once second clone cells lines have been established and are seen to be stable by continuing to grow well and produce the desired antibody, backup cells from previous stages can be discarded.

For storage by freezing, cells should be healthy and in their exponential growth phase (at a density of about 2×10^5/ml), with at least 5×10^6 cells per vial

(*Protocol 15*). Because the viability of cells can change, it is important to freeze cells in different batches (at least three vials per batch) on separate days. Approximately 1 week after freezing, the viability of each batch should be checked by thawing one vial and growing up the cells. In addition, and very importantly, cell lines should be kept at two different locations in case of freezer breakdown. It is wise to freeze enough vials at this stage to meet foreseeable needs (usually about 10 are sufficient).

Cells stored in liquid nitrogen will normally remain viable for many years (we have successfully grown up cells stored untouched for more than 10 years). Periodically, however, cells should be thawed (*Protocol 16*) and their viability checked (*Protocol 12*). If the viability has dropped appreciably (to $< 50\%$ viability), the cells should be expanded and grown for approximately 2 weeks, checked for antibody production, re-cloned, if necessary, and re-frozen. Ideally this should be carried out annually.

When expanding the scale of cell culture from wells in 96-well plates, to wells in 24-well plates, to small tissue culture flasks (25 cm^2) to medium flasks (80 cm^2), a slowing of growth can occur. We have sometimes found that it is quite difficult to grow some cell lines in 'jumbo' size tissue culture flasks (200 cm^2). This may be due to a dilution of the growth factors in the medium or the cells may have overgrown at the previous stage. It is thus vital that hybridoma cells should be at their exponential growth stage when the scale of their culture is being increased. If cell growth is slow or if, under the microscope, they do not appear as healthy (not as bright, more granular) as in the previous stage, it may be necessary to reintroduce growth factors (e.g. HES, spleen lymphokine, feeder cells, etc.).

Protocol 15
Freezing cells

Materials

- Cell suspension (approximately 2×10^5 cells/ml)
- Freezing medium (*Table 2*)
- Cryotubes
- Ice
- $-80°C$ freezer
- Polystyrene box
- Liquid nitrogen in suitable container

Procedure

1. Use only cells that are healthy and rapidly dividing., i.e. at a density of about 2×10^5 cells/ml on day of freezing. If freezing rat splenocytes, the cells from the spleen are prepared as if a fusion is to be carried out.

2. Take a 30-ml volume of cells (since the final cell concentration should be at least 5×10^6 cells/vial) or a third of the cells prepared from one rat spleen and centrifuge at 1500 **g** for 5 min at 4°C.

Protocol 15 continued

3. Decant medium and resuspend each pellet in 1 ml ice-cold freezing medium. Dispense the 1 ml into a sterile cooled cryotube. (Note: cells must be kept on ice once suspended in freezing medium.)

4. Place the cryotube in a polystyrene container or insulating bag or container and keep at −80°C for 24–72 h before transferring the cryotube to liquid nitrogen.

Footnote: Insulating the cryotube ensures that the temperature fall is gradual and reduces the likelihood of intracellular ice formation.

Protocol 16
Thawing cells

Materials

- Frozen vial
- Regular culture medium (*Table 1*)
- Water-bath, 37°C

Procedure

1. Remove vial of cells from liquid nitrogen store. **Liquid nitrogen can cause severe burns so wear suitable protective clothing.**

2. Rapidly thaw by placing in a disposable glove and plunging into a water-bath at 37°C.

3. Remove from water-bath before ice has fully melted. Drench the outside of the vial with 70% alcohol, transfer contents to a 50-ml centrifuge tube and wash with 50 ml growth medium (warmed to 37°C) by centrifugation at 1000 g for 3 min at room temperature.

4. Resuspend pellet in 12 ml of growth medium warmed to 37°C and dispense 2 ml/well of a 24-well multi-dish. Place in a CO_2 incubator.

5. Expand to flasks (5, 10, 30 ml volume) as cell density increases and use as required or freeze down for long term storage in liquid nitrogen.

5.5 The production of monoclonal antibodies

5.5.1 Ascites tumours

Previously, small- and even medium-scale production of monoclonal antibodies for diagnostic applications was achieved by the induction of ascites tumours in mice with the antibody-secreting hybridoma cell line. This involved the injection of hybridoma cells into the peritoneum, where the cells grew in high densities and eventually yielded about 10 ml of ascitic fluid per mouse, which contained specific antibody at concentrations of between 1 and 10 mg/ml. Although quite large quantities of antibodies can be obtained in this way, this procedure is not recommended as the animal is put under undue stress, and particularly as alternative and easier *in vitro* methods are now available. In addition, in many countries (including the UK and Ireland) it is, understandably, becoming more difficult to obtain a licence for the production of ascitic fluid and the procedure is likely to be banned in the EU. For these reasons, no protocol for this procedure is given here.

5.5.2 Conventional cell culture

For most if not all purposes, including immunoassay development, hybridoma culture supernatants are a suitable source of monoclonal antibody and can have yields of up to about 50 µg/ml. After second cloning, or the thawing of a storage vial, culture of the cells should be expanded from wells of 96- or 24-well plates to tissue culture flasks of progressively increasing size. This is achieved by allowing cell densities to rise and then transferring the total volume of the culture as a starter to the next stage. For example, when expanding from a well in a 24-well plate, the cells in the 2 ml of medium (inoculum) are mixed by gently drawing up and expelling with a pipette. The inoculum is then transferred to a small tissue culture flask (25 cm^2) and fresh growth medium is added to a total volume of 10 ml. Because antibodies are resistant to the proteases from dying cells, hybridomas in the final tissue culture flasks should be allowed to grow until they die. The cell debris can be removed by centrifugation (1000 *g* for 10 min) and the supernatant containing the antibody collected. High yields of antibody can be obtained with much less effort if, when the cells cover approximately 90% of the flask surface, the flask is filled completely with fresh medium and left standing upright (instead of the normal horizontal position) in the incubator for up to 1 month (41). The final concentration of antibody in the medium is similar with both methods but almost 10 times more medium is generated per flask (250 ml versus 25–30 ml) with the upright method, representing a significant saving in materials.

5.5.3 Alternative methods

There are a number of more recently developed cell culture techniques and systems that allow the attainment of much higher hybridoma cell densities and antibody concentrations.

Even with 'standard' culture vessels, the use of simple electrically driven roller or spinner systems allows cell densities to be increased from 1×10^6 to about 2×10^6 cells/ml with antibody concentrations of about 170 µg/ml in a 1-l flask (42). Cell densities up to 1×10^8 cells/ml and antibody concentrations up to 5 mg/ml can be obtained with special culture flasks that have integral membranes (Integra Biosciences). In these flasks, the cells are separated by a double membrane system with the upper membrane allowing diffusion of nutrients and the lower membrane allowing gas exchange. The addition and renewal of media is done manually but the cells can be easily viewed under a microscope.

Hollow-fibre cell culture systems (e.g. Technomouse, Integra Biosciences) allow the attainment of hybridoma cell densities of up to 1×10^9 cells/ml and antibody concentrations of up to 5 mg/ml in up to five separate chambers or cassettes. A single bench-top culture system of this kind, equipped to allow continuous operation, can make possible the production of 10 mg of antibody per day (when running at full capacity with all five cassettes containing the same cell line), according to data provided by the manufacturer. However, the speed of cell growth varies and generally not all of the cassettes are used at the same time so, in our experience, actual yields are often much lower. Separation of cultivation, nutrient and oxygenation chambers is by means of hollow fibres in combination with gas-permeable membranes. Nutrients are pumped through the hollow fibres which allow low molecular mass components (< 10 kDa) to diffuse through and supply the cells. In the same way, metabolic waste products can diffuse through to the circulating medium and be removed. These systems have a high degree of automation and several cell lines can be grown at the same time in separate 'cassettes' with only the need for replenishing medium reservoirs.

All the above commercial systems are supplied with full operating instructions.

6 Antibody purification

The extent to which antibodies need to be purified depends on their intended use. For many immunoassay applications, the antibody-containing serum, culture supernatant or ascites fluid can be diluted to the required concentration with a suitable buffer and used without treatment or fractionation. This is particularly true with high titre antibody preparations as the required dilution effectively reduces the possibility of interference by other components in the matrix to a negligible level. However, where the application necessitates the binding of the antibody in high concentration to a solid phase or where an antibody conjugate is required, at least partial purification is necessary.

Luckily, most antibodies are relatively stable proteins, although repeated freezing and thawing should be avoided. This simplifies the purification procedure considerably as common purification steps may be carried out at room temperature, thus benefiting from the extra speed at which separations take place at higher temperatures. Generally, similar procedures are used for the purification of polyclonal and monoclonal antibodies. However, when embarking on the purification of a newly-produced monoclonal antibody, it is normal to start by determining its isotype unless the screening assay was designed to detect antibodies only of a specific class. The easiest procedure is to use one of the several commercial ELISA (e.g. Sigma-Aldrich) or membrane-based (e.g. Stratagene) kits which are now available for isotyping mouse monoclonal antibodies. Tissue culture supernatant from fairly densely-grown hybridoma cells should be used in the test.

The standard procedures for antibody purification which are widely described usually refer to the purification of polyclonal antibodies and are based on the behaviour of the bulk of the antibody molecules in the antiserum. However, for any particular polyclonal antiserum, small modifications may be necessary to maximize the recovery of the antibody populations of most interest. If such selective purification occurs, the specificity and/or affinity of the purified poly-clonal 'antibody' may be significantly different from the original antiserum. The necessity to modify standard antibody purification procedures from application to application is particularly true for monoclonal antibodies. The method chosen very much depends on the isotype involved and also, because each is a unique molecular entity, general purification methods may have to be modified considerably for each one.

It may also be desirable to improve the specificity of a polyclonal antiserum by eliminating antibodies with high affinity for a particular crossreactant, or to eliminate immunoglobulins that do not bind the antigen. In such cases, affinity methods employing immobilized crossreactant or antigen may be used. Most frequently, this involves the immobilization of the antigen or crossreactant onto cyanogen bromide-activated Sepharose 4B (Pharmacia) following the manufacturer's instructions, and preparation of an affinity column (5). The antiserum is then passed over the column and antigen-specific or cross-reactant-binding antibodies retained depending on which is immobilized on the solid phase. In the case of the former, a change of mobile phase leads to elution of the desired antibody (43). When crossreactant is immobilized, the desired antibody is in the unbound fraction.

The most common procedure used for the initial purification of antibodies from serum, tissue culture supernatant and ascites is ammonium sulfate pre-cipitation (*Protocol 17*). Immunoglobulins precipitate out of solution when the ammonium sulfate concentration is raised to between 30% and 50% saturation. Most commonly, 40% saturation is used to precipitate IgG; if IgM is also needed a 50% ammonium saturation is used. The precipitate is recovered by centrifugation and is then extensively dialysed after redissolution. This is a very useful way of concentrating the antibody, especially when tissue culture supernatant, which usually has a very low antibody concentration (1–10 μg/ml), is the starting point. Although still impure, the product of ammonium sulfate precipitation often shows considerably improved performance in assay systems and further purification is not necessary.

A variety of column chromatography steps have been used for further purification of antibodies. Common among these are anion-exchange chromato-graphy with DEAE-modified resin and a high pH for isolation of IgG, and hydroxyapatite chromatography for the isolation of various immunoglobulin classes (*Protocol 18*). Gel filtration can also be used to isolate IgM class antibodies, which, because of their large size (≈ 970 kDa) can be readily separated from other proteins.

Affinity chromatography on columns of gels derivatized with the bacterial proteins, Protein A or Protein G, is perhaps the most useful method for the

Table 2. Reactivities of Proteins A and G with IgG from different species

Antibody	Protein A	Protein G
Rabbit IgG	+ +	+ +
Sheep IgG	–	+ +
Goat IgG	+	+ +
Horse IgG	–	+ +
Rat IgG	–	+
Mouse IgG1	–	+
Mouse IgG2a	+ +	+ +
Mouse IgG2b	+ +	+ +
Mouse IgG3	+ +	+ +
Chicken IgG	–	–

purification of IgG (*Protocol 19*). These proteins bind the Fc portion of many IgG subclasses from many species, albeit with varying affinities (*Table 2*), and can give good yields of purified IgG. One advantage of these methods is that they can be used directly with serum, tissue culture supernatant or ascites fluid, thus considerably simplifying the purification procedure.

Protocol 17

Purification of rabbit IgG by ammonium sulfate precipitation

Materials

- Saturated ammonium sulfate solution (1 g/ml distilled water, stirred well for at least 24 h; ensure some crystals remain undissolved)
- PBS

Procedure

1. Place a known volume of serum into a glass beaker and stir gently with a magnetic bar.

2. Add a volume of saturated ammonium sulfate solution, equal to two-thirds the volume of serum, very slowly to the serum to bring the solution to 40% saturation. It is important that the ammonium sulfate solution be mixed thoroughly with the serum as it is added, otherwise pockets of higher concentration will result in precipitation of extra serum proteins and a less pure product will result.

3. Continue stirring for 30 min.

4. Centrifuge at 10 000 g for 15 min at 4°C.

5. Carefully remove the supernatant and resuspend the pellet in 5 ml of PBS.

6. Dialyse exhaustively against at least three changes of PBS.

Protocol 18

Hydroxyapatite purification for IgM (and other Igs)

Materials

- Hydroxyapatite (Biogel-HT, Biorad)
- 10 mM sodium phosphate buffer, pH 6.8
- 120 mM sodium phosphate buffer, pH 6.8
- 300 mM sodium phosphate buffer, pH 6.8
- Basic liquid chromatography equipment with UV monitor and fraction collector.

Procedure

1. Pack a 25-ml column with hydroxyapatite.

2. Set up the chromatography equipment according to the manufacturers' instructions with a flow rate of about 1.0–1.5 ml/min and a fraction size of about 2 ml.

4. About 10 ml of ammonium sulfate-precipitated serum proteins (*Protocol 17*) are washed onto the column with 10 mM sodium phosphate buffer until the baseline is stable (about 0.5 h).

5. Change the buffer to 120 mM and continue until 2 peaks have been eluted (these should be proteins from the tissue culture medium).

6. Step to 300 mM sodium phosphate buffer, start the fraction collector and collect the next peak, which will be the elution of Ig.

7. Bulk the fractions containing Ig and dialyse with PBS.

8. The column can be regenerated with 1 M NaCl.

Protocol 19

Purification of a mouse monoclonal IgG antibody by Protein G affinity chromatography

Materials

- Prepacked Protein G column
- Antibody solution to be purified
- PBS
- 0.1 M glycine-HCl (pH 2.7)
- 2 M Tris–HCl, pH 8.0
- Dialysis tubing
- Spectrophotometer

Procedure

1. Pass two column volumes of PBS through the column.

2. Pass the antibody solution to be purified (which should be in buffer at neutral pH and physiological ionic strength) through the column, retaining the eluate. This may contain some residual IgG which can be purified later.

Protocol 19 continued

3. Wash the column by passing PBS through it until the eluate is free of protein. This is confirmed by collecting 1 ml fractions and checking the absorbance at 280 nm.

4. Elute the bound IgG with glycine-HCl buffer, continuing to collect 1 ml fractions until the protein peak has been completely eluted. The pH of the eluted protein should be neutralized as quickly as possible following elution to avoid damage to acid-labile proteins. This can best be achieved by adding 100 μl of 2 M Tris–HCl, pH 8.0 to each fraction tube before eluting the IgG.

5. Dialyse the eluted IgG exhaustively against PBS.

6. Regenerate the column by washing with two to three bed volumes of elution buffer followed by re-equilibration with two to three bed volumes of PBS.

7 Emerging technologies

7.1 *In vitro* immunization

The *in vitro* immunization of spleen cells prior to fusion with myeloma cells and subsequent monoclonal production was described several years ago (44) but has now become much more feasible with the availability of commercial kits for this purpose (Immune Systems Ltd). There are three stages in the process. First, a monolayer of support cells is established and primed with immunogen. Second, a suspension of spleen cells is prepared and these are incubated in the immunization medium with the immunogen and the pre-primed support cells. The fusion is then performed in the usual manner, with the whole process taking about 5 days. In addition to the speed of the process, other stated advantages are that less than 30 μg of antigen is required in total and that it may induce cells secreting antibodies with a specificity not found on *in vivo* presentation of the immunogen. In addition, the technique can be used to generate antibodies against immunogens that are toxic *in vivo* yet have negligible toxicity *in vitro*. The use of *in vitro* immunization systems offers the possibility of an alternative to the use of hyperimmune animals but the full potential of this has probably still to be realized.

7.2 Recombinant antibody techniques

The first recombinant antibodies were derived from the cloning of genes from specific antibody-producing hybridomas. The cloned genes were inserted into a vector and expressed as whole antibodies in mammalian cells or as antibody fragments in bacteria, such as *Escherichia coli*. The antibody genes and, hence, the structure of the resulting antibodies could be altered as required, either to change their specificity, increase their affinity or give them new properties (45–48). The immortalization of antibody genes in bacteria made it feasible to produce large quantities of antibody fragments from bacterial culture. In theory this was much quicker and easier than with mammalian cell culture, although the effort involved was highly dependent on the antibody in question. Since this initial approach still necessitated immunization, the use of animals and fusion techniques, it offered few, if any, advantages over existing methods of mono-clonal antibody production except that it could be used to rescue failing or contaminated cell lines.

Advances in recombinant DNA and gene expression technology have since allowed the immortalization of large repertoires of antibody genes derived initially from the selected cells of a hyperimmune spleen (thus bypassing the fusion process) or from the lymphocytes of unimmunized individuals (49, 50). With the addition of phage display technology (51), these antibody libraries have been expressed on the surface of filamentous bacteriophage, such as M13, simplifying the screening for specificities of interest. These exciting develop-ments have opened up new possibilities for antibody specificities not available using conventional approaches.

For example, large, combinatorial, single-chain variable-fragment (sFv) phage display libraries have been created by amplifying the variable regions (corres-ponding to V_H and V_L) of human immunoglobulin genes. These contain up to 6.5×10^{10} variables (52, 53). From one of these libraries, a number of immune reagents have been isolated (for review see 54). This approach has also been used successfully to produce antibodies to a number of plant pathogens (e.g. potato virus Y) for use in ELISA at one of our laboratories (CSL) (55).

References

1. Kohler, G. and Milstein, C. (1975). *Nature* **256**, 495.
2. Owens R. J. (1997). In *Immunochemistry 1: a practical approach.* (eds A. P. Johnstone and M. W. Turner), p. 27. IRL Press, Oxford.
3. Melamed, M. D., Thompson, K. M., Gibson, T., and Hughes-Jones, N. C. (1987). *J. Immunol. Methods* **104**, 245.
4. Ekins, R. and Newman, B. (1970). In *Steroid assay by protein binding* (eds E. Diczfalusy and A. Diczfalusy), p. 11. WHO/Karolinska Institut, Stockholm.
5. Goding, J. W. (ed.) (1996). *Monoclonal antibodies: principles and practice*, 3rd edn, p. 327. Academic Press, London.
6. Pettersson, K. and Soderholm, J. (1991). *Clin. Chem.* **37**, 333.
7. Banks, J. N., Cox, S. J., Northway, B. J., and Rizvi, R. H. (1994). *Food Agric. Immunol.* **6**, 321.
8. Banks, J. J., Chaudhry, M. Q., Matthews, W. A., Haverley, M., Watkins, T., and Northway, B. J. (1998). *Food Agric. Immunol.*, **10**, 349.
9. Adib-Conquy, M., Avrameas, S., and Ternynck, T. (1993). *Mol. Immunol.* **30**, 119.
10. Shamim, M., Ghosh, D., Baig, M., Nataraju, B., Datta, R. K., and Gupta, S. K. (1997). *J. Immunoassay* **18**, 357.
11. Thakkar, H., Newman, D. J., Holownia, P., Davey, C. L., Wang, C. C., Lloyd, J., Craig, A. R., and Price, C. P. (1997). Clin. Chem., **43**, 109.
12. Yarmush, M. L., Gates, F. T., Weisfogel, D. R., and Kindt, T. J. (1980). *Proc. Natl Acad. Sci. USA* **77**, 2899.
13. Shulman, M., Wilde, C. D., and Kohler, G. (1978). *Nature* **276**, 269.
14. Harlow, E. and Lane, D. (eds) (1988). *Antibodies: a laboratory manual*. Cold Spring Harbor Laboratory Press, New York.

15. Bazin, H. (ed.) (1990). *Rat hybridomas and rat monoclonal antibodies.* CRC Press, Boca Raton.

16. Galfre, G. C., Milstein, G. W., and Wright, B. (1979). *Nature* **277**, 131.

17. Smith, H. G., Barker, I., Brewer, G., Stevens, M., and Hallsworth, P. B. (1996). *Eur. J. Plant Pathol.* **102**, 163.

18. Jensenius, J. C. and Koch, C. (1997). In *Immunochemistry 1: a practical approach* (eds A. P. Johnstone and M. W. Turner), p. 89. IRL Press, Oxford.

19. Boulard, C. and Lecroisey, A. (1982). *J. Immunol. Methods* **50**. 221.

20. Whalen R. (1999). *The DNA vaccine web-site.*
http://www.genweb.com/Dnavax/dnavax.html

21. O'Rorke, A., Kane, M., Gosling, J. P., Tallon, D. F., and Fottrell, P. F. (1994). *Clin. Chem.* **40**, 454.

22. Laakel, M., Bouchard, M., and Lagace, J. (1996) *J. Immunol. Methods* **190**, 267.

23. Stollar, B. D. (1989). *Int. Rev. Immunol.* **5**, 1.

24. Stollar, B. D., Zon, G., and Pastor, R. W. (1986). *Proc. Natl Acad. Sci. USA* **83**, 4469.

25. Mantero G., Zonaro, A., Albertini, A., Bertolo, P., and Primi, D. (1991). *Clin. Chem.* **37**, 422.

26. Spitz M. (1986). In *Methods in enzymology* (ed. J. J. Langone and H. van Vanukis) ,Vol. 121, p. 33. Academic Press, New York.

27. Kenney, J. S., Hughes, B. W., Masada, M. P., and Allison, A. C. (1989). *J. Immunol. Methods* **121**, 157.

28. Vogel, F. R. and Powell, M. F. (1995). In *Vaccine design: the subunit and adjuvant approach* (eds M. F. Powell and M. Newman), p. 141. Plenum Publishing, New York.

29. Colwell, D. E., Michalek, S. M., and McGhee, J. R. (1986). In *Methods in enzymology* (eds J. J. Langone and H. van Vanukis), Vol. 121, p. 42. Academic Press, New York.

30. Dean, C. J., Gyure, L. A., Hall, J. G., and Styles, J. M. (1986). In *Methods in enzymology* (eds J. J. Langone and H. van Vanukis), Vol. 121, p. 52. Academic Press, NY.

31. Voller, A., Bidwell, D. E., and Bartlett, A. (1979). *The Enzyme linked immunosorbent assay (ELISA),* Dynatech Europe, Guernsey, UK.

32. Tijssen, P. (ed.) (1985). *Practice and theory of enzyme immunoassays. Vol. 15, Laboratory Techniques in Biochemistry and Molecular Biology* (eds R. H. Burden and P. H. van Knippenberg). Elsevier Science Publishers, Amsterdam.

33. Kemeny, D. M. and Challacombe, S. J. (eds) (1988). *ELISA and other solid phase immunoassays.* John Wiley & Sons, Chichester, UK.

34. Banks, J. N. and Cox, S. J. (1992). *Mycopathologia* **120**, 79.

35. Briand, J. P., Muller, S., and van Regenmortel, M. H. V. (1985). *J. Immunol. Methods* **78**,59.

36. Banks, J. N., Rizvi, R. H., Barker, I., Turner, J. A., Northway, B. J. and Rahman, S. (1996). Food Agric. Immunol. **8**, 249.

37. Freshney, R. I. (ed.) (1994). *Culture of animal cells: a manual of basic technique.* Wiley-Liss, Chichester.

38. Metcalf, D. (1977). *Recent Res. Cancer Res.* **61**, 1.

39. Kohler, G. (1979). In *Immunological methods* (ed. I. Lefkovits and B. Pernis), p. 397. Academic Press, New York.

40. Cook, W. D. F. and Scharff, M. D. (1977). *Proc. Natl Acad. Sci. USA* **74**, 5687.

41. Ker-hwa Ou, S. and Patterson, P. H. (1997). *J. Immunol. Methods* **209**, 105.

42. Reuveny, S., Velez, D., Miller, L., and Macmillan, J. D. (1986). *J. Immunol. Methods* **86**, 61.

43. Tsang, V. C. and Wilkins, P. P. (1991). *J. Immunol. Methods* **138**, 291.

44. Hengartner, H., Luzzati, A. L., and Schreier, M. (1978). *Curr. Top. Microbiol. Immunol.* **81**, 92.

45. Yang, W. P., Green, K., Pinz-Sweeney, S., Briones, A. T., Burton, D. R., and Barbas, C. F. (1995). *J. Molec. Biol.* **254**, 392.

46. Whitlow, M., Filpula, D., Rollence, M. L., Feng, S. L., and Wood, J. F. (1994). *Prot. Engineer.* **7**, 1017.

47. Holliger, P., Prospero, T., and Winter, G. (1993). *Proc. Natl Acad. Sci. USA* **90**, 6444.

48. Queen, C., Schneider, W. P., Selick, H. E., Payne, P. W., Landolfi, N. F., Duncan, J. F., Avdalovic, M. M., Levitt, M., Junghans, R. P., and Waldmann, T. A. (1989). *Proc. Natl Acad. Sci. USA* **86**, 10029.

49. Huse, W. D., Sastry, L., Iverson, S. A., Kang, A. S., Alting-Mees, M., Burton, D. R., Benkovic, S. J., and Lerner, R. A. (1989). Science, **246**, 1275.

50. Marks, J. D., Hoogenboom, H. R., Bonnert, T. P., McCafferty, J., Griffiths, A. D., and Winter, G. (1991). *J. Molec. Biol.*, **222**, 581.

51. Hoogenboom. H. R., Griffiths, A. D., Johnson, K. S., Chiswell, D. J., Hudson, P., and Winter, G. (1991). *Nucl. Acids Res.* **19**, 4133.

52. Nissim, A., Hoogenboom, H. R., Tomlinson, I. M., Flynn, G., Midgley, C., Lane, D., and Winter, G. (1994). *EMBO J.* **13**, 692.

53. Griffiths, A. D., Williams, S. C., Hartley, O., Tomlinson, I. M., Waterhouse, P., Crosby, W. L., Konteemann, R. E., Jones, P. J., Low, N. M., and Allison, T. J. (1994). *EMBO J.* **13**, 3245.

54. Winter, J. (1994). *Drug Devel. Res.* **33**, 64.

55. Boonham, N. and Barker, I. (1998). *J. Virol. Methods* 74, 193.

Chapter 3
Choosing and characterizing antibodies

A. _____ and J. Coley[†]

_____ entre, National University of Ireland Galway, Galway,
_____ esearch Colworth, Colworth House, Sharnbrook,
_____

1. Introduction

Choosing an antibody for immunoassays is usually the most important preliminary to developing any immunoassay. The assay developer may have just raised antibodies for the particular application, or candidate antibodies may have been obtained from one of the many commercial and noncommercial organizations that produce antibodies. In either case, the best must be selected, or they all must be rejected and the search continued.

An immunoassay is defined primarily by its analyte molecule, which can range in size from an intact cell such as a microorganism, to a natural antigen (which could be almost any size above about 2 kDa), to a specific antibody and to a peptide or small organic molecule. In all immunoassays, the specificity or uniqueness of just one, or at most two, key components determine(s) the properties of the molecules that will be detected, be they antigens or specific antibodies. In reagent limited (competitive) assays and Western blot analysis of antigens, a single reagent antibody determines specificity, whereas in sandwich assays for antigen the analyte is defined by two complementary antibodies. In addition, in many assays for specific antibodies anti-Ig antibodies are used to define the class(es) or subclass(es) of antibodies that are detected, and the specificities of these antibodies are critical to the discriminating power of the assay. Antibodies acting as key reagents in these ways may be defined as primary antibodies.

1.1 Secondary antibodies

Secondary antibodies are used for many purposes. Anti-species Ig antibodies that bind to primary antibodies are especially useful for indirect labelling and for indirect immobilization, and these may be raised against the Fc fragment of the target Ig to improve the configuration of the resultant complexes. With the widespread use of monoclonal antibodies, polyclonal anti-mouse IgG antibodies are especially important.

Secondary antibodies are particularly useful in assay development as, by means of a labelled secondary antibody, one can assess a panel of antibodies for their suitability for labelling without having to conjugate each antibody to the reporter molecule. Indirect labels of this kind also allow alternative reporter molecules (radioactive, enzymatic or fluorimetric, etc.) to be evaluated for their effect on sensitivity.

Often, alternative binding proteins are used instead of secondary antibodies. For example, a number of immunodiagnostic companies (e.g. Roche–Boehringer, Amersham) now coat solid-phase supports with strepavidin to indirectly immobilize any of a range of biotinylated antigens or antibodies. The biotin–strepavidin combination also figures in the most common kind of ligand labelling, in which streptavidin conjugated to a reporter is used to quantify biotinylated antibody or antigen. However, biotin may also be quantified with labelled anti-biotin antibodies, just as antibodies conjugated to FITC are quantified by means of high-affinity labelled anti-FITC antibodies. All of these are readily available from commercial suppliers (Roche-Boehringer, Sigma, Dako, Biogenesis, Serotec, AaltoBio, etc.).

In effect, no immunology laboratory could operate without a range of secondary antibodies used as general purpose reagents, and they are widely available commercially. Secondary antibodies already conjugated to reporter molecules are also obtainable from many commercial sources and are available for a range of antibody classes and species. However, if resources and suitable facilities are available, the preparation of secondary antibodies (and related reagents) 'in-house' may provide improved quality and continuity of supply. If they are needed in large quantities or can be sold on, this can also be cost effective.

To produce anti-Ig secondary antibodies, an Ig preparation is used as immunogen in another animal species and the exact Ig preparation used may be critical to the usefulness of the resulting antiserum. A gross Ig preparation with all IgG subclasses, IgA and IgM could give a reagent that is useful for the monitoring of total immune response, and an individual IgG subclass will give a much more selective antibody. Alternatively, an Fc preparation from total IgG may give a more general-purpose antibody that forms immune complexes with more desirable configurations. The antiserum produced is then tested for reactivity, titre and crossreactivity, purified and, if needed, conjugated to a labelling substance or immobilized on a solid phase.

The most essential precaution is to determine the suitability of the secondary antibody in the assay system under development. For example, in an indirect sandwich immunoassay for the measurement of an antigen (solid phase-GAb–**Analyte**-MAb-RAb-enzyme) the primary antibodies are from two different species. A goat antibody (GAb) is used as capture antibody and a murine antibody (MAb) is the potential reporting antibody, and all potential secondary antibody conjugates (e.g. rabbit anti-mouse Ig conjugated to enzyme, RAb-enzyme) should be checked before use for crossreactivity to the goat antibody.

The finding of any significant crossreactivity is grounds for rejecting use of the reagent. However, if the conjugate is being prepared 'in house' and cross-reactivity caused by a minor subpopulation of antibodies is found, these may be removed by passing the polyclonal rabbit antibody through a column with immobilized goat Ig.

1.2 Specificity

Immunoassays depend on the reversible binding of an antigen to the binding site of an antibody. When antigens are being measured, immunoassay specificity is related to the degree to which compounds other than the antigen participate in the binding reaction, thereby appearing to be molecules of analyte and causing a falsely high reading or a false positive result. Such compounds, if present, are termed interferants or crossreactants and contribute to low assay specificity. Assay specificity is thereby dependent on both the exclusivity of the antibody-binding site and on the degree of availability of crossreactants within the assay. In characterizing the specificity of an antibody for an antigen, only binding specificity may be of direct interest, whereas when validating the specificity of an immunoassay (as in Chapter 7) both binding specificity and the degree to which crossreactants are removed from samples before they are analysed are relevant.

Binding specificity is never absolute and no matter how specific an antibody may appear to be, compounds undoubtedly exist that would crossreact if tested. Crossreactants, although often close structural relatives of antigen, may have totally different general physiochemical properties. Binding specificity can also vary, depending on pH, ionic strength, and the relative concentrations of antigen and crossreactant, and on the degree to which binding equilibrium is attained. Specificity in the context of assay optimization and validation is discussed further in Chapters 7 and 8, respectively.

1.3 Epitope mapping

Epitope mapping is the use of a panel of monoclonal antibodies to investigate the immunochemical structure of an antigen. With a sufficient number of different antibodies, which bind to a variety of epitopes that may or may not overlap and are more or less evenly spaced over the surface of the antigen, a comprehensive three-dimensional epitope map or model of the antigen can be constructed. Testing the same antibodies against a panel of synthetic peptides that represent different portions of the antigen polypeptide chain can help to relate the epitope map to the antigen sequence and, if it is available, to the three-dimensional structure of the antigen. A wide variety of other methods have also been used in epitope mapping studies. X-ray diffraction crystallography can visualize the antigen–Fab complex. Alternatively, the protein can be modified by chemical, enzymatic or recombinant DNA methods to help define epitopes.

Epitope mapping is a powerful tool in the investigation of the structures of proteins (1), and when a protein has been comprehensively mapped, potentially suitable antibody pairs from the panel of antibodies used to perform the mapping can be selected with confidence. For example, if it has been reported that a certain epitope is subject to genetic variation and that some variants are not recognized by antibodies to that epitope, then such antibodies can be avoided (2).

However, for practical immunoassay development, less sophisticated and less ambitious methods may be adequate. The Ouchterlony method can provide sufficient information to identify complimentary pairs of antibodies suitable for a typical sandwich assay, while basic ELISA techniques can compliment this method to further define epitopes (3).

1.4 Affinity

1.4.1 Background

Affinity and avidity are two different terms used to describe the tendency of antibodies to bind to antigens and the durability of this binding, and, although they may be difficult to separate experimentally, they should not be confused with each other. Affinity is a precise term borrowed from chemical kinetics. It represents the balance between the ease with which an interaction occurs and the probability that the complex will dissociate, and is a measure of the overall strength of the interaction. Avidity has no precise thermodynamic meaning but is useful because it expresses the 'total tightness' of binding when bivalent or multivalent antibodies make multiple interactions with large multivalent anti-gens. Avidity is very important biologically, because it is much greater than the simple affinity of each interaction multiplied by the number of links formed. The terms intrinsic affinity and functional affinity are also used (4). Intrinsic affinity refers to the overall or average affinity of a polyclonal antibody, whereas functional affinity is somewhat equivalent to avidity.

Antibody-binding affinity is most easily explained if it is taken as a measure of the strength of the interaction between one binding site of an antibody and its monovalent antigen. The formation of the antibody-antigen complex is reversible and the equilibrium reaction can be written as:

$$Ab + Ag \longleftrightarrow AbAg$$

where k_a and k_d are the association and dissociation rate constants, respectfully. At equilibrium and applying the law of mass action:

$$k_a[Ab][Ab] = k_d[AbAg]$$

Rearranging gives an equation defining the ratio of the rate constants, and, by definition, this ratio is equal to the equilibrium (affinity) constant, K_a,

$$K_a = \frac{k_a}{k_d} = \frac{[AbAg]}{[Ab][Ag]}$$

When half of the antibody-binding sites are occupied by antigen, then:

$$[Ab] = [AbAg]$$

and

$$K_a = \frac{1}{[Ag]}$$

Thus, at equilibrium when half the antibody-binding sites are occupied, K_a is equal to the reciprocal of the concentration of free antigen. The units of K_a are, therefore, M^{-1} or l/mol.

1.4.2 Data analysis

Three methods for calculating affinity constants from binding data are commonly employed and each can be used with or without knowledge of the absolute concentration of antibody used. One of these methods were developed in an attempt to take into account the heterogeneous nature of polyclonal antisera, which normally contain antibodies with a wide range of affinities, equivalent to K_a values spread over two orders of magnitude. Monoclonal antibodies, on the other hand, are homogeneous with respect to affinity.

The following symbols are used for all the methods:

i = concentration of antibody, expressed in M units

n = valency of antibody

ni = concentration of antibody binding sites, M

x = concentration of bound antigen, M

a = concentration of free antigen, M

r = ratio of concentrations of bound Ag/and antibody ($= x/i$)

K_a = association equilibrium affinity constant, M^{-1}

K_d = dissociation equilibrium affinity constant ($= 1/K_a$), M

K_0 = intrinsic association affinity constant, M^{-1}

α = heterogeneity index

1.4.2.1 Scatchard plot

This method is commonly used to characterize molecular binding events throughout biology (5). When a fixed concentration of a homogeneous 'binder' is incubated with a carefully selected range of ligand concentrations until equilibrium is reached, plotting the ratio of bound and free ligand concentrations (x/a) versus the concentration of bound ligand (x) yields a straight line. If the molar concentration of the 'binder' is known, this method can yield its valency and the equilibrium affinity constant.

To obtain Scatchard plots, (a) if the antibody concentration is known, r/a is plotted against r (*Figure 1A*) according to the equation:

$$\frac{r}{a} = K_a (n - r)$$

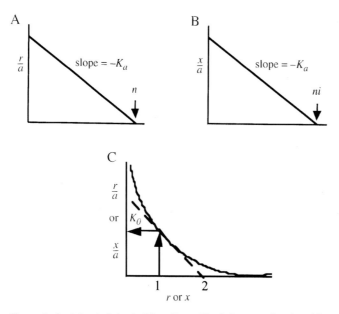

Figure 1. Scatchard plots. A. When the antibody is monoclonal and its concentration is known r/a may be plotted against r to give a straight-line plot and the valence of the antibody estimated. B. When an unknown concentration of a monoclonal antibody is analysed x/a is plotted against x allowing the total binding site concentration to be estimated. In both cases, K_a is estimated from the slope of the line. C. When the antibody is polyclonal the fitted line is curved and concave. The average or intrinsic affinity (K_o) is estimated from the slope of the tangent to the curve at the mid-point, when about half the sites are occupied.

and (b) when the antibody concentration is unknown x/a is plotted versus x (*Figure 1B*) according to the equation:

$$\frac{x}{a} = K_a\,(ni - x)$$

Whereas a Scatchard plot is a straight line for monoclonal antibodies, it is a curved line for polyclonal antisera (*Figure 1C*). The affinity of a polyclonal antiserum, often referred to as its intrinsic affinity constant (K_0), is measured at the point in which half the antibody-binding sites are occupied. Since divalent antibodies react with monovalent antigens when $n = 2$, $r = 1$ and $K_0 = 1/a$, some idea of the range of affinities of the constituent antibodies in a polyclonal mixture can be gained by taking tangents to the curve along its length (low affinity at $r = 2$, intrinsic or average affinity at $r = 1$, and high affinity when r is small). IgM antibodies have a theoretical valency of 10, but in practice this tends to be about 5.

1.4.2.2 Langmuir plot

The Langmuir plot is a variant of the Scatchard plot. As described here, the equilibrium binding data (which give a hyperbolic saturation curve when r or x

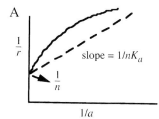 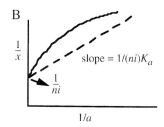

Figure 2. Langmuir double reciprocal plots are linear with monoclonal antibodies but curved with heterogeneous populations of binding sites. The two plots represent the cases when the antibody concentration used is known (A) and unknown (B).

is plotted against a) are 'linearized' by plotting the reciprocals $1/r$ or $1/x$ against $1/a$ (6), corresponding to the situations when the antibody concentration is known (*Figure 2A*):

$$\frac{1}{r} = \frac{1}{n} \cdot \frac{1}{K_a} \cdot \frac{1}{a} + \frac{1}{n}$$

and when the antibody concentration is unknown (*Figure 2B*):

$$\frac{1}{x} = \frac{1}{ni} \cdot \frac{1}{K_a} \cdot \frac{1}{a} + \frac{1}{ni}$$

For an homogeneous population of binding sites either plot gives a straight line. Extrapolation of this line to infinite free antigen ($1/a = 0$) gives an estimate of the valency of the antibody (*Figure 2A*) or of the total concentration of the antibody binding sites (*Figure 2B*). The association constant is derived from the slope.

As with the Scatchard plot, polyclonal antibodies give a curved plot, making graphical extrapolation uncertain. The presence of even a small amount of high-affinity antibody can result in significant underestimation of the concentration of low-affinity antibody. In addition, saturation of low-affinity binding sites requires high concentrations of antigen, which is often impractical.

1.4.2.3 Sips plot

The Sips plot was derived to try to describe more fully the heterogeneity of mixed populations of binding sites (7), of which polyclonal sera are good examples. To obtain Sips plots, (a) when the antibody concentration is known $\log (r/[n - r]$ is plotted against $\log a$ (*Figure 3A*) according to the equation:

$$\log \frac{r}{n - r} = \alpha(\log K_0 + \log a)$$

and (b) when the antibody concentration is unknown $\log (x/[ni - x])$ is plotted versus $\log a$ (*Figure 3B*) according to the equation:

$$\log \frac{x}{(ni) - x} = \alpha(\log K_0 + \log a)$$

65

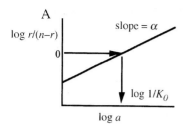 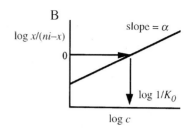

Figure 3. Sips plots are complex and are designed to characterize the heterogeneity of polyclonal antisera. When the antibody concentration is known (A) or unknown (B), the intrinsic affinity constant is interpolated at log $(r/[n - r]) = 0$ or $\log(x/[ni - x]) = 0$, respectively. The slope α represents the heterogeneity index of the antibody population and would be 1.0 for a monoclonal antibody.

The derivation assumes a distribution of affinity constants around a mean value that is close to a normal distribution, which, however, is unlikely to be true in practice. The double log plot is also a relatively insensitive method of plotting data. Nevertheless, a plot of log $(r/n - r)$ versus log a should produce a straight line as shown.

As α approaches 1.0, the antibody population approaches homogeneity with regard to affinity constants. Log $1/K_0$, the intrinsic affinity constant, is given by log a when log $(r/n - r) = 0$, this is also the peak of the presumed normal distribution. There appears to be no advantage in its use for monoclonal antibodies, since homogeneity is more easily demonstrated by Langmuir or Scatchard plots (8).

1.4.3 Factors affecting affinity

While the binding of antibodies and antigens can occur over quite a wide range of environmental conditions, relatively small variations in pH, ionic strength and temperature may significantly affect the affinity of binding. In immunoassays, binding may occur in solution or with the antibody or antigen bound to a solid surface, which may also introduce differences in apparent or real affinity. This may be due to restricted diffusion (thereby decreasing the probability of association), to orientation and steric effects, and to denaturation of the immobilized reactant. Epitope density on the immobilized antigen will also affect antibody binding to the solid phase. Most often, immobilization of a reactant can be expected to lower affinity and this was found by Underwood *et al.* (9). Here, an antibody to haemagglutin from the influenza virus had a lower affinity constant for the solid-phase antigen than for the antigen in solution. However, Nygren *et al.* found the converse for antibodies to the hapten, 2-phenyloxazolone coupled to BSA as a carrier protein (10). The high epitope density (molar ratio of 2-phenyloxazolone to BSA of 19:1), would have resulted in the antibody having a higher functional affinity for the immunogen-coated solid phase.

Most methods used to estimate the affinity of an antibody require the use of labelled antibody or antigen. Any form of labelling can alter the binding characteristics of a molecule, but most especially if it is conjugated to a separate label molecule. Labelling can also lead to damage of the labelled molecule and hence affect its binding affinity. To minimize the effects of labelling for proteins, radioactive iodine-125 is often used, since it is small, and low substitution ratios do not appear to greatly affect binding. For haptens, tritiated derivatives may be commercially available that are chemically almost identical to the unlabelled molecule.

Consequently, since quite different conditions may have been applied, the estimates of antibody affinity given by commercial suppliers may be inappropriate to the assay being developed. Serious inaccuracies can also result from procedural design, the need to make corrections for the sometimes very large fraction of labelled proteins which are not 'bindable', and deficient methods of data manipulation. For all of the above reasons, estimates of affinity supplied by different suppliers cannot be compared with confidence.

2 Sourcing antibodies

In the absence of a proven track record, or of any innovative strategy, for obtaining antibodies with exceptional properties, antibodies obtained elsewhere may be just as good or better than those that might reasonably be expected to be raised 'in-house'. It is often also less costly to obtain antibodies externally.

To supply the most suitable antibody, the vendor must understand the requirements of the assay developer, but the first prerequisite is that the actual buyer, such as the materials manager in a company, be supplied with a detailed account of the product to be identified and purchased.

Companies supplying antibodies typically supply a data sheet for each antibody product outlining its characteristics (*Figure 4*). This data sheet or product information leaflet usually includes the title of the product, the standard unit for sale and specific information on the characteristics of the antibody. But the requirements of the assay developer may be quite specific and involve information not always, or even normally given.

Therefore, the assay developer should list the minimum specifications of the required antibody. The antigen must be defined. Can it be a natural preparation, or must it be recombinant? Is there a further specification on the actual preparation of antigen used or on epitope recognition? Can the antibody be polyclonal, and if so which species are acceptable? If it must be monoclonal, could it be a rat antibody, and is the class or subclass of antibody important? How much will be required for the project? This sometimes can be defined as weight (mg) of a freeze-dried preparation or as a titre or dilution of a liquid sample. Is the thermal stability of the product known?

Choosing antibodies may be simplified if they have been used in an epitope-mapping exercise or otherwise characterized as part of a scientific study. Antigens that have been subjected to relevant detailed studies include all the dimeric glycoprotein hormones and prostate-specific antigen. Laboratories that carry out such studies may be willing to supply particular antibodies in small

The Antibody Company Inc.

Product Specification Sheet

Product:	Antibody to (antigen)
Clone No.:	234X
Batch No.:	12345 abc
Description:	Purified murine monoclonal, by salt fractionation and ion-exchange chromatography. The product is supplied as salt-free, (less than 0.9% sodium), lyophilized powder.
Immunogen:	ABX, from bovine muscle.
Reconstruction/volume:	1 mg/ml in saline solution (150 mM NaCl).
Protein Concentration:	10.0 mg/ml in ammonium sulphate solution dilute in 0.01 M phosphate buffer, pH 7.4 (0.1% azide) at 1/600 for EIA.
Storage:	Store at 0-5°C.
	After reconstitution, store aliquots at −20°C
	Repeating freezing and thawing is not recommended
Specificity:	The antibody reacts with bovine (antigen), and cross-reacts with equine (antigen) (50%). It also reacts with human (antigen) (10%) and has not been tested with other animal species. Epitope mapping tudies suggest that the epitope contains the amino acid sequence [ ]. The specificity was ascertained as follows:
	Cross-immunoelectrophoresis
	Immunohistochemistry.
Applications:	The product is suitable for use in immunohistochemistry: 1:200
	EIA at a dilution 1:10,000
	RIA at a dilution 1:20,000
	Recommended as a capture or reporter antibody.
	Not recommended for competitive assays.

For *in-vitro* research and manufacturing of diagnostic kits only.

Figure 4. Model antibody specification sheet for a commercially supplied antibody.

quantities for the purpose of basic research, or be willing to enter into a commercial agreement.

Linscotts Directory (William D. Linscott, 4877 Grange Rd., Santa Rosa, California 95404, USA) is a source of comprehensive information on commercially available antibodies. This is an international catalogue of antibodies, antigens, assay kits and other reagents, together with contact names and addresses. It includes polyclonal antibodies, monoclonal antibodies, hybridoma cell lines, tissues, blood products, biochemicals, cytokines, enzymes, lectins and venoms. Also listed are living organisms and their derivatives, and cell cultures. Immunoassay kits and contract testing services are also included. The suppliers' addresses, telephone and fax numbers are given and, in some cases, the distributors of the original suppliers in various countries are provided. If a particular antibody or antigen is not listed, it is still advisable to contact some suppliers with ranges of similar products, as the material required may have just come into stock or another supplier may be recommended.

The World Wide Web is now an excellent source of information on components for immunoassay development. Most relevant companies and organizations have a web page dedicated to the products they supply and in many cases information on the characteristics of individual antibodies is immediately accessible (11).

These are some initial sites that can be used as starting points:

www.antibodyresource.com

www.wenet.net/~sjdanko/biotech.html

www.researchd.com

They provide not only information on the products but may also have links to research topics of interest.

There are also individual company sites on the web, detailing the products they produce. Finally, it should be noted that many of these companies have distributors in numerous countries and your local suppliers of laboratory reagents may be of help in obtaining the required materials.

It is recommended that the buyer obtain a number of samples from different suppliers to enable a through evaluation to be carried out. In addition, antibodies, and antibody-conjugates, may be substituted because of improvements in general quality, or price, or as a consequence of failures to meet required specifications during the optimization and validation processes. The novice immunoassay developer should be aware that a final, fully validated test system may contain few or none of the initial components.

3 Exploring specificity

Information on conducting a specificity study is given in Chapter 8 and it can be readily adapted to the purposes of the preliminary screening of a panel of antibodies. Antibody and assay specificity are also discussed in Chapters 2 and 7.

3.1 Specificity, as assessed by suppliers

It is impractical for suppliers of antibodies to determine the full extent to which each antibody that they market binds to potential crossreacting substances under all likely conditions. In practice, specificity is generally characterized by testing a relatively small number of potential crossreactants in just one of a number of common assay formats. Well-chosen potential crossreactants may be closely related to antigen and are found in significant concentrations in the kinds of samples most tested for the antigen in question, or be known to be frequent crossreactants with antibodies against the particular antigen. The number of compounds tested will also depend on the antigen and in some cases when very few compounds are tested, it is because they are difficult or impossible to obtain in pure form, or even to identify. However, the selection of compounds to be tested may be haphazard and limited.

Therefore, for these and other reasons explained below the potential buyer can use the specificity data supplied with commercial antibodies as only a rough guide. In practice, the user should endeavour to obtain samples of potentially useful antibodies from several commercial suppliers and undertake a carefully designed and controlled comparative evaluation to identify those which may be suitable for the application in question.

3.2 Specificity and the assay developer

Whether obtained commercially or raised 'in house', it is essential that the final selection of an antibody be based on a method that is as close to the final assay design as possible. This is because compounds that bind to antibodies in one type of assay system may have little or no affinity in another.

Gani *et al.* (12) subjected a panel of 78 anti-hCG monoclonal antibodies that had been selected by a standard EIA to further testing in haem-agglutination assay and RIA systems. For the EIA the hCG had been adsorbed onto a polystyrene surface, for the haemagglutination assay sheep red blood cells were coated with hCG (in the presence of 15% glutaraldehyde), and for the RIA ^{125}I-hCG was used. The reaction pattern (*Table 1*) clearly showed the influence of assay format on hCG binding because, while the majority of clones were positive in all three systems, some were positive in only one or two, probably because of differences in the accessibility of specific epitopes. Lack of binding could also have been due to differences in incubation conditions between the assays. What applied to antigen in this experiment can apply also to any crossreactant.

Most primary antibodies fall into one of two categories: those used in competitive assays and those used in two-site immunometric assays. While competitive binding assays can be developed for both high and low molecular weight antigens, in practice they are most commonly used to measure haptens.

3.2.1 Antibodies for competitive assays

The overriding concern in the selection of an antibody for a hapten assay is usually specificity, particularly in the case of steroids, where many structurally similar metabolites occur in samples. Assessing the specificity of anti-hapten antibodies is complicated by the fact that, in the preparation of immunogen, the way hapten is coupled to carrier protein can have a determining effect on crossreactivity (13). Specificity depends both on the nature of the hapten link to the protein carrier and on the position of the linking site on the hapten molecule. In addition, if the assay in which the antibody is used involves a

Table 1. Reaction pattern of HCG antibodies in three different HCG assays

Number of clones	ELISA[a]	HA[b]	RIA[c]
48	+	+	+
10	+	–	+
14	+	+	–
6	+	–	–

[a] Standard enzyme-linked screening assay.
[b] Haemagglutination assay with hCG-coated cells.
[c] Competitive RIA with ^{125}I-hCG.

Table 2. The binding of anti-progesterone monoclonal antibodies to homologous and heterologous progesterone-enzyme conjugates

Antibody code	Immunogen[a]	Conjugate[b]		
		Prog-3-CMO-AP	Prog-6-HS-AP	Prog-11-HS-AP
3562	Prog 3-CMO-BSA	+[c]	—	—
3568	Prog 6-HS-BSA	+ +	+ + +	—
2533	Prog 11-HS-BSA	+ +	+	+ + +
4159	Prog 11-HS-BSA	+ +	—	+ +

[a] The immunogens used to raise the antibodies were coupled via carbon 3, 6 or 11 on the steroid nucleus with either CMO or HS bridging molecules to BSA.

[b] The enzyme conjugates were coupled via a variety of positions and bridges to AP.

[c] The scores represent optical density readings at 280 nm that indicate the degree of conjugate binding to immobilized antibody: $+++$, > 1; $++$, 0.6–1; $+$, < 0.6 and greater than background.

conjugate label (e.g. enzyme–hapten), the linkage position in this conjugate will also have a major influence on the crossreactivity and sensitivity of the resulting assay.

Table 2 shows how four anti-progesterone monoclonal antibodies raised to immunogens in which the carrier protein was coupled to progesterone at position 3, 6 or 11 interacted with different progesterone–enzyme conjugates, again coupled through positions 3, 6 or 11. One antibody (3562) was apparently specific to its homologous conjugate, and it bound even this with relatively low affinity. Two antibodies (3568 and 4153) had dual reactivity, and antibody 2533 could bind to all three conjugates, although clearly discriminating among them. *Table 3* shows the results of a detailed crossreactivity study in which the same four antibodies were each tested in combination with up to three different conjugates against a panel of 13 steroids. The results clearly demonstrate that the steroid coupling site has a determining effect on the crossreactivity of the antibodies obtained, with about 100% or greater crossreactivity always being found when the steroid used in the immunogen (with or without the bridge attached) is tested. However, there are otherwise no guidelines as to which coupling positions should be used initially. In most cases it simply depends on the sites of available reactive groups.

Homologous combinations of antibody and conjugate, i.e., same coupling position etc. for both immunogen and conjugate, should always be investigated initially. Provided that assay sensitivity and crossreacting are acceptable then there is nothing to be gained by investigating other combinations. However, a heterologous combination (i.e. different coupling position or orientation – e.g. linkage via an α- or β-hydroxyl – on the hapten, or different spacer groups in the immunogen compared with the conjugate) will occasionally give an improvement in sensitivity or specificity. In the case referred to above, antibody 4159 bound progesterone 3–alkaline phosphatase and progesterone 11–alkaline phosphatase conjugates with similar affinities, but its heterologous combination

Table 3. Crossreaction studies with monoclonal anti-progesterone antibodies (*Table 2*), in homologous and heterologous combinations with progesterone-enzyme conjugates

Steroids	% Crossreactivity[a] (antibody code and immunogen/conjugate[b])							
	3562 **I-3/C-3**	**3568** **I-3/C-6**	**3568** **I-6/C-6**	**2533** **I-11/C-3**	**2533** **I-11/C-6**	**2533** **I-11/C-11**	**4159** **I-11/C-3**	**4159** **I-11/C-11**
Progesterone	100	100	100	100	100	100	100	100
Progesterone-11α-HS	0.0	0.0	0.0	100	103	600	100	100
Progesterone -6β-HS	0.0	600	1650	0.0	9.0	0.0	4.0	0.0
Progesterone-3-CMO	633	517	1320	13	22	100	32	42
Pregnenolone	13	46	71	1.0	0.6	0.0	4.1	30
11α-Hydroxyprogesterone	0.0	0.0	0.0	100	100	380	100	91
17α-Hydroxyprogesterone	0.0	0.0	0.0	1.0	0.5	0.0	5.9	34
6β-Hydroxyprogesterone	0.0	150	132	3.0	2.0	5.0	16	42
5β-Pregnan-3α-ol-20-one	0.0	65	73	1.0	1.0	0.0	4.7	33
5β-Pregnan-3α,20α-diol	0.0	0.0	0.0	1.0	0.0	0.0	4.0	31
5α-Pregnan-3,20-dione	66	78	94	44	32	46	22	40
5β-Pregnan-3,20-dione	0.0	50	71	17	12	33	71	81
5α-Androstan-3α-ol-17-one	0.0	4.0	0.0	1.0	0.3	0.0	6.0	33

[a] Defined as $X \times 100/Y$, where X is the concentration of progesterone and Y the concentration of steroid being tested, both being the concentrations required to produce 50% inhibition of the binding of conjugate.

[b] Both the immunogens (I) and conjugates (C) are the same as for the experiment in *Table 2*. The immunogens are coded as follows: Prog 3-CMO-BSA (I-3), Prog 6-HS-BSA (I-6), Prog 11-HS-BSA (I-11); and the conjugates as Prog 3-CMO-AP (C-3), etc.

with a conjugate linked via carbon 3 was more specific with respect to the steroids tested.

3.2.2 Antibodies for two-site assays

The main preliminary criteria for selecting a monoclonal antibody for optimum performance in a two-site assay are usually the ability to bind simultaneously to antigen with the 'other' antibody, retention of binding activity and stability on the solid phase and retention of activity upon labelling. The specificity of the final assay is governed by the combined interactions of a pair of antibodies.

These criteria are exemplified in the selection of antibodies for the detection of intact complex proteins such as the bi-subunit hormone hCG (14). *Table 4* shows the antibody pairing matrix for four antibodies against α-hCG and seven against β-hCG, used both as solid-phase antibodies and as antibody–enzyme conjugates (15). The data also clearly demonstrate that not every α-specific antibody will pair with every β-specific antibody, and that not every antibody performs equally well as a capture antibody and as a detector antibody. The suitability of pairs of monoclonal antibodies for use in such assays cannot be predicted with confidence and must be established by carrying out such a 'matrix' experiment. Some combinations of α-specific antibodies used both on solid phase and in conjugate also gave sandwich formation and, if used in an assay, would probably measure both intact hCG and free α subunit.

Table 4. Sandwich formation when a panel of 11 anti-hCG monoclonal antibodies (four anti α-subunit and seven anti β-hCG) are used as both capture antibodies and in enzyme conjugates in two-site immunometric assays.

Capture antibody[b]	Degree of sandwich formation[a] (conjugate antibody[b])										
	β1	β2	β3	β4	β5	β6	β7	α1	α2	α3	α4
β1	−	−	−	−	−	−	−	++	+++	+++	+++
β2	−	−	−	−	−	−	−	++++	++++	++	++
β3	−	−	−	−	−	−	−	+	+	−	+
β4	−	−	−	−	−	−	−	+	+	−	−
β5	−	−	−	−	−	−	−	+	+	++	++
β6	−	−	−	−	−	−	−	+++	++++	+++	++
β7	−	−	−	−	−	−	−	++++	++++	+++	+++
α1	++	++++	++++	++++	++++	++	++++	−	−	++++	+++
α2	+	++++	++++	++++	++++	++	++++	−	−	++	+
α3	+	++	+	+	++	−	+++	+++	+	−	−
α4	+	+++	++	+++	++++	+	++++	+++	+	−	−

[a] The scores represent optical density readings at 280 nm that indicate the degree of conjugate binding via hCG standard to capture antibody: ++++, > 1.5; +++, 1.0−1.5; ++, 05−1.0; +, < 0.5 and greater than background.

[b] Antibodies: α1 to α4, α-subunit-specific antibodies; β1 to β7, β-hCG subunit-specific antibodies.

The criteria for selecting a polyclonal antibody for a two-site immunometric assay are dependent on whether the antibody is to be paired with itself, with another polyclonal antibody or with a monoclonal antibody. Its individual specificity will depend largely on the antigen preparation used. To influence specificity, highly purified intact antigen, a subunit, a fragment obtained by partial digestion, or a peptide representing part of the antigen may have been used for immunization. The specificity of a polyclonal antibody may also be 'improved' be selective absorption with excess crossreactants or by affinity chromatography on immobilized 'pure' antigen. Affinity purification of a polyclonal antibody, by removing nonspecific antibodies, should also give higher coating densities on a solid phase and higher specific activity conjugate. Also, because of its heterogeneous nature, a polyclonal antibody is less likely to exhibit marked instability than a monoclonal antibody.

With Ouchterlony immunoprecipitation, the interaction of at least two monoclonal antibodies with antigen are needed to form precipitin lines and this can be exploited to identify matched pairs of monoclonal antibodies for use in a sandwich assay system (*Protocol 1*).

Suitable pairs of polyclonal, monoclonal or mixed antibodies can also be identified by a means of one of a number of standard immunoassay procedures employing microtitre wells and enzymatic labels, although alternative solid-phase types and labels are also used.

In one approach each antibody from the panel of n antibodies is coated onto the solid phase, saturated with antigen and the ability of a labelled antibody (Ab$_1$–enzyme, previously selected from the panel) to bind is tested (sp-**Ab$_n$** –Ag–

Ab$_1$-enzyme). Another antibody is then chosen (Ab$_2$), labelled, tested against the full panel, and so on. In a variant of this approach a limited amount of the labelled antibody (Ab$_1$) is incubated with immobilized antigen (sp-Ag or sp-[Ag]) and each of the panel members (**Ab$_n$**) in excess. The binding of the labelled antibody to the solid phase indicates simultaneous binding of both antibodies to the antigen (**Ab$_n$**–[sp-]Ag–Ab$_1$-enzyme). Both of these may require that a considerable number of different antibodies be purified and labelled. These methods were used in thorough and systematic epitope mapping studies before the advent of optical immunosensor systems.

Protocol 1

Selection of pairs of monoclonal antibodies by Ouchterlony immunoprecipitation

Equipment and reagents

- Antigen (Higher Mr e.g. hCG, osteocalcin, etc.) in PBS or other suitable buffer
- Anti-antigen antibodies to be tested
- Buffer (015 M NaCl, 0.005 M EDTA, 0.01% NaN$_3$, 0.01 M Tris, pH 7.6)
- Plastic disposable Petri dishes (60 mm)

Method

1. Prepare 100 ml 1% (w/v) agarose in the buffer with gentle boiling on a hot plate while continuously stirring. Place in water-bath at 60 °C.

2. Add ≈ 12 ml hot agarose solution to eight Petri dishes, allow to cool on a level surface, cap plates and store at 4 °C.

3. Carefully punch a hole in the centre of an agarose plate with the cork borer. Punch further holes in a circle around the centre hole, ≈ 5 mm from each other. Carefully remove the agarose 'plugs' with a spatula or other pointed instrument.

4. While on a level surface, add antigen solution to the centre hole and, for each antibody, a range of dilutions to the surrounding holes (100 μl), and incubate at room temperature, or at 37°C to speed up diffusion. Determine dilutions that produce precipitin lines approximately midway to the centre wells. Note: If a sample is very dilute, it is possible to refill (two to three times) each hole as the antibody diffuses away.

5. Repeat steps 1–3. Add antigen to the centre hole of a new plate and potential pairs of antibodies to the outer wells (100 μl), ensuring that adjacent wells contain different antibodies. Incubate as above.

6. Check for precipitin lines after 6–8 h, and leave over night for further examination. A dark background and a source of light will facilitate the detection of faint bands.

Results: Precipitin lines which cross with no interaction, or produce a spur, indicate the pairs of antibodies that are able to bind to two different and spatially orientated epitopes on the antigen. Precipitin lines which produce a continuous arc (line of identity) indicate antibodies that are binding to the same epitopes. With antigens that are not very large and have only one copy of each specific epitope per molecule (e.g. osteocalcin) it may be necessary to include PEG at up to 20% in the agarose buffer to help visualize the precipitin lines.

In the more convenient method described in *Protocol 2* the antigen is labelled (Ag-enzyme or Ag[-enzyme]) and, therefore, only one labelling procedure is necessary. The labelled antigen is preincubated with each of the panel members (Ab_n) before being tested for its ability to bind to each of the panel (Ab_1 to Ab_n) previously coated onto a solid phase. Again, the binding of the label to the solid phase indicates simultaneous binding of both antibodies to the antigen (sp-Ab_1–Ag[-enzyme]–Ab_n).

Protocol 2

Selection of antibody pairs by labelled-antigen ELISA

Equipment and reagents

- Panel of monoclonal antibodies that is to be screened
- Conjugate: antigen labelled with enzyme or alternative
- Coating buffer (0.1 M Na carbonate, pH 9.6)
- Wash buffer: PBS-Tween
- Blocking solution: PBS–BSA
- Microtitre plates or strips (or alternative solid phase)
- Microtitre plate reader or alternative

Method

1. To test one pair of monoclonal antibodies, coat microtitre wells (or alternative solid phase) with a preselected antibody at about 1 μg/ml) in coating buffer (200 μl per well) overnight at 4°C or for at least 1 h at 37°C.

2. Empty wells, wash three to four times with 300 μl wash buffer, and add 250 μl blocking solution for 1 h at 37 °C. Empty and wash as before.

3. Add 100 μl of labelled antigen dilutions (0, 1/20, 1/40, 1/80, etc) to the coated wells, incubate at 37°C for 1 h, empty, wash and determine endpoints. Plot endpoint reading against antigen dilution. A limiting concentration of labelled antigen is that equivalent to 60% of the maximum reading (the asymptote).

4. Repeat steps 1 and 2.

5. Preincubate at 37°C for 30 min 100 μl labelled antigen (at twice the limiting concentration determined in step 3) with 100 μl buffer as control or with 100 μl of a range of dilutions of a second antibody from the panel (1/1000, 1/500, 1/100, 1/10, 1), some dilutions giving excess antibody.

6. Add 100 μl of pre-equilibrated conjugate-antibody mixtures to the coated wells and incubate for 1 h at 37 °C.

7. Empty wells and wash as step 2.

8. Estimate antibody–antigen binding by an appropriate detection system.

9. Interpretation of results: If the antigen-conjugate binds to the capture antibody after it has been exposed to high concentrations of the other antibody, this pair of antibodies is a potential choice for a sandwich assay. However if the second antibody inhibits the binding of the antigen-conjugate, it is likely that the capture and second antibodies both recognize the same epitope or adjacent epitopes.

10. To identify all potential pairs, repeat the procedure from step 5 with the other antibodies in the panel, including the coated antibody as a negative control. If the panel is not large (five or less antibodies) it should be feasible to repeat the whole process five times with each of the antibodies used to coat the solid phase to confirm the valid pairs.

Notes

1. All the monoclonal antibodies on the panel being tested should previously have been shown to be capable of binding to the antigen, by means of a standard screening assay with antigen-coated wells and anti-mouse antibody conjugate.

2. A positive control, i.e. labelled antigen alone without the 'second' antibody, should be included in all test runs.

3. It is advisable to use the first antibody as the soluble competitor to determine concentrations of labelled antigen and test antibodies for the above protocol in a checker board titration experiment.

4 Estimating affinity

4.1 Approaches

Two strategies are open to the assay developer who wishes to assess a panel of antibodies for affinity. If the assay to be developed is a competitive assay, and especially if it is a solid phase assay with immobilized antibody and a complex conjugate as label, affinity may be taken as being functionally equivalent to sensitivity and assessed by comparing the errors and slopes of standard curves. To take a more theoretical approach would be experimentally very complex. Even then, the very highest affinity antibody (highest K_a in liquid phase with near-'native' antigen) may not give the greatest sensitivity (O'Connor and Gosling, unpublished). This is particularly relevant when a solid-phase reactant and/or a complex label is used (if only because the rate association and dissociation constants – k_a and k_d – are also important). As in the assessment of specificity, the conditions used should be as similar as possible to those that will be used in the final assay format. However, the systematic estimation of the affinities of candidate antibodies to tritiated analyte may be useful as it can allow the prior elimination of low-affinity antibodies.

If the assay to be developed is a reagent-excess assay, standard curves do not give a clear measure of the affinities of individual antibodies. Despite this, low-affinity antibodies are best avoided as they may require longer incubation times for optimum assay performance and are subject to leaching during thorough and repeated washing steps. Therefore, especially if an unusually low detection limit is required or if a high-volume, commercial assay is under development, a methodical assessment of the affinity of each candidate antibody may be beneficial. Under these circumstances, accurate estimates of affinity are most useful and methods based on the solution interaction of antibody and antigen, with minimal interference from the effects of labelling and immobilization, are the most appropriate. Such effects can be estimated separately.

4.2 Methods

The methods discussed and described below will be adequate for most purposes related to the development of immunoassays. More detailed accounts of measuring antibody affinity in solution by means of ELISA or RIA (16) and with a biosensor instrument (17,18) may be found in recent volumes in the *Practical Approach Series*.

4.2.1 Equilibrium dialysis

This is the classical method for the determination of the affinity of the inter-action between an antibody and its homologous hapten in solution (19). Because it involves use of a dialysis membrane to partition antibody-bound antigen and free antigen, it is not appropriate for antibodies against higher molecular weight antigens or hapten conjugates.

Antibody is placed inside a dialysis sac and allowed to dialyse against a large volume of buffer containing tritiated antigen until equilibrium is attained (*Figure 5*), and this procedure is performed with a range of different antigen concentrations. Other kinds of label, including radio-iodinated derivatives, may be used provided that they are of sufficiently low weight that their diffusion is unimpeded by the membrane. At equilibrium, the concentration of antigen out-side the membrane is a measure of the concentration of free antigen, while the concentration inside is greater, and is a measure of the free plus bound antigen concentrations. The optimum concentration of antibody to use is the reciprocal of its K_a. Since, a priori, this is unknown it is recommended that the total anti-

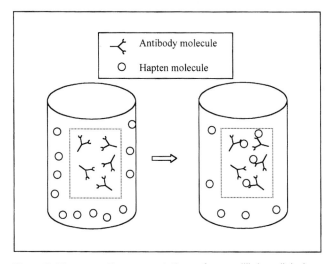

Figure 5. Diagrammatic representations of an equilibrium dialysis procedure to estimate antibody affinity, showing the relative distributions of the hapten and antibody molecules at time zero and after equilibrium has been established

body concentration chosen be as small as possible, and that the procedure be repeated when an initial estimate is obtained. The range of antigen concentrations used should give an antigen excess, if possible, of from one to 20.

Protocol 3

Estimating antibody affinity by equilibrium dialysis

Reagents

- Tritiated hapten diluted with unlabelled hapten of the same molarity to give a working solution with a specific activity of about 10^{10} Bq/mmol. (In one actual experiment, the label was supplied with a cited specific activity of 750×10^9 Bq/mmol at a concentration of 51 μM. To allow it to be counted without undue wastage of the stock material, it was diluted 1/50 with unlabelled hapten of the same molarity to give a working solution with a specific activity of 1.5×10^{10} Bq/mmol)

- Buffer: 50 mM tris, 0.1 mg/ml ovalbumin, 0.1 M NaCl, 0.05% sodium azide, pH 8.0

- Monoclonal antibody (purified, $E_{280\,nm}$ = 1.4, (concentration equivalent to about $1/K_a$ or, when starting, in the range 10^{-7}–10^{-9} M)

- Narrow dialysis tubing (10 mm or 'half-inch'), previously boiled in 2 l 0.1 M NaHCO$_3$, 10 mM EDTA, pH 7.5 for 20 min and rinsed three times, each time in 3 l of high quality deionized water

- Liquid scintillation counter, vials and scintillation fluid

Method

1. Prepare 8×50 ml solutions of tritiated hapten covering the concentration range 1×10^{-7} M to 5×10^{-9} M in tris buffer (the concentrations are chosen to span the expected value for the affinity constant).

2. For each of the eight concentrations of hapten to be used, prepare dialysis sacs (in triplicate) containing 0.5 ml of each of the following: test antibody (5×10^{-8} M); normal IgG (5×10^{-8} M) (control for nonspecific binding of hapten to antibody) and buffer (control to check that equilibrium is attained). Ensure the end of each dialysis sac is clearly coded, e.g. with coloured cotton.

3. Place the nine dialysis sacs in each of the eight 50 ml hapten solutions and leave to mix gently (end-over-end mixer or equivalent) for 48–72 h at room temperature.

4. Count triplicate 0.1 ml samples of each solution from inside and outside all dialysis sacs, collecting 5000 or 10 000 counts for each to standardize counting errors.

5. Estimate the affinity constant by means of one of the methods described in section 1.4.

Data from an equilibrium dialysis experiment with a monoclonal antibody against oestrone at a concentration of 1×10^{-7} M with a valency of 2 is shown in *Table 5*. Plotting these data and metameters will give Scatchard (8.96×10^7), Langmuir (8.5×10^7) and Sips plots (8.2×10^7) from which the affinity constants

Table 5. Data and metameters derived by transforming this data from an equilibrium dialysis experiment with a monoclonal antibody against a hapten

Variable	Symbol[a]	Data						
Ag (M)		1.76×10^{-7}	8.81×10^{-8}	4.44×10^{-8}	2.25×10^{-8}	1.15×10^{-8}	5.84×10^{-9}	2.86×10^{-9}
Bound Ag (M)	x	8.2×10^{-8}	8.34×10^{-8}	7.21×10^{-8}	5.82×10^{-8}	4.23×10^{-8}	2.54×10^{-8}	1.47×10^{-8}
Free Ag (M)	a	1.47×10^{-7}	7.66×10^{-8}	3.69×10^{-8}	1.85×10^{-8}	8.67×10^{-9}	4.21×10^{-9}	2.14×10^{-9}
$1/[Ag]_{bound}$ (/M)	$1/x$	1.22×10^{7}	1.20×10^{7}	1.39×10^{7}	1.72×10^{7}	2.36×10^{7}	3.94×10^{7}	6.80×10^{7}
$1/[Ag]_{free}$ (/M)	$1/a$	0.68×10^{7}	1.31×10^{7}	2.71×10^{7}	5.41×10^{7}	11.42×10^{7}	23.75×10^{7}	46.73×10^{7}
$[Ag]_{bound}/[Ag]_{free}$	x/a	0.56	1.09	1.95	3.15	4.83	6.03	6.87
$Log[Ag]_{free}$	$Log(a)$	−6.83	−7.12	−7.43	−7.73	−8.06	−8.38	−8.67
$Log[Ag]_{bound}/[Ab_t] - [Ag]_{bound}$	$Log(x/[ni\text{-}x])$[b]	0.793	0.849	0.494	0.197	−0.097	−0.439	−0.738

[a]For definitions of symbols see Section 1.4.2.

[b]The concentration of antibody used (i) was 1×10^{7} and n was taken to be 2.

in parentheses can be interpolated and calculated. The heterogeneity index (α) as estimated from the Sips plot is 0.88.

4.2.2 ELISA

The ELISA method of Friguet et al. (20) is a well-accepted method for estimating solution affinity values for antibodies (21, 22). The method is simple: it involves no labelling of antibody or antigen and is equally applicable to antibodies against both small and large molecular weight antigens. In brief, a fixed concentration of antibody and a range of concentrations of antigen are mixed and allowed to come to equilibrium. Samples of the incubation mixtures are then taken and the concentrations of free antibody are measured by means of an ELISA under conditions in which the equilibrium is not significantly disturbed. This is confirmed experimentally (see measurement of f-value, Protocol 4). The difference between the total antibody (no antigen) and free antibody gives the bound antibody concentration.

The ELISA used employs immobilized antigen and an enzyme-labelled antibody reagent to measure the free antibody in the equilibrium mixtures. The affinity values that can be measured are limited by the specific activity of the labelled antibody and the highest affinities measurable are about 10^9–10^{10} l/mol when a chromogenic enzyme substrate is used for determination of the endpoint. A fluorogenic substrate can enable affinities of up to 10^{12} l/mol to be estimated.

Assuming there is no significant change in the equilibrium of the antibody–antigen mixture during its incubation in the coated wells ($f < 10\%$), then the concentration of free antibody sites (ni_f) is related to the absorbance (A_f) measured in the ELISA by the equation:

$$\frac{ni_f}{ni} = \frac{A_f}{A} \tag{1}$$

where ni is the total antibody site concentration (as defined in Section 1.4.2), and A is the absorbance measured in the absence of antigen. At equilibrium:

$$x = ni - ni_f \text{ and } a = a_t - x \tag{2}$$

where x is the concentration of bound antigen, a_t is the total concentration of antigen and a is the free antigen concentration. The variables x, a and ni are related to the association constant K_a of the equilibrium by the Scatchard equation:

$$\frac{x}{a} = K_a(ni - x) \tag{3 (as in Section 1.4.2).}$$

However, combining equations [1] and [2], x can be related to the absorbances measured in the ELISA:

$$x = ni\frac{(A - A_f)}{A}$$

or setting the fraction of bound antibody,

$$V = \frac{A - A_f}{A}$$

$$x = niV$$

Now the equation [3] can be rewritten as:

$$\frac{niV}{a} = K_a(ni - niV)$$

or, simplifying, as:

$$\frac{V}{a} = K_a(1 - V)$$

and a plot of V/a versus V will ideally yield a straight line with the slope $= -K_a$

Protocol 4 describes how the affinity of an antibody may be estimated in this way and is in three parts. The first part is necessary to choose an antibody concentration for the saturation experiment, and to establish that the (immobilized) antigen concentration and incubation time are suitable for the ELISA to be used to measure the free antibody concentrations. The second part consists of the antibody saturation experiment, which involves a series of tubes with a constant antibody concentration and a range of antigen concentrations, and the subsequent measurement by ELISA of the free antibody concentrations in these tubes. The third part is concerned with calculations, plotting the results and interpolating the affinity constant.

Protocol 4

Estimating antibody affinity by indirect ELISA

Reagents

- Microtitre plates (Dynatech or equivalent) coated with antigen (pure protein antigen or hapten-carrier protein conjugate) Typical concentrations of antigen used are 0.25–1 µg/ml.

- Antibody-enzyme conjugate: anti-mouse IgG (whole molecule) conjugated to alkaline phosphatase (Sigma) (Use appropriate conjugates for antibodies from other species.)

- PBSTA: 10 mM sodium phosphate, 0.15 M NaCl, 0.15% Tween 20, pH 7.1, 10 mM sodium azide

- DEA substrate buffer: 1 tablet of PNPP substrate (Sigma 104 phosphatase substrate tablets, code 104-105) in 5 ml 1 M aqueous DEA, 1 mM MgCl2, pH 9.8

- 0.5 ml glass test tubes

A. Calibration curves to establish initial requirements

1. Prepare two series of antigen-coated microtitre wells on separate plates.

2. Prepare a series of dilutions of the antibody being characterized in PBSTA, i.e. typically eight dilutions spanning the linear region of the antibody dilution curve, as established by a preliminary experiment. Add 200 µl antibody solution (in duplicate) to the first series of wells and incubate for 1 h. All incubations are at room temperature.

3. Remove the contents of each well and add to the corresponding well of the second series of coated wells and incubate for 1 h.

Protocol 4 continued

4. In the meantime, wash the first series of wells four times with PBSTA and then add 200 μl anti-mouse conjugate (use the dilution recommended by Sigma, typically 1/1000). Incubate for 1 h. Wash the wells as before with PBSTA. Add 200 μl substrate solution and incubate for a further hour. Measure the OD at 405 nm.

5. Repeat the washing, conjugate and substrate incubation steps for the second series of wells. Ensure that the incubation times are the same as for the first series of wells. Measure the OD as before.

6. Calculate the *f* value for each concentration of antibody (c) where $A_1(c)$ and $A_2(c)$ are the optical densities for the first and second series of Ag-sensitized wells, and where:

$$f = \frac{A_1(c) - A_2(c)}{A_1(c)}$$

7. All the *f*-values should be low (< 10%), indicating that the amount of antibody captured by the solid phase represents only a small fraction of the free antibody, and should not, therefore, perturb the antibody–antigen binding equilibrium (see below). If some or all of the *f*-values are > 10% the experiment must be repeated (with less antigen in the coating step and/or a shorter incubation time) until this requirement is satisfied.

8. Plot the OD readings for each series against antibody concentration and choose an antibody concentration from the linear portion of the plot for use (x 2 to allow for dilution) in Step 2 below. The concentration chosen should also be the lowest concentration that gives a reasonable range of OD readings (up to 1.0 if possible) in the ELISA after a reasonable enzyme assay incubation time.

B. Antibody–antigen saturation curve

1. Prepare a series of 11 antigen solutions in PBSTA covering the concentration range 10^{-8}–10^{-10} M plus a zero control (PBSTA only).

2. Add 400 μl of each antigen concentration to 12 400-μl aliquots of a fixed concentration of antibody (as determined above) in test tubes and leave the mixture to equilibrate overnight at room temperature.

3. Transfer 200 μl of each mixture to the wells (in triplicate) of an antigen coated microtitre plate and incubate for 1 h (as for step A1). (The concentration of antigen and incubation time were shown to be suitable above.)

4. Wash the plate four times with PBSTA, add 200 μl of anti-mouse alkaline phosphatase conjugate at the dilution as in step A2. Incubate for 1 h. Wash the wells as before with PBSTA. Add 200 μl of substrate solution and incubate for a further h. Measure the OD at 405 nm.

C. Calculation of the affinity constant

1. Construct a table with the following four headings; antigen concentration (*a*), mean OD, *V*, and *V*/*a*.

Protocol 4 continued

2. Calculate V and V/a for each antigen concentration used.

3. Plot V/a versus V.

4. Calculate the slope of the best straight line by means of the least squares method (e.g. with the 'LINEST' function in Microsoft Excel®). The slope $= -K_a$.

Tables 3.6 and 3.7, and *Figure* 6 present the results obtained from an indirect ELISA procedure to measure the affinity constant of a steroid-specific antibody. After *Protocol 4A* was carried out, a final antibody concentration of 3×10^{-11} M was chosen (*Table* 6 and Calibration curve of *Figure* 6) for use in the saturation curve experiment (*Protocol 4B*). This concentration was on the linear part of the antibody calibration curve, and, to meet the condition that the antibody concentration should be close to or lower than its affinity constant (K_d), it was also as low as was practically possible. (The optical density reading given by the chosen antibody concentration [$A = 0.667$] was a little lower than ideal in this particular experiment.) The data shown in *Table* 7 gave the Scatchard plot of *Figure* 6.

4.2.3 Surface plasmon resonance

Biosensor technology based on either surface plasmon resonance (SPR, BIAcore™, Pharmacia) or a resonant mirror (IAsys, Affinity Sensors) is increasingly used to study the kinetics and binding affinities of bimolecular interactions (23). BIAcore instruments are more widely available and will be discussed here.

The BIAcore instrument measures changes in refractive index close to the sensor surface (24), and changes in this are proportional to changes in the mass immobilized on that surface, allowing binding phenomena to be monitored in 'real time'. The actual sensor is a gold-coated chip with a hydrogel coat (carboxymethyl dextran covalently linked to the gold surface) on which reactants can be immobilized, and to which ligates can be delivered by a microfluidic flow system. Molecular binding interactions on the dextran layer affect the angle of incidence of a beam of reflected monochromatic light. The changes in

Table 6. Data for the calibration curves obtained when establishing the initial requirements for determining the affinity of an anti-steroid antibody by ELISA (Protocol 4A) (see also Table 7 and Figure 6)

	Antibody concentration ($\times 10^{-11}$ M) and OD at 405 nm								
Series of wells	8.0	7.0	6.0	5.0	4.0	3.0	2.0	1.0	0
1	1.621	1.437	1.251	1.113	0.883	0.740	0.497	0.264	0.020
2	1.527	1.402	1.272	1.082	0.854	0.704	0.496	0.246	0.012
Difference (1-2)[a]	0.094	0.035	-0.021	0.031	0.029	0.036	0.001	0.020	

[a] All the differences when expressed as percentages of the optical densities in the Series 1 wells are $< 10\%$.

Table 7. Initial and transformed data for the saturation curve obtained when estimating the affinity of an anti-steroid antibody by indirect ELISA (*Protocol 4B*) (see also *Figure 6*) (ni = 3 × 10^{-11}, A ni = 0.667)

	Hapten concentration M × 10^{-11} (*a*)										
	3.45 **× 10^{-8}**	**8.63** **× 10^{-9}**	**2.16** **× 10^{-9}**	**1.08** **× 10^{-9}**	**5.39** **× 10^{-10}**	**2.70** **× 10^{-10}**	**1.80** **× 10^{-10}**	**1.20** **× 10^{-10}**	**7.99** **× 10^{-11}**	**5.32** **× 10^{-11}**	**3.55** **× 10^{-11}**
Mean optical density (A)	0.032	0.037	0.054	0.073	0.107	0.142	0.185	0.222	0.285	0.350	0.467
V	0.952	0.945	0.919	0.891	0.840	0.787	0.723	0.668	0.573	0.476	0.301
V/a × 10^8	0.276	1.099	4.317	8.474	16.35	32.00	45.76	66.97	91.43	122.2	113.7

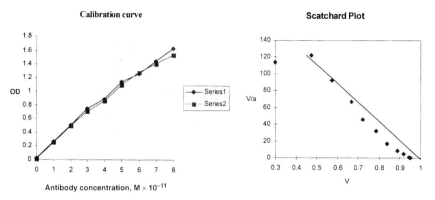

Figure 6. Plots of data (*Tables 6* and *7*) from an indirect ELISA procedure to estimate the affinity of an anti-steroid antibody (*Protocol 4*). The units for the *V/a* scale on the Scatchard plot are $\times\ 10^8$. It was estimated from the Scatchard plot that $K_a = 2.55 \times 10^{10}$.

angle caused by SPR are measured by means of a two-dimensional detector array and are expressed as resonance units (RU). A value of 1000 RU corresponds to ≈ 1 ng of protein bound/mm^2 of the sensor surface (25). The data are presented on a computer screen as a 'sensorgram' showing RU plotted as a function of time.

Briefly, the system comprises a pumping system, a robotic injector, an integrated fluidic cartridge, a sensor chip and a surface resonance detector. The sensor chip consists of an optically flat glass slide coated on one side with a thin layer of gold ≈ 50 nm thick to which is bound a hydrophilic dextran matrix (24). Protein is coupled to the dextran surface by N-hydroxysuccinimide/carbodiimide-mediated amine coupling and Pharmacia supply an 'Amine Coupling Kit' for this purpose. To maximize sensitivity, it is normal practice for the smaller of the two interacting species under study to be coupled to the dextran surface. Numerous examples on the use of the BIAcore™ instrument have been described (26–28).

Purified rabbit anti-mouse Fc (RAMFc, also available from Pharmacia) is normally coupled to the biosensor surface to immobilize monoclonal antibodies under study. Presensitized RAMFc sensor chips ready for investigating mouse monoclonal antibodies are also available. Monoclonal antibodies are thereby selectively adsorbed, and the preparations used do not need to be purified in advance, allowing antibodies in unfractionated supernatants to be used directly. Measurements of affinity constants for hapten-specific antibodies are undertaken with the hapten coupled to the surface, via a hapten–carrier protein conjugate, so the natures of this conjugate and of the immunogen used to raise the antibodies must be kept in mind.

No protocols on the use of BIAcore or IAsys instruments for the exploring antibody affinity are given here because these are included in the accompanying manuals and (for BIAcore) are to be found in two other volumes of the *Practical Approach Series* (17, 18).

5 Conclusion

A suitable antibody cannot be considered to be such until the assay of which it is a component has been assembled, fully optimized and validated. Even then, routine operation may disclose problems that could require that the antibody be changed. However, careful design of the preliminary specifications and thorough initial characterization of all the reagent antibodies will increase the probability of success and, on average, reduce development time and costs.

Acknowledgements

I thank Dr R. A. Badley for providing examples of antibody binding data and Dr S. Howell for information on the use of the BIAcore.

References

1. Bidart J. M. (1993). In *Immunotechnology* (eds J. P. Gosling and D. J. Reen), p. 77. Portland Press, London.
2. Pettersson, K., Ding, Y. Q., and Huhtaniemi, I. J. (1992). *J. Clin. Endocrinol. Metab.* **72**, 164.
3. Morris, G. E. (ed.). (1996). Epitope mapping protocols, methods in molecular biology. Humana Press, New Jersey, USA.
4. Devey, M. E. and Steward, M. W., (1988). In *ELISA and other solid phase immunoassays* (eds D. M. Kemeny and S. J. Challacombe), p. 135. John Wiley & Sons, Chichester.
5. Scatchard, G. (1949). *Ann. NY Acad. Sci. USA* **51**, 660.
6. Stanley, C., Lew, A. M., and Steward, M. W. (1983). *J. Immunol. Methods* **64**, 119.
7. Sips, R. (1948). *J. Chem. Phys.* **16**, 490.
8. Pinkard, R. N. and Weir, D. M. (1978). In *Handbook of experimental Immunology* (ed. D. M. Weir), p. 493. Blackwell Scientific Publications, Oxford.
9. Underwood, P. A., (1985). *J. Immunol. Methods* **85**, 309.
10. Nygren, H., Kaartinen, M., and Stenberg, M. (1986). *J. Immunol. Methods* 92, 219.
11. Francisco, M. (1998). *Nature Biotechnol.* **16**, 788.
12. Gani, M., Coley, J., and Porter, P. (1987). *Hybridoma* **6**, 637.
13. Gani, M., Coley, J., Piron, J., Humphreys, A. S., Arevalo, J., Wilson, I. A., and Taussig, M. J. (1994). J. *Steroid Biochem. Molec. Biol.* **48**, 277.
14. Kofler, R., Berger, P., and Wick, G. (1982). *Am. J. Reprod. Immunol.* **2**, 212.
15. Porter, P., Coley, J., and Gani, M. (1988). In *Non-radiometric assays; technology and application in polypeptide and steroid hormone detection* (eds B. D. Albertson and F. P. Haseltine), p. 181. Alan R. Liss, New York.
16. Djavadi-Ohaniance, L., Goldberg, M. E., and Friguet, B. (1996). In *Antibody engineering a practical approach* (eds J. McCafferty, H. R. Hoogenboom, and D. J. Chiswell), p. 77. IRL Press, Oxford.
17. Hefta, L. J., Wu, A. M., Neumaier, M., and Shively, J. E. (1996). In *Antibody engineering a practical approach* (eds J. McCafferty, H. R. Hoogenboom, and D. J. Chiswell), p. 99. IRL Press, Oxford.
18. Saunal, H., Karlsson, R., and van Regenmortel, M. H.V. (1996). In *Immunochemistry a practical approach* (eds A. P. Johnstone and M. W. Turner), Vol. 2, p. 1. IRL Press, Oxford.
19. Eisen, H. N. and Karush, F. (1949). *J. Am. Chem. Soc.* **71**, 394.

20. Friguet, B., Chaffotte, A. F., Djavadi-Ohaniance, L., and Goldberg, M. E. (1985). *J. Immunol. Methods* **77**, 305.

21. Goldberg, M. E. and Djavadi-Ohaniance, L. (1993). *Curr. Opin. Immunol.* **5**, 278.

22. Azimzadeh, A. and van Regenmortel, M. H. V. (1990). *J. Molec. Recogn.* **3**, 108.

23. van Regenmortel, M. H. V. (1995). *J. Immunol. Methods* **183**, 3.

24. Karlsson, R., Michaelsson, A., and Mattsson, L. (1991). *J. Immunol. Methods* **145**, 229.

25. Stenberg, E., Persson. B., Roos, H., and Urbaniczky, C. (1991). *J. Colloid Interf. Sci.* **143**, 513.

26. Pellequer, J. L. and van Regenmortel, M. H. V. (1993). *J. Immunol. Methods* **166**, 133.

27. Zeder-Lutz, G., Altschuh, D., Geysen, H. M., Trifilieff, E., Sommermeyer, G., and van Regenmortel, M. H. V. (1993). *Molec. Immunol.* **30**, 145.

28. Schofield, D. J. and Dimmock, N. J. (1996). *J. Virol. Methods* **62**, 33.

Chapter 4
Labels and endpoints

Wajdi Abdul-Ahad* and Martin Brett†

*Beckman Coulter, Inc., 200 South Kraemer Boulevard, Brea, CA 92822, USA, and †Sierra Biomedical, 10326 Roselle Street, San Diego, CA 92121, USA

1 Labelling substances

The sophistication of current immunoassay methodology allows the assay developer a wide choice of labelling substances and assay endpoints, so that it is not usually difficult to find a combination that well suits the specification required for a new assay. This chapter will deal primarily with the three major kinds of labels and endpoints that are used when immunoassays for research purposes are being developed, i.e. radioisotopic (1), enzymatic (2) and fluorescent (3). Information on the preparation of ligand labels containing biotin and fluorescein (4) is also given.

Chemiluminescent labels (5–8) are also used for high-performance immunoassays, but will not be covered here because the better labelling reagents of this type are not generally commercially available. (Acridinium ester labelling reagent is now available from Assay Designs Inc. and Biotrend Chemikalien GmbH.)

Table 1 lists a selection of general-purpose labelling substances (including atoms, ions, small and large molecules, and chelates) and some of the methods used for measuring them. References to these applications can be found in review articles (9,10).

1.1 Radioisotopic labels

The major advantages of radioisotopic labels are that the basic labelling procedures for proteins can be simple, and that the radioisotopic parts of radiolabels are totally impervious to environmental factors. The disadvantages are the associated hazards, the expensive facilities required, and the availability of better alternatives when either convenience or a very low detection limits is required. In addition, some of the radiation energy emitted may cause damage to the labelled compound (radiolysis). However, when radioisotopic atoms are substituted into molecules, labels that are chemically almost identical are possible, unlike other labelling methods (*Figure 1*).

The radioisotopes commonly used for immunoassay are iodine-125 (^{125}I), which emits gamma rays and has a half-life of 60 days, and tritium (^{3}H), which emits weak beta particles and has a half-life of 12.26 years.

Table 1. Some substances used for labelling and methods used to measure them

Type	Substance	Endpoint
Enzyme	Acetylcholinesterase	Colorimetric
	Alkaline phosphatase	Amplified colorimetric
		Colorimetric
		Electrochemical
		Enhanced luminometric
		Time-resolved (TR) fluorimetric
		Visual assessment
	β-D-Galactosidase	Colorimetric
		Fluorimetric
		Luminometric
	Horseradish peroxidase	Colorimetric
		Fluorimetric
		Luminometric
	β-Lactamase	Colorimetric
Fluorescent	Fluorescein	Fluorimetric
	Eu^{3+}	TR fluorimetric
	Eu^{3+} chelate or cryptate	TR fluorimetric
Ligand	Biotin derivative	Avidin–acridinium ester, luminometry
		Avidin–enzyme, colorimetry
		Avidin-Eu^{3+} chelator, TR fluorimetric
		Avidin-^{125}I, solid scintillation counting
(SSC)		
	FITC	Anti-FITC–enzyme
Luminescent	Acridinium ester	Luminometry
	Isoluminol derivatives	Luminometry
Microparticle	Colloidal gold	Visual assessment
	Coloured latex	Visual assessment
	Latex, etc.	Particle counting
	Stained bacteria	Visual assessment
Radioisotopic	[57]Co	Solid scintillation counting (SSC)
	[3]H	Liquid scintillation counting (LSC)
		Scintillation proximity assay and LSC
	[125]I,	SSC
	^{125}I-Bolton and Hunter reagent	SSC
Vesicle	Liposome	Entrapped enzyme or dye, colorimetry

With radioisotopic labels, the endpoint is measured with a scintillation counter, in which ionizing radiation is detected by means of a scintillant. The weak β particles emitted by tritium require a liquid scintillant to be mixed in solution with each sample to be counted. For gamma rays, the scintillant crystal surrounds the counting well. Photomultiplier tubes convert the light flashes into electric pulses that are proportional to the energies of the decay events. Most laboratories that carry out radioimmunoassays now have multi-well γ-counters and some of these are capable of counting samples in microtitre wells.

The rate of radioactive decay is given in disintegrations/min (d.p.m.). Counting efficiency is the percentage of disintegrations detected, measured in counts/min (c.p.m.), and for ^{125}I and ^{3}H it is typically about 80% and 50%, respectively.

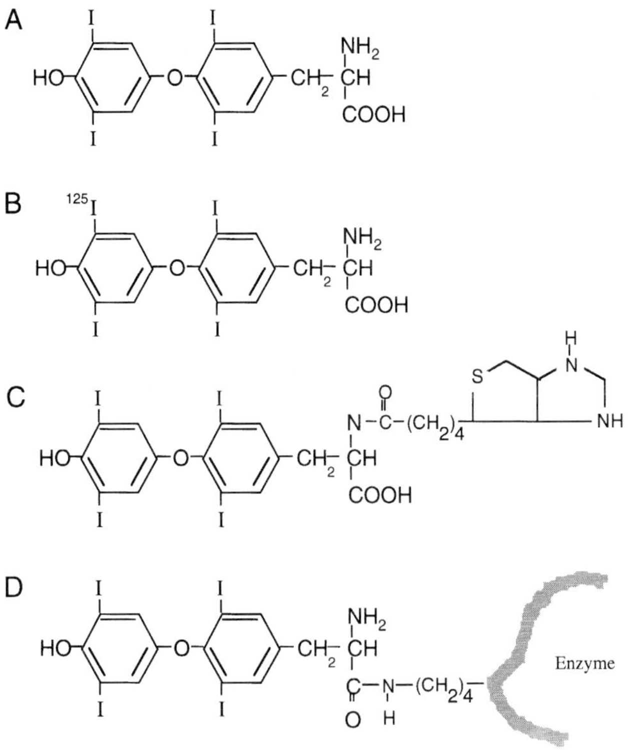

Figure 1. The hormone thyroxine (A) and three ways it could be labelled for the development of an immunoassay. A single substitution of ^{125}I for one of the I atoms would give a label (B) of reasonable specific activity (e.g. Bq/pmol or c.p.m./pg) and multiple substitution could greatly increase this. A biotinylation reagent such as NHS-biotin could be used (*Protocol 15*) to give biotinylated thyroxine (C), which can be titrated with labelled avidin or streptavidin. (Fluorescent or luminescent molecules could be attached in similar ways.) Alternatively, thyroxine could be directly conjugated (via the ε-amino group of a lysine residue) to an enzyme (D), perhaps by means of a procedure with carbodiimide (Section 3.2.2). However, greater distances between the thyroxine and biotin or enzyme tags would probably be beneficial (Section 3.4). The alternative biotinylation reagent NHS-LC-Biotin (Pierce Chemical Co.) has a bridging arm that is five carbons longer, and the thyroxine could be derivatized to add a bridging group before conjugation (as with 11α-hydroxyprogesterone in *Figure 2*).

Because disintegration is a random process, the error in any estimated count rate is dependent on the total number of counts detected, so that low count rates estimated quickly may be subject to considerable errors. For example, sufficient counting time needs to be allowed for each sample to generate about 10 000 counts to give a counting error of 1%. (Discounting the background count, which is valid if it is much less that 10% of the total count, the percentage error is about 100 divided by the square root of the total count.) However, while this approach is safe, it can lead to a highly significant waste of counter time (1, 11). The solution is to focus on the error in the final assay measurement. This is easily achieved if the software that controls the counter and processes the immunoassay data allows the user to terminate automatically each measurement when the counting error has reached a user-definable proportion of the error for the appropriate part of the standard curve (11).

High background counts increase counting errors, while high and variable background counts can completely destroy the validity of an experiment. Contamination of the counting chamber of a multi-well counter is particularly serious.

Some general points relevant to the choice and use of radioisotopic labels are:

- Radioisotopic immunoassays are only relevant in appropriately equipped and licensed laboratories. In house radioiodination is hazardous and requires special care and facilities

- Carefully estimate all amounts of radioisotope used to avoid unnecessary hazards and to ensure that all endpoint count rates are sufficient for good precision

- Use good procedures and adequate equipment to avoid contamination and adopt a strict routine of laboratory contamination testing. Routinely check the scintillation counter for counting efficiency and background, and all tube carriers for contamination

- Count samples to an adequate fixed total count, to a fixed error or, if feasible, to a specified proportion of the 'total' error at the appropriate point on the precision profile for the assay standard curve (see the counter manual).

1.2 Enzyme labels

Enzyme labels are used widely and in a variety of assay formats because they are detectable down to very low concentrations through the generation of easily visible, coloured, fluorescent or luminescent products from neutral substrates. Conjugates between suitable enzymes and antibodies or antigens are easily prepared and, with reasonable care, can be extremely stable and of very high quality.

The main disadvantages of immunoassays with enzymatic labels are that there are at least two incubation stages, antibody–antigen binding and signal generation, and each needs to be controlled, optimized and kept free from interfering substances. Enzymes also make for very large labels with slow diffusion rates.

Factors affecting the selection of an enzyme for use in immunoassay labels include high catalytic turnover number, the availability of simple and sensitive assay methods, the possession of reactive groups for coupling, long-term stability and high retention of activity after coupling.

Two enzymes dominate enzyme immunoassays. Horseradish peroxidase is an inexpensive, 44000 Da glycoprotein with four lysine residues available for conjugation without any loss of enzyme activity. Peroxidase reacts with the substrate hydrogen peroxide, becoming oxidized. It then oxidizes the second substrate, forming a coloured, fluorescent or luminescent derivative, depending on the substrate used. Alkaline phosphatase is a 140 000 Da dimeric glyco-protein containing many free amino groups that can be used for conjugation. It catalyses the hydrolysis of a very wide range of phosphate esters of primary alcohols, phenols and amines, facilitating the development of a wide variety of methods for the detection and measurement of its activity. Multistage, amplified assay methods that allow the measurement of very low activities of phospha-tase have been developed with colorimetric, fluorimetric and amperometric endpoints (2). β-D-Galactosidase is also used in the development of 'in house' immunoassays.

Other general tips relevant to enzymatic labels are:

- An enzymatic label is a reasonably safe choice for most applications and the necessary equipment for colorimetric microtitre plate assays is widely avail-able. Horseradish peroxidase can give more sensitive simple colorimetric assays, while alkaline phosphatase is usually chosen for qualitative assays when the endpoint is assessed visually

- High-quality enzyme conjugates, with good retention of enzymatic and immunological activities and little tendency to bind nonspecifically, are pre-requisites to the development of immunoassays with low inherent non-specific binding, which resist general interference and have low detection limits

- For most purposes, and particularly with competitive enzyme immuno-assays, the colorimetric measurement of endpoint can give sufficiently low detection limits

- Because of the inherent limitations of colorimetry and to ensure optimum precision, assays with colorimetric endpoints should be designed so that all readings fall within the optical absorbance range 0.1–1.6

- With reagent-excess assays, fluorimetric or luminometric measurements of enzyme activity enable wide analytical ranges and the lowest detection limits.

1.3 Fluorescent labels

Certain molecules, called fluorophores, absorb light at one wavelength and be-come excited, resonating with the frequency of the light applied. The molecule soon returns to the ground state by emitting light at a lower energy, i.e. a longer wavelength. This wavelength difference (the Stokes' shift) is 25–50 nm for most fluorescent organic molecules, including fluorescein (28 nm). However, it is greater than 200 nm for organic chelates of lanthanide ions such as europium (12, 13).

Another important variable is the average time between excitation and decay. Decay times for lanthanide chelates (10^{-5}–10^{-2} s) are much longer than for fluorescent organic molecules such as fluorescein (4.5×10^{-9} s). Fluorescent compounds also differ in quantum yield (the ratio of absorbed to emitted light energy). The efficiency of fluorescence emission is highly dependent on the presence and concentration of quenching compounds. In particular, nonspecific binding of the fluorophore to serum proteins can quench the signal, and molecules such as bilirubin and haemoglobin, if present in serum samples, can absorb excitation and/or emission light energies.

Time-resolved fluorescence spectrophotometry and exploitation of the long decay times of the lanthanide chelate labels make possible the development of highly sensitive immunoassays. By delaying measurements until the background has decayed, this approach can completely eliminate interference from sample constituents that give rise to significant and variable levels of short-lived fluorescence.

General tips relevant to fluorescent immunoassays include:

- An appropriate fluorimeter or time-resolved fluorimeter is a prerequisite

- They are preferable to enzymatic assays when the relative fragility or bulk of enzyme labels is undesirable

- Reagent excess sandwich assays with very low detection limits are more feasible with europium chelate labels and time-resolved measurement

- The manufacturers of the DELFIA time-resolved fluorescence system (Wallac OY) supply to developers of 'in-house' assay systems all necessary equipment, reagents and support.

1.4 Ligands and indirect labelling

The label determined at the end of an immunoassay for antigen may be a secondary label. For example, a labelled 'second' antibody (e.g. radioiodinated rabbit anti-mouse IgG, RAb-^{125}I) may be added to immobilized mouse 'first' antibody (solid phase-[ ]–MAb) in order to measure it (solid phase-[ ]–MAb–RAb-^{125}I). Here, the constant region of the mouse IgG can logically be said to be the primary label. Alternatively, labelled protein A can be used.

Also widely used is biotin conjugated to the anti-analyte antibody (or antigen) as primary label in combination with labelled avidin as secondary label (e.g. solid phase-[ ]–Ab-biotin–avidin-enzyme or solid phase-[ ]–Ag-biotin–avidin-enzyme). However, streptavidin is often preferred to avidin because it has a lower pI (5.5–6.5) and is not glycosylated, both of which properties help to decrease nonspecific binding. The biotin binding site of avidin can be sterically hindered when certain amino acids or glycosylated residues are present nearby on the biotinylated protein and improved binding capabilities are found when a biotin derivative that has an extended spacer arm is used.

Fluorescein is also used as primary label in this way, the concentration of label being determined with anti-fluorescein antibodies linked to secondary label (4) (e.g. solid phase-[ ]–Ab-fluorescein–Ab-enzyme).

Some general points related to choosing an indirect labelling method are:

- Indirect labelling with a second antibody is particularly useful when a number of anti-analyte antibodies are being evaluated. It is also useful when an anti-analyte antibody is in short supply or is susceptible to damage during conjugation

- Indirect labelling allows the use of a single secondary label for a range of assays (sometimes termed a universal label)
- Conjugates with biotin and fluorescein are easily prepared and stable, and are much less bulky than enzyme conjugates.

2 Enzyme measurement methods

Apart from assays carried out on membranes, the volumes and procedures outlined below apply to the measurement of enzyme activity bound to the lower parts of microtitre wells (equivalent to the area covered by 150 μl of buffer when the wells were being coated with antibody or antigen). The volumes of the total immunoassay mixture and of the buffered substrate for the enzyme assay are assumed to be 200 μl and 150 μl, respectively. Controlling the temperature during the assay incubation step (which should be in the dark if any component is light sensitive) is necessary for good precision.

For peroxidase assays, many of the cosubstrates are light sensitive and should be added just before use, while the H_2O_2 substrate diluted in substrate buffer is generally stable for up to 1 year. Add the buffered substrate solution to microtitre wells in a fixed sequence, mix thoroughly with a multivortex mixer and, after incubation, stop the reaction by adding stopping solution (normally 50 μl) in the same sequence and at the same rate.

2.1 Methods with chromogens

There are two general approaches to measuring enzyme activity with chromogenic substrates. For assays carried out in microtitre wells or tubes, a substrate that is converted to a soluble coloured product is used and the intensity of the colour developed is measured colorimetrically. For assays carried out on membranes, a substrate that yields an insoluble coloured product at the site of the reaction is used and the result is evaluated by visual inspection or quantified by reflection densitometry.

2.1.1 Horseradish peroxidase

2.1.1.1 ABTS

To prepare substrate solution, dissolve 100 mg ABTS (Boehringer or Sigma A1888, powder or preweighed tablets) in 100 ml of 100 mM phosphate–citrate buffer, pH 4.0. Add 10 μl 30% w/w H_2O_2 (Sigma, H1009) and mix thoroughly.

Add 150 μl per microtitre well. Incubate in the dark for 15–30 min. Stop reaction by addition of 50 μl 0.01% w/v sodium azide in 0.1 M citric acid. The green colour is measured at 415 nm. Alternatively, the reaction could be stopped with 10% dodecyl sulfate.

'Ready to use' one-component' ABTS Peroxidase systems may be obtained from Kirkegaard & Perry Laboratories, Inc.

2.1.1.2 OPD

Dissolve 200 mg OPD (*o*-phenylenediamine dihydrochloride) (Sigma, powder or tablets) in 100 ml 100 mM sodium citrate, pH 5.0 and protect from light by covering the flask or dispenser bottle with aluminium foil. Just before use add 66 μl H_2O_2 (30% w/w) or 55 mg urea hydrogen peroxide (Sigma, U1753) and mix thoroughly.

Add 150 μl per microtitre well and incubate in the dark for 15–30 min. Stop reaction with 50 μl of 2 M H_2SO_4 or 2.5 M HCl. Read optical absorbance at 492 nm.

2.1.1.3 TMB

Dissolve 10 mg TMB (Sigma, T2885) in 1 ml DMSO. Add 99 ml 0.1 M sodium acetate buffer, pH 6.0. Add H_2O_2 as with OPD.

Use as above. The addition of 50 μl 2 M H_2SO_4 as stopping reagent produces a bright yellow colour which is read at 450 nm. If a stopping reagent is not used the blue colour can be measured at 650 nm, but make sure to mix thoroughly before reading as the colour is likely to be stronger near the walls.

As with other peroxidase substrates, care should be taken to minimize the possibility of contamination of solutions with airborne particles. Ensure that solid peroxidase is not exposed in the vicinity of TMB preparation.

One milligram TMB tablets are available from Sigma. Ready-to-use one-component TMB peroxidase substrate systems may be obtained from Kirkegaard & Perry Laboratories, Inc. and Sigma (T8540).

2.1.1.4 DAB

DAB gives a brownish-black product that is insoluble in water and alcohol and is often used to detect enzyme that is immobilized on a membrane. Dissolve 6 mg DAB tetrahydrochloride (Sigma, D5637) in 9 ml 0.05 M Tris buffer, pH 7.6. Add 1 ml of a 0.3% w/v stock solution of nickel chloride or cobalt chloride in water. Remove precipitate, if present, by filtering through Whatman No. 1 filter paper or equivalent and add 10 μl 30% H_2O_2.

Apply reagent to membrane and incubate for 1–20 min at room temperature. To stop the reaction, rinse the membrane with PBS.

DAB is also available in a liquid substrate system from Kirkegaard and Perry and Sigma (D7304).

2.1.1.5 Chloronaphthol

4-Chloro-1-naphthol gives a blue-black product that is also insoluble in water. It gives an assay that is less sensitive than with DAB and the product is soluble in alcohol. Prepare stock solution by dissolving 0.3 g chloronaphthol (Sigma, C8890) in 10 ml absolute ethanol. The stock solution is stable if stored at −20°C. Just before use, add 100 μl of chloronaphthol stock, with stirring, to 10 ml 0.05 M Tris buffer, pH 7.6. Remove any precipitate by filtering through Whatman No. 1 filter paper or equivalent and add 10 μl of 30% H_2O_2.

Apply reagent to the immobilized enzyme and incubate for 10–40 min. To stop the reaction, remove remaining substrate by rinsing with PBS.

2.1.2 Alkaline phosphatase

2.1.2.1 PNPP

Dissolve 100 mg PNPP (Sigma, powder or capsule) in 100 ml 10 mM diethanol-amine, 0.5 mM $MgCl_2$, pH 9.8. Add 150 μl substrate to the microtitre well and incubate for 10–30 min at room temperature. Stop reaction with 50 μl 3 M NaOH or 0.1 M EDTA. A bright yellow colour due to *p*-nitrophenol appears when activity is present. Read the absorbance at 405 nm.

2.1.2.2 BCIP/NBT

BCIP/NBT generates an intense black-purple precipitate where molecules of enzyme are bound, and is the most commonly used substrate for assays carried out on membranes. Combined BCIP/NBT in tablet form is available (Sigma, B5655).

Prepare two reagent stock solutions: (a) Dissolve 0.5 g NBT (Sigma, N6876) in 10 ml 70% dimethlyformamide; (b) Dissolve 0.5 g BCIP, p-toluidine salt (Sigma, B8503) in 10 ml 100% DMF. Both stocks are stable for 1 year at 2–8 °C. Add 66 μl NBT stock to 10 ml 100 mM Tris buffer or ethanolamine solution containing 5 mM $MgCl_2$, and 100 mM NaCl, pH 9.5. Mix well and add 33 μl BCIP stock. Use within 1 h.

Apply reagent and incubate for 5–20 min. Stop reaction by rinsing with PBS containing 20 mM EDTA.

2.1.3 β-D-Galactosidase

2.1.3.1 ONPG

Dissolve 70 mg ONPG (Sigma, N1127) in 100 ml 0.1 M potassium phosphate, 1 mM $MgCl_2$, 0.01 M 2-mercaptoethanol, pH 7.0. Stop the reaction after 30 min by adding 2 M sodium carbonate. Read the absorbance of the yellow product at 405 nm.

2.1.3.2 BCIG

BCIG (Sigma B4252 or Boehringer) gives an insoluble blue-purple end product on hydrolysis. Dissolve 5 mg of BCIG in 0.1 ml dimethylformamide. Add 0.1 ml of BCIG solution to 10 ml 50 mM PBS (pH 7.8) containing 1 mM $MgCl_2$, 3 mM potassium ferrocyanide. Filter through Whatman No. 1 filter paper or equivalent and apply reagent to site of immobilized enzyme and incubate for 30 min. Stop reaction by rinsing with PBS containing 20 mM EDTA.

2.2 Methods with fluorogens

Fluorogenic substrates release a fluorescent product upon reaction with enzyme. Spectrofluorimeters for 96-well plates are now available from a number of manufacturers and the use of fluorogenic substrates may allow the measurement of femtomolar or even attomolar levels of enzyme.

2.2.1 Horseradish peroxidase

2.2.1.1 HPAA

To the tube containing the peroxidase to be measured, add 250 μl of 0.5% HPAA (Sigma, H4377) in 0.1 M sodium phosphate buffer, pH 7.0 at 30°C for 5 min. Start the reaction by adding 50 μl 0.03% hydrogen peroxide and incubate for 90 min at 30°C. Stop the reaction with 2.5 ml 0.1 M glycine–NaOH buffer, pH 10.3. The fluorimeter can be adjusted to a suitable range by adjusting the scale to give a reading of 100 with 1 μg/ml quinine dissolved in 0.1 N H_2SO_4. The wavelengths used for excitation and emission are 320 and 405 nm, respectively (14).

2.2.1.2 HPPA

Prepare the initial substrate solution by adding 0.5 g HPPA (Sigma, H6380) to 100 ml 100 mM sodium phosphate buffer, pH 8.0 (pH falls to 7.0). Add 100 μl to the well containing the enzyme (washed previously with 100 mM sodium phosphate buffer, pH 7.0). After 5 min at 30°C, add 20 μl 0.03% H_2O_2 and continue to incubate for the desired period (10–100 min). Stop the enzyme reaction by adding an equal volume of 200 mM glycine–NaOH, pH 10. Use 320 nm as the excitation wavelength and 405 nm as the emission wavelength. Adjust instrument intensity scale as described above.

2.2.2 Alkaline phosphatase

2.2.2.1 4-MUP

Add 2.6 mg 4-MUP (Sigma, M8883) to 33.3 ml 0.1 M glycine-NaOH, 1 mM $MgCl_2$, 0.1 mM $ZnCl_2$, 0.5 g/l NaN_3, pH 10.3. Start the enzyme reaction by adding the 4-MUP substrate solution and incubate for 10–60 min. Stop the reaction by adding 0.5 M potassium phosphate buffer, 10 mM EDTA, pH 10.4. Use 10–1000 nM 4-methylumbelliferone in the same buffer as a standard to measure fluorescence intensity using 360 nm for excitation and 450 nm for emission.

Fluorogenic substrates that yield 4-methylumbeliferone give enzyme assays with 100-fold lower detection limits than those that yield a coloured product, such as p-nitrophenol.

2.2.3 β-Galactosidase

2.2.3.1 4-MU-Gal

Dissolve 10 mg of 4-MU-Gal (Sigma, M1633; Boehringer) in 2 ml DMF by shaking at 37°C for 4–5 h and add 98 ml of deionized water. Start the enzyme reaction by adding the 4-MU-G substrate solution and incubating for 10–60 min. Stop the reaction by adding 100 mM glycine buffer, pH 10.3 and measure the fluorescence intensity as above.

2.3 Methods that generate luminescence

In chemiluminescent reactions, chemical energy generated as a result of the decomposition of a weak bond produces excited-state intermediates that decay to a ground state with the emission of light, which is detected using a lumino-meter. Microtitre plate luminometers require the use of white opaque plates or strips to prevent 'cross-talk' between wells. The overall quantum yield of a chemiluminescent reaction is generally in the range of 1–10%. There are two main approaches to the measurement of enzyme activity with a chemilumin-escence endpoint, one applicable to horseradish peroxidase and one to alkaline phosphatase.

2.3.1 Horseradish peroxidase

2.3.1.1 Enhanced chemiluminescence

Horseradish peroxidase, in the presence of hydrogen peroxide, catalyses the chemiluminescent oxidation of luminol. In the presence of p-iodophenol, the signal-to-blank ratio for detection is increased several-thousandfold over the reaction in the absence of an enhancer, resulting in a dramatic increase in the signal-to-noise ratio.

The enhanced chemiluminescent assay based on luminol and a phenolic primary enhancer (e.g. 4-iodophenol, 1,6-dibromo-2-naphthol, 6-hydroxybeno-thiazole, 4-methoxy-aniline) is the most sensitive assay for HRP with a detection limit < 25 attomoles. Various enhancers e.g. 6-hydroxybenzothiazole derivatives, including some non para-substituted phenols, produce greater enhancement re-actions and some of these have been adapted for use with microtitre plates. Enhanced luminescence is a glow rather than a flash of light, which persists for hours, although the signal is usually read within 2–20 min (15, 16). Prepared reagent mixtures are available commercially (e.g. SuperSignal® LBA, Pierce Chemical Company).

2.3.2 Alkaline phosphatase

2.3.2.1 Activated dioxetanes

The substrate is usually the adamantane 1,2-dioxetane phosphate derivative AMPPD (17). On enzymatic cleavage of the phosphate group, the dioxetane moiety is destabilized and decomposes via an intermediary anion, which is moderately stable with half-life of 2–180 min, depending on its environment. The wavelength of maximum emission is 470 nm, and the background due to the nonenzymatic hydrolysis of AMPPD is very low at alkaline pH. An equiva-lent substrate for β-D-galactosidase has also been developed (17).

3 Labelling and conjugation

3.1 Radiolabelling

All iodination methods are chemically similar. ^{125}I ions are oxidized to form free radicals that spontaneously insert into tyrosyl or histidyl residues. With Bolton–Hunter reagent (1) this step has already been carried out by the manufacturer, giving a radioiodinated entity that is capable of linking to free amino groups. Tritiated labels are almost always purchased from specialized commercial laboratories or custom-synthesized by the same laboratories. Two practical and efficient radioiodination procedures (*Protocols 2 and 3*) are described here, a 'solid phase' chemical method with iodogen (an insoluble derivative of chloramine T), and an enzymatic method with lactoperoxidase.

3.1.1 Safety procedures

Radioiodination is the most potentially hazardous radioactive procedure in wide-spread use in biological laboratories, but with care, attention to detail, good facilities and good practices it need not represent any risk to health (*Protocol 1*). It is most important to avoid the escape of iodine vapour and to systematically check for contamination.

Protocol 1
Safety procedure for radioiodinations

Equipment and reagents

- A laboratory fitted, equipped and licensed to the standards of a 'medium hazard' radioactive facility for the manipulation of unsealed sources. (The whole area used must be clearly identified with appropriate signs to prevent inadvertent access of unauthorised personnel)

- A suitable fume hood

- Light lead blocks or, preferably, a transparent lead-containing acrylic shield (e.g. from Scie-Plas Ltd, UK).

- Personal dosimeters for each person involved, a properly maintained contamination monitor (freshly swathed in cling-film) and a small radioactive source for checking its function

- Two to four shallow trays on which all manipulations will be carried out

- Laboratory coats and disposable aprons, over-shoes, head-covering of suitable standard, safety glasses

- Generous supplies of latex gloves (to be worn two per hand), disposable plastic aprons, paper tissues and absorptive paper suitable for lining trays, covering work surfaces and floors

- Equipment for taking 'swipes' to check for contamination, including suitable forceps, a wash bottle for wetting surfaces, counting tubes and pieces of absorptive material that fit easily into the tubes

- A suitable form for recording the completion of each stage of the safety procedure and with space for the results of all contamination checks and rechecks.

Procedure

1. Reserve an easily isolated section of the laboratory with a fume hood (if possible the whole laboratory room) for the full duration of the procedure, and post notices restricting access.

Protocol 1 continued

2. Appoint an 'iodinator' and an assistant, both of whom will be present all of the time, and check that both are free from contamination (including thyroid checks with suitable equipment).

3. Take measures to avoid any necessity to leave the area before the whole procedure is completed, and put on protective clothing.

4. Take swipes from sufficient sites to ensure that the whole area is free from contamination.

5. Set out trays and absorptive coverings and set up the equipment. Locate the site where the iodination is to be carried out and place the separation column in the fume hood behind suitable shielding.

6. Place the contamination monitor in a convenient location where the background count is low. Take small items to the monitor to check them for contamination and do not move the monitor unnecessarily. This approach avoids the confusion caused by the necessarily highly variable background counts in the work area, and reduces the risk of the monitor itself becoming contaminated.

7. Throughout the iodination and separation steps, the hands of the operators should be regularly checked for contamination and, when any is found, the outer glove (at least) should be changed immediately. If a spill is suspected, take a swipe with a piece of tissue and bring it to the monitor to check. Keep the plate-glass sash of the fume hood as low as is comfortable at all times to provide extra shielding to the head and upper body, and fully down when immediate access is not needed.

8. When the iodination procedure is complete, tidy up the whole work area immediately and dispose of all radioactive waste and contaminated items according to the official local procedures. Minimize the volume of such waste by use of the contamination monitor.

9. Take swipes from at least all the same sites as before to ensure that the whole area is free from contamination. If any contamination is found, wash and check again, until clean.

10. Remove all nondisposable protective clothing and check for contamination.

11. Report all serious spills, and all contamination that is difficult to remove to the radiological protection officer.

12. Check that both iodinator and assistant are free from contamination, immediately after the procedure and next day. Report any significant contamination found and seek medical advice.

Protocol 2

Radioiodination of IgG with iodogen

Equipment and reagents

This procedure must be carried with institute-approved monitoring of radiation exposure and waste disposal. The precautions detailed in *Protocol 1* should be followed.

- 0.1 M sodium phosphate, pH 7.4
- 10 µg IgG (molecular weight 150 000 Da) in 25 µl phosphate buffer, pH 7.4, giving a concentration of 400 µg/ml or 2.7 µM. For other proteins, adjust the amount in accordance with their molecular sizes (e.g. 2 µg for a 30 000 Da protein).
- 500 µCi Na^{125}I (Amersham Pharmacia Biotech)
- 20 µg/ml iodogen (Pierce Chemical Company) in dichloromethane
- 0.1 M PBS, pH 7.4: 0.1 M sodium phosphate, 0.15 M NaCl, pH 7.4
- PBS-BSA: 0.1 M PBS, pH 7.4 containing 1% BSA

- Sephadex G-25, fine grade (Pharmacia) or Biogel P-10 gel, fine grade (BioRad) column (1 cm diameter × 60 cm long). To minimize losses through nonspecific binding of the iodinated protein, prewash with 10 column-volumes of 1% BSA in PBS, and then wash with 10 volumes of PBS
- Cylinder of compressed nitrogen gas
- Stop buffer: 10 mg/ml tyrosine in PBS
- 10 × 75 mm plastic tubes compatible with solvent
- Pasteur pipette and rubber teat
- Vortex mixer
- Other equipment and materials specified in *Protocol 1*

Procedure

1. Prepare iodogen-coated tubes by dispensing 100 µl aliquots of 20 µg/ml iodogen into 1.5 ml conical polypropylene tubes. For proteins that are susceptible to denaturation use a 4 µg/ml iodogen solution. Allow the dichloromethane to evaporate in a fume hood, fill the tubes with nitrogen gas, cap and store desiccated at room temperature (stable for 2 years).

2. To an iodogen-coated tube add 25 µl PBS followed by 25 µl 0.1 M sodium phosphate pH 7.4 containing the 10 µg of the IgG to be iodinated.

3. Add 500 µCi Na^{125}I (5 µl) to the iodogen tube. Vortex.

4. Incubate for 2 min.

5. With a Pasteur pipette, transfer the contents of the iodogen tube to 0.5 ml PBS in a clean tube (include a rinse of the reaction vial).

6. Stop the reaction by adding 50 µl Stop buffer.

7. Separate the iodinated protein from the free iodine on the G-25 column.

8. To establish the elution profile, which will have two distinct peaks if a column-volume or more of buffer is eluted, check each sample with the contamination monitor at a fixed distance and/or by counting 5- or 10-µl aliquots in the scintillation counter. The fractions of the first peak should contain the iodinated protein and should be pooled.

9. If necessary, estimate the specific activity of the radioiodinated IgG by the self-displacement method, whereby two sets of tubes are put through a standard RIA procedure (18, 19). The tubes in the first set contain a constant concentration of an antibody against the iodinated IgG (sufficient to bind about 33% of label in zero tubes i.e. without IgG) and a constant (about 60 000 c.p.m. per tube) concentration of the iodinated IgG with zero or increasing amounts of unlabelled IgG. The range and spacing of concentrations should be equivalent to that used for a standard curve, giving < 10% displacement at the lowest concentration and full displacement of label at the highest concentration. The tubes in the second set contain an identical concentration of antibody and increasing amounts of iodinated IgG only (60 000 up to at least 1×10^6 c.p.m. per tube). Plot the two (parallel) curves obtained (total/bound counts versus concentration of unlabelled protein, and total/bound versus radioactivity) on the same graph with duplicate x-axes. At a higher, medium and lower bound/total value, estimate the amount of radioactivity (c.p.m., d.p.m., Ci or Bq) equivalent to a quantity of standard (g or mol) by interpolation from the plots. Take the average of the three and calculate the specific activity (c.p.m./μg, Bq/mol or Ci/mol).

10. Store the iodinated protein at 2–8 °C and use it within six weeks of preparation.

Protocol 3

Radioiodination of IgG with lactoperoxidase

Equipment and reagents

- 10 μg IgG in 25 μl 0.1 M sodium phosphate, pH 7.4 (2.7 μM IgG). For other proteins, adjust the amount in accordance with their molecular weights
- Lactoperoxidase (Sigma, L8257), 1 unit/ml in 0.1 M PBS, pH 7.4 from *Protocol 2*

- Hydrogen peroxide (30%) (Sigma, H1009) diluted 1 in 20 000 with PBS
- See *Protocols 1* and *2* for other requirements

Radioiodination

1. To 25 μl of protein (e.g. IgG) in buffer add 10 μl lactoperoxidase solution and then 5 μl Na^{125}I (500 μCi).

2. Start the reaction by adding 1 μl H$_2$O$_2$ solution then mix gently. Add a further four 1-μl aliquots of H$_2$O$_2$ at 1-min intervals.

3. Terminate the reaction by adding 25 μl of Stop buffer.

4. Separate the iodinated protein on the gel filtration column. Pool the fractions containing the iodinated protein and estimate specific activity as described in *Protocol 2*: step 9.

5. Store the iodinated protein at 2–8 °C and use it within 6 weeks of preparation.

3.2 The chemistry of conjugation

Certain pairs of functional groups spontaneously condense at moderate temperatures and under near-physiological conditions to give covalent bonds that are stable or that can be stabilized under similarly mild conditions. To prepare a conjugate for use as an immunoassay label it is necessary to ensure that the antibody or antigen has at least one such group that is suitably located, and that this group is complementary to a reactive group on the labelling substance. Some such groups are common in biomolecules, others can be induced by chemical alteration of existing groups, or can be introduced by means of special reagents.

The most common starting groups in the molecules to be conjugated are amino, carboxyl, sulfhydryl, and carbonyl, but all of the common conjugation procedures involve amino groups on one or both of the molecules to be linked. Amino groups may be linked to other amino groups, to carboxyl groups or to sulfhydryl groups with the help of a range of reagents (20, 21). (There are also discussions on conjugation methods and some equivalent protocols in Chapters 5 and 6.)

3.2.1 Amino groups to amino groups

Free amino groups are common in biomolecules. In most proteins the terminal amino group is free and many proteins are rich in lysine, which has a free ε-amino group.

3.2.1.1 With glutaraldehyde

Glutaraldehyde is a very simple, five carbon, homo-bifunctional molecule with two aldehyde groups that readily react with amino groups, and it is very widely used to link pairs of proteins together. The coupling may be carried out in one step, with the formation of undesirable products being minimized by the judicious limitation of concentrations and reaction time, or over two steps, with one protein being treated with glutaraldehyde to introduce aldehyde groups before the introduction of the second protein. Separation of the reactions gives more control over the conjugation ratio and reduces polymerization.

Glutaraldehyde coupling is relatively crude, and may give significant amounts of homodimers or polymers and low yield of product (often just 5–25%). It also may give poor retention of the original biological activities and is difficult to control. However, it (especially the one-step procedure) is simple, cheap and appears to be adequate for many applications. It may be quite appropriate when a peptide or other hapten containing only a single free reactive amino group is to be coupled.

3.2.1.2 With hetero-bifunctional reagents

Many such reagents have been developed and are commercially available, and only a selection are listed in *Table 2*.

SAMSA reacts with amino groups to give available acetylmercaptan groups

Table 2. Reagents for protein–protein coupling and for inserting sulfhydryl groups into proteins. These are available from various suppliers, including Boehringer Mannheim, Pharmacia and Pierce Chemical Company

Acronym	Name	Group1 reacts with	Group 2 reacts with
ABDP	N-(4-aminobenzoyl)-N′-(pyridyldithiopropionyl)-hydrazine	-SH	-OH (tyrosine)
DPEM	N-[β-(4-diazophenyl)ethyl]maleimide (reference 99)	Phenol and imidazole	-SH
	Glutaraldehyde	-NH$_2$	-NH$_2$
HSAB	N-hydroxysuccinimidyl-4-azidobenzoate	-NH$_2$	-unspecific
MBS	m-Maleimidobenzoyl-N-hydroxysuccinimide ester	-NH$_2$	-SH
SMCC	Succinimidyl 4-(N-maleimidomethyl) cyclohexane-1-carboyylate	-NH$_2$	-SH
SATA	N-hydroxysuccunimide S-acetylthioacetic acid (inserts protected -SH)	-NH$_2$	
SPDP	N-Succinimyl 3-(2-pyridyldithio) propionate (inserts protected -SH)	-NH$_2$	
	2-Iminothiolane (Traut's reagent) (inserts -SH)	-NH$_2$	

that can be easily treated to expose free sulfhydryl groups. SPDP reacts with amino groups to introduce pyridyldithio groups that react readily with sulfhydryl groups allowing conjugation with molecules treated with SAMSA. SAMSA and SPDP (22, 23) are two of a wide, and initially bewildering, range of specially designed reagents for the introduction of reactive groups and for coupling. For example, SPDP itself can be cleaved to expose sulfhydryl groups, so that the above procedure can be carried out with SPDP for both of the initial derivatization steps.

Such reagents are useful when linking one protein to another, or a hapten to a protein or when coupling two small molecules. In the last case, the 'link' introduced may dominate the chemical nature of the resulting conjugate and lead to problems such as insolubility. However, many such reagents are available in more water-soluble sulfated forms, or with connecting groups of different lengths.

Hetero-bifunctional reagents are (collectively) highly versatile and the linking and de-blocking reactions can be carried out under quite mild conditions, but the overall conjugation procedures are sometimes long and complex, with many chromatographic separation steps (24–26).

3.2.2 Amino groups to carboxyl groups

Although the free carboxyl groups of aspartates and glutamates are common in proteins, the most common situation of this kind is where the molecule with the carboxyl group is of low molecular weight and is a hapten and the molecule with the amino group(s) is a protein. The original hapten may have a free hydroxyl group and a carboxyl group can be introduced by reacting it with succinic, glutaric or maleic anhydride. Alternatively, a free carboxyl group may be available and the carboxyl can be introduced by a reaction with O-(carboxy-methyl) hydroxylamine. Both of these derivatization methods have the added advantage of introducing a spacer arm between the hapten and what is often an enzyme.

3.2.2.1 Mixed anhydride procedure

The carboxyl group of the hapten is first converted to an acid anhydride, by a reaction at low temperature in organic solvent with isobutyl chloroformate in the presence of N-ethylmorpholine and is then allowed to react with the molecule carrying the amino group(s) (27, 28). This procedure is widely used and can give very good-quality enzyme–hapten conjugates.

3.2.2.2 Carbodiimide procedure

This procedure consists of condensation between an amino group on a protein and a carboxyl group on a hapten, previously activated with carbidiimide to form an o-acyl-isourea intermediate. However, the quality of enzyme conjugates may be inconsistent.

3.2.2.3 Active ester procedure

Carbodiimide is also used in this procedure (*Figure 2*), but here it enables the formation of an active N-succinimidyl ester from the carboxyl-containing hapten and N-hydroxysuccinimide. The active ester can then be used directly or, more effectively, isolated in solid form. This procedure allows the removal of residual carbodiimide, which could deactivate the protein during the second step, and also facilitates the adjustment of the molar ratio of hapten to enzyme or other amino group-containing molecule (29). A range of such activated derivatives of some steroid and thyroid hormones is available commercially from Boehringer Mannheim (Now Roche Diagnostics; ask for their special 'Immuno-logicals for the Diagnostic Industry' Catalogue).

3.2.3 Amino groups to sulfhydryl groups

Although cysteine residues are common constituents of proteins, they usually participate in disulfhydryl linkages, making proteins with free sulfhydryl groups suitable for conjugation reactions quite rare. However, β-D-galactosidase has a number of such groups and, in normal pure preparations of the enzyme, up to four free sulfhydryls are available. In addition, while intact immunoglobulins have no free sulfhydryls, Fab' fragments have at least one near the carboxy terminal. Alternatively, sulfhydryl groups may be inserted by the derivatization of free amino groups (see Section 3.2.1).

3.2.3.1 With hetero-bifunctional reagents

It is the possession of reactive groups such as maleimide or pyridyldithio that makes a hetero-bifunctional reagent reactive with sulfhydryl groups, and many such reagents also have a succinimidyl group for reacting with amino groups. SPDP is one such reagent, but perhaps the most often mentioned is SMCC. A more water-soluble, sulfated derivative of SMCC (sulfo-SMCC) is also available.

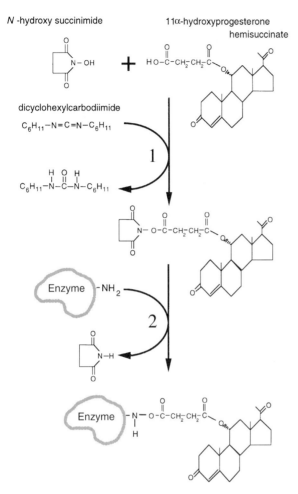

Figure 2. Active ester procedure for the conjugation of steroid hapten to molecule with free amino groups such as an enzyme. The procedure is carried out in two steps, the first to generate the active ester derivative of the carboxyl-containing hapten, which can then be used directly or stored until needed, and the second for the reaction of the activated hapten with the protein. 1. 11α-Hydroxyprogesterone hemisuccinate, the steroid to be conjugated, is reacted with N-hydroxy succinimide in the presence of DCCD in dioxane at room temperature (14–20°C) for at least 2 h, with stirring. As the carbodiimide is transformed to N,N'-dicyclohexyl urea, the NHS active-ester of the 11-α-hydroxyprogesterone hemisuccinate is formed. The NHS ester is then isolated after dilution with water and extraction with ethyl acetate, and can be stored until needed. This procedure also removes residual carbodiimide, which could deactivate the protein during step 2, and facilitates the adjustment of the molar ratio of hapten to enzyme for step 2. 2. The active ester and enzyme are mixed together in 10 mM phosphate buffer, pH 7.0 and allowed to react at 4°C overnight, before the conjugate is separated from the reactants by means of dialysis (with removal of precipitate by centrifugation) and gel filtration chromatography on Sephadex G25.

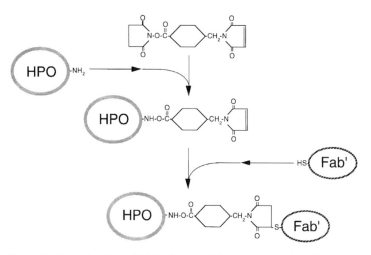

Figure 3. The conjugation of Fab' to horseradish peroxidase with SMCC. The cyclohexane bridge gives stability to the maleimide group. A sulphonated derivative of SMCC with improved water solubility is available (Pierce Chemical Co.). m-Maleimidobenzoyl-N-hydroxysuccinimide ester (MBS) has the same reactive groups but a benzoyl bridge. Firstly SMCC is reacted with a protein containing available free amino groups, and no free sulfhydryl group, in this case HRP (the abbreviation HPO is used above). The consequent maleimide-substituted HRP is then reacted with the sulfhydryl-containing protein, in this case Fab'. Both reactions proceed efficiently under mild conditions which facilitates full retention of enzyme and antigen-binding activities.

SIAB is yet another such reagent that is highly effective (30). All may be used with small molecules as with large, provided that the necessary groups are available, or have been inserted previously.

Fab'-enzyme conjugates prepared with SMCC (*Figure 3*) normally retain full immunological activity because of the favourable geometry of the linkage, and full enzymatic activity because of the mildness of the reaction conditions. They also have little tendency to bind nonspecifically because of the absence of the Fc and their relatively low molecular weight.

3.2.4 Amino groups to carbohydrate side-chains

Because the carbohydrate side-chains of most glycoprotein enzymes and of many other glycoproteins are not required for full activity, and because they seldom occlude active sites, they are very useful attachment points for conjugations. While glycoproteins are common in biology, it is the fact that horseradish peroxidase, the most popular enzyme used for labelling, has eight O-linked chains that has made this approach to the preparation of enzyme conjugates popular, and vice versa. Glucose oxidase, another glycoprotein, and the low molecular weight drug digoxin can also be conjugated in this way.

3.2.4.1 With periodate oxidation

Briefly, the peroxidase, or another sugar-containing molecule, is subjected to mild oxidizing conditions by exposing it to sodium periodate, causing cleavage of vicinal glycols in carbohydrate residues to generate dialdehydes. These can then react with free amino groups on other protein molecules to form Schiff base linkages. These linkages can then be stabilized by reduction with sodium borohydride or cyanoborohydride. When the method is well executed up to 90% coupling efficiency and up to 90% retention of horseradish peroxidase activity are feasible.

3.3 Protein–protein conjugation

Often, these procedures involve linking an enzyme to an antibody, but they are also used with fluorescent proteins, and with antigens. The most popular include the one- and two-step glutaraldehyde methods (useful when raw materials are plentiful and high-specification conjugate is not needed, *Protocols 4* and *5*) and, with horseradish peroxidase, the periodate procedure (relatively simple and adequate for most application, *Protocol 6*). The enzyme to antibody ratio should be optimized, higher ratios may lead to polymerization while lower ratios may be required for proteins that are susceptible to inactivation.

Protocol 4

One-step glutaraldehyde method for IgG and alkaline phosphatase

Equipment and reagents

- Phosphate buffer: 100 mM sodium phosphate buffer, pH 6.8 (without added preservative)
- Alkaline phosphatase suspension (Sigma, Type VII-N, P2276). (Alkaline phosphatase is usually supplied as a suspension in 65% ammonium sulfate. Calculate the amount of alkaline phosphatase based on the specific activity of the enzyme. Clarify by centrifugation in the cold, discard supernatant and mix the pellet with 0.1 ml phosphate buffer. Dialyse against a suitable buffer to get rid of ammonium sulfate.)
- IgG to be conjugated

- 1% glutaraldehyde (Sigma EM grade I: 25% aqueous solution, G5882) in phosphate buffer
- 1 M ethanolamine in water, pH 7.0 or 1 M Lysine in 0.1 M phosphate buffer, pH 7.5
- Dialysis tubing
- Elution buffer: 0.05 M Tris–HCl, 1 mM $MgCl_2$ pH 8.0
- Sephacryl S-200 (Pharmacia) or Ultrogel AcA44 (Biosepra) column (2.6 cm diameter $\times$ 100 cm long)
- Magnetic stirrer and small stirring bar
- Diaflo ultrafilter concentrator unit using YM10 membrane (Millipore)

Procedure

1. Add 5 mg of alkaline phosphatase enzyme to 5 mg antibody (IgG or 2.5 mg Fab′) in a total volume of 2 ml to give an approximately equimolar ratio.

2. Dialyse the enzyme/antibody solution for 18–24 h against two 1-l volumes of phosphate buffer, changing the buffer twice.

Protocol 4 continued

3. Slowly add 0.05 ml 1% glutaraldehyde solution to the dialysed protein mixture with constant gentle mixing.

4. After 5 min switch off the stirrer.

5. Incubate at room temperature for 2–3 h then overnight at 2–8 °C.

6. Stop reaction by blocking glutaraldehyde with 0.1 ml ethanolamine solution or 1 M lysine.

7. Incubate for 1 h at room temperature.

8. Separate the conjugate from unconjugated proteins and large aggregates by means of the Sephacryl or Ultrogel column and the elution buffer at a flow rate of 0.3–0.5 ml/min with 1-ml fraction volumes.

9. Read absorbance of fractions collected at 280 nm. Measure the enzymatic and immunological activity of each fraction. Pool those fractions with enzyme and antibody label and concentrate to 2–3 ml with the Diaflo concentrator unit.

10. Add 0.5% BSA, 0.1% sodium azide and an equal volume of glycerol to the conjugate solution. Store at −20 °C.

Protocol 5

Two-step glutaraldehyde method for IgG and alkaline phosphatase

Equipment and reagents

- Alkaline phosphatase, phosphate buffer, column for purification step as in *Protocol 4*

- 0.15 M NaCl (saline)

- 5 mg/ml immunoglobulin for conjugation in saline

- Glutaraldehyde diluted to 10% with 100 mM phosphate buffer, pH 6.8

- Sephadex G-25 (F) column (1 × 60 cm) (Pharmacia) equilibrated with saline

- 500 mM sodium bicarbonate buffer, pH 9.5

- Centriprep-10 concentrators (Millipore)

- 1 M L-lysine in 0.1 M phosphate buffer, pH 7.5

Procedure

1. Dialyse 5 mg of enzyme in 100 mM phosphate buffer, pH 6.8 for 18–24 h against two 1-l volumes of phosphate buffer, changing the buffer twice.

2. Activate the enzyme by slowly adding 0.1 ml 10% glutaraldehyde with constant mixing.

3. Incubate for 30 min at room temperature.

4. Remove excess glutaraldehyde by passing through Sephadex G-25 column equilibrated with normal saline

5. Concentrate the pooled fractions that contain enzyme–antibody label to 2 ml with a Centriprep-10 concentrator (Millipore)

6. Add 1 ml of antibody (5 mg IgG or 2.5 mg Fab') equilibrated with normal saline to the activated enzyme. Add 0.2 ml bicarbonate buffer pH 9.5 and mix gently.

7. Incubate for 24 h at 2–8 °C.

8. Block the remaining activated groups by adding 0.1 ml 1 M L-lysine. Adjust the pH to 7.0 and incubate for 2 h at 2–8 °C.

9. Separate the conjugate protein from unconjugated by gel filtration and store as in *Protocol 4*.

Protocol 6

Periodate coupling for IgG and HRP

Equipment and reagents

- HRP type IV (Sigma, P8375)
- Purified immunoglobulin preparation
- 0.1 M PBS, pH 7.5
- 15 mM sodium metaperiodate (freshly prepared in deionized water)
- Acetate buffer: 1 mM acetate buffer, pH 4.4
- Sephadex G-25 (F) column (1.0 cm diameter × 45 cm long; Pharmacia) equilibrated with acetate buffer
- 100 mM carbonate buffer, pH 9.2
- 5 mg/ml sodium borohydride in deionized water (freshly prepared)
- Gel filtration column as in *Protocol 4* but equilibrated with PBS
- Diaflo ultrafilter concentrator unit using YM10 membrane (Millipore)
- Centriprep-10 concentrators (Millipore)

Procedure

1. Dissolve 5 mg of HRP in 0.5 ml deionized water in a small tube.

2. Add 0.5 ml of 15 mM $NaIO_4$, close tube, mix gently and incubate at 20 °C for 2 h in the dark.

3. Separate oxidized HRP from reactants on Sephadex G-25 column by eluting with acetate buffer and pool HRP-containing fractions. Concentrate fractions to 2 ml using a Centriprep-10 concentrators (Millipore)

4. Add 20 µl carbonate buffer to HRP followed immediately by 5 mg (1 ml) of IgG and mix gently.

5. Incubate for 3 h at room temperature (without stirring).

6. Add, with mixing, 50 µl sodium borohydride.

7. Incubate for 1 h at 2–8 °C.

8. Purify the conjugate as in *Protocol 4*, eluting with 0.1 M PBS, pH 7.5.

9. Read absorbance of collected fractions at 280 nm and 403 nm. Measure the enzymatic and immunological activity of each fraction.

10. Estimate the HRP/IgG ratio in the solution of conjugate spectrophotometrically as follows: HRP (mg/ml) = $A_{403}/2.25^a$; IgG (mg/ml) = $(A_{280} - (A_{403}/\text{RZ of initial HRP}))/1.4$; HRP/IgG ratio (mol/mol) = [HRP (mg/ml)/IgG (mg/ml)] $\times$ (M_r IgG/M_rHRP).

11. Pool fractions with highest enzyme–antibody activity and concentrate by means of Diaflo concentrator unit to 2–3 ml.

12. Add 0.01% thimerosal, 0.5% BSA and an equal volume of glycerol to the conjugate solution. Store at −20°C.

[a] The optical absorbance at 403 nm (A_{403}) for a 1 mg/ml solution of HRP is 2.25. A_{280} for IgG at 1 mg/ml is 1.4. RZ is the absorbance ratio A_{403}/A_{280} for the HRP preparation used. M_r for HRP is 44 000 Da and for IgG is 150 000 Da.

3.3.1 Fab′–enzyme conjugates

The use of intact IgG molecules as reagents in immunoassays is not always ideal as IgG is a large molecule with a range of binding functions associated with its constant regions. These include sites for components of the complement system and for macrophage receptors, and epitopes recognized by auto-antibodies.

Conjugates with Fab′ rather than whole IgG have inherent properties conducive to low nonspecific binding and, because of the conjugation methods usually used for their preparation, often have very high retention of binding activity. In addition, the free sulfhydryl group(s) in Fab′ fragments are in a portion of the heavy chain polypeptide that form part of the hinge region in the intact molecule. Importantly, this allows conjugation at a site that is distant from the antigen-binding site.

The main disadvantage of conjugates with Fab′ is the length and relative complexity of the preparation procedure, which here, starting with a pure preparation of IgG, is separated into four protocols (see also Figure 3). None of these are more difficult than the more common protocols described above, but special care must be taken to monitor and to ensure good recovery at every step, as cumulative losses can easily become important. The overall procedure is as follows:

- *Protocol 7*: prepare F(ab′)$_2$ by pepsin digestion
- *Protocol 8*: activate enzyme with SMCC
- *Protocol 9*: prepare Fab′ from F(ab′)$_2$
- *Protocol 10*: conjugate activated enzyme to Fab′.

3.3.1.1 Planning and executing Protocols 7–10

To prepare conjugates of the highest quality with good yield a number of precautions should be taken. In the overall planning and execution of the combined protocols, careful forward planning and speed and efficiency are important, since thiol groups and other properties of the intermediate products are more labile at low concentrations. Use very high purity water and degas all buffers before use with columns. Do not use NaN_3 as a preservative in buffers, since it accelerates the decomposition of maleimide groups and inactivates peroxidase. Ultrogel AcA 44 provides a sharper separation of F(ab')$_2$ than Sephadex G-150 (Pharmacia), which could be considered as an alternative.

In the preparation of F(ab')$_2$ digestion time may be significantly species and subclass specific and optimization experiments are recommended. Washing columns with a buffer containing BSA before use helps to increase the recovery of smaller quantities of F(ab')$_2$ and other products. With IgG from goat, sheep, guinea pig and probably other animals except for rabbit, the Ultrogel column should be equilibrated, and the F(ab')$_2$ eluted with 0.1 M phosphate buffer, pH 6–7 since its elution is retarded at pH 8. For rabbit antibodies use the borate buffer, pH 8.0.

3.3.1.2 F(ab')$_2$ preparation

Mouse monoclonal antibodies of different IgG subclasses show a wide degree of variation in their susceptibility to proteolysis by pepsin in the order IgG2b > IgG3 > IgG2a > IgG1.

Preliminary tests to assess the efficiency of the pepsin digestion protocol may be very important. These would involve varying the pH of the reaction (maximum 5.5, minimum 2.5), the amount of pepsin added (1:10 to 1:200 ratio of pepsin to antibody) and the length of the incubation (from 10 min to 18 h for monoclonals compared with 18–24 h for rabbit or goat antibodies). Each set of conditions can be verified on SDS–polyacrylamide gels (31) with samples being run with and without reduction using dithiothreitol. One convenient electrophoresis system that may be employed is the Amersham Pharmacia Biotech Phast™ system.

Protocol 7

Preparation of rabbit F(ab')$_2$

Equipment and reagents

- Acetate buffer: 0.1 M sodium acetate, pH 4.5
- Rabbit IgG, 5 mg/ml in acetate buffer (see text for advice if an antibody from another species is to be fragmented)
- 3200–4500 units pepsin (Sigma, P 6887)
- TBS: 0.1 M Tris-HCl, 0.15 M NaCl, 2 mM EDTA, pH 7.7

- Borate buffer: 0.1 M sodium borate, pH 8.0
- Ultrogel AcA44 column (1.5 cm diameter × 45 cm long for a 1.0–1.5 ml sample or 2.0 cm diameter for up to 2–3 ml; Biosepra Inc.), equilibrated with borate buffer
- Diaflo ultrafilter concentrator unit with YM10 membrane (Millipore)

Procedure

1. Weigh sufficient crystalline pepsin to give a 1:40 pepsin/antibody (w/w) ratio and dissolve in a small amount of acetate buffer.

2. Add the pepsin solution into the antibody solution, mix well and incubate for 18–24 h at 37°C. (see section 3.3.1.2)

3. While mixing, stop digestion by the addition of small crystals of Tris salt to raise the pH to 8.0 for rabbit antibody, or to pH 7.0 for other antibodies (section 3.3.1.1).

4. Apply digested IgG solution to the Ultrogel column. The first peak absorbing at 280 nm will normally be F(ab')$_2$, the second the Fc fragment and the third broad peak peptide fragments.

5. Calculate the amount of F(ab')$_2$ obtained from its absorbance at 280 nm (extinction coefficient 1.48/g.l^{-1}.cm[a], M_r 92 000). Concentrate to 1 mg/ml using a Diaflo ultrafilter concentrator.

[a] i.e. a 1 mg/ml solution with a path length of 1 cm has an absorbance of 1.48 at 280 nm.

Nonreduced IgG migrates as a 150 000 Da band, F(ab)$_2$ as a 110 000 Da band, and nonreduced Fc fragment as an $\approx$ 25 000 Da band, or as a smear representing a mixture of low molecular weight fragments. Under reducing condition, IgG migrates as two bands, at about 50 000 and 25 000 Da, and (F(ab')$_2$ fragments give a doublet of bands at about 25 000 Da. Conditions that minimize the amount of whole IgG remaining and the amount of degraded lower molecular weight material, while maximizing the nonreduced 110 000 Da band and the reduced 25 000 Da doublet, are to be preferred.

Protocol 8

Activation of HRP with SMCC

Equipment and reagents

- SMCC (M_r 334.33) (Calbiochem, Sigma, Pierce Chemical Co.)
- HRP type IV (Sigma, P8375) or other enzyme
- DMF (Sigma)
- 0.1 M sodium phosphate buffer, pH 7.0
- Sephadex G-25 (F) column (1.0 cm diameter $\times$ 45 cm; Pharmacia) equilibrated with phosphate buffer pH 6.0

- 0.1 M sodium phosphate buffer, pH 6.0
- 0.1 M 2-mercaptoethylamine-HCl (M_r 113.6) (11.36 mg/ml), freshly prepared
- 0.05 M EDTA, adjusted to pH 6.0 with 1 M NaOH
- 5 mM 4,4'-dithiodipyridine in methanol, M_r 220.32 (1.10 mg/ml)
- Centriprep-10 concentrators (Millipore)

A. Activation procedure

1. Dissolve about 6 mg (150 nmol) of HRP in about 1 ml phosphate buffer, pH 7.0. Estimate its concentration from the absorbance at 403 nm and adjust to 150 nmol/ml (extinction coefficient 2.275 g.l.cm, M_r 44 000 Da).

2. Dissolve 1.5 mg (4500 nmol) of SMCC in 50 µl DMF. If sulfo-SMCC is used, dissolve in 0.1 ml phosphate buffer, pH 7.0.

Protocol 8 continued

3. Add SMCC solution (prewarmed to about 30 °C to prevent precipitation when added) to 1 ml of peroxidase solution, mix and incubate the mixture at room temperature for 2 h with gentle mixing approximately every 30 min.

4. Centrifuge the reaction mixture briefly to remove excess precipitated reagent and apply the clear supernatant to Sephadex G-25 column and elute with phosphate buffer, pH 6.0.

5. Pool peak fractions absorbing at 403 nm and concentrate using a Centriprep-10 concentrator (Millipore).

B. Measurement of maleimide groups on treated protein[a]

1. Dilute a small aliquot of the treated peroxidase with phosphate buffer, pH 6.0 to give a total volume of 0.45 ml, with an OD at 403 nm of 0.7–1.0 (0.31–0.44 g peroxidase/l, 7.7–11 μM). Record the OD reading. Use 0.45 ml of the same buffer as a control.

2. Mix 0.01 ml 0.1 M 2-mercaptoethylamine and 2.0 ml 0.05 M EDTA, giving a final concentration of 0.5 mM.

3. Add 0.05 ml of this 2-mercaptoethylamine–EDTA to the 0.45 ml of treated peroxidase, mix and incubate at 30 °C for 20 min. Add 0.02 ml 5 mM 4,4″-dithiodipyridine, mix and incubate at 30 °C for 10 min.

4. Read the absorbance at 324 nm of the test and control. Calculate the average number of maleimide groups introduced per peroxidase molecule with the molar extinction coefficient of pyridine-4-thione ($19\ 800\ M^{-1}.cm^{-1}$) and the concentration of peroxidase.

[a] The number of maleimide groups introduced into the protein is determined by first reacting it with a known amount of 2-mercaptoethylamine. The remaining 2-mercaptoethylamine is in turn determined by reaction with 4,4′-dithiodipyridine to produce pyridine-4-thione, the absorbance of which is measured. The reduction in absorbance compared to a control is used to calculate the number of maleimide groups introduced.

Protocol 9

Preparation of Fab′

Equipment and reagents

- 0.1–3 mg of F(ab′)$_2$ from *Protocol 7* and phosphate buffer, pH 6.0 from *Protocol 8*
- Sephadex G-25 (F) column (1 cm diameter × 45 cm long; Pharmacia) equilibrated with EDTA phosphate buffer
- 5 mM 4,4″-dithiodipyridine in methanol
- EDTA phosphate buffer: 0.1 M sodium phosphate buffer, 5 mM EDTA, pH 6.0 (freshly prepared)
- 0.1 M 2-mercaptoethylamine (Sigma, M9768) in EDTA phosphate buffer

Protocol 9 continued

A. Preparation of Fab′

1. Prepare 0.1–3 mg of F(ab′)$_2$ in 0.45 ml phosphate buffer.

2. Add 0.05 ml (1/9 volume) 2-mercaptoethylamine. Incubate at 37 °C for 1.5 h.

3. Apply to Sephadex G-25 column, elute and pool the 280 nm peak fractions.

4. Calculate the amount of Fab′ obtained from its extinction coefficient at 280 nm (1.48 g.l.cm) and M_r (46,000).

B. Measurement of thiol groups in Fab′

1. Dilute a small aliquot of the Fab′ with phosphate buffer, pH 6.0 to give a total volume of 0.5 ml, with an absorbance at 280 nm of 0.2–1.0 (0.13–0.67 g/l, 2.9–14 μM). Use 0.5 ml of the same buffer as a control.

2. Add 0.02 ml 5 mM 4,4′-dithiodipyridine.

3. Incubate at room temperature for 10–20 min. Read absorbance at 324 nm.

4. Estimate the number of thiol groups per Fab′ molecule with the molar extinction coefficient at 324 nm of pyridine-4-thione (19 800/M.cm) and the concentration of Fab′. The number of thiol groups per Fab′ should be at least one. Thiol groups are stable in the presence of EDTA at 23 °C for at least 4 h.

Protocol 10

Conjugation of Fab′ with activated enzyme

Equipment and reagents

- Buffers and starting materials from *Protocols 8* and *9*
- 100 mM N-ethylmaleimide in phosphate buffer, pH 6.5
- 0.1 M sodium phosphate buffer, pH 6.5
- Ultrogel AcA 44 column from *Protocol 7* re-equilibrated with phosphate buffer, pH 6.5

A. Procedure

1. Prepare about 1.8 mg (45 nmol) of the maleimide-activated peroxidase in 0.2–0.4 ml phosphate buffer, pH 6.0.

2. Prepare about 2.0 mg (43 nmol) of Fab″ in 0.2–0.4 ml EDTA phosphate buffer.

3. Add the two solutions together, mix gently and incubate at 4 °C for 20 h or at 30 °C for 1 h (without stirring).

4. Block remaining thiol groups with 20 μl N-ethylmaleimide.

5. Apply the reaction mixture to Ultrogel AcA 44 column and elute with phosphate buffer, pH 6.5. Adjust the flow rate to 0.3–0.5 ml/min and collect fractions with a volume of about 1.0 ml.

6. Read the absorbance of each fraction at 280 and 403 nm and measure the peroxidase activity of each fraction (see *Protocol 6* for details)

7. Store the Fab′-peroxidase conjugate at 4°C with 0.1 g/l thimerosal (**not** azide) as preservative.

3.4 Enzyme–hapten coupling

The chemistry of linking small nonpeptide molecules to proteins for use as immunogens (Chapter 6), or to enzymes (or other labelling substances) for use as labels may be exactly the same, but the desired substitution ratios may be much higher in the case of immunogens. The choice of procedure for coupling is dependent on the functional groups available on the molecules. The most common procedures link haptens to free α- or ε-amino (lysine) or sulfhydryl (cysteine) groups on the enzyme or other protein.

A spacer group four to six carbon or oxygen atoms long between the hapten and the enzyme is usually necessary to allow adequate immunological recognition and this is normally added to the hapten before conjugation. In such cases, a suitable group is required on the hapten to which the spacer arm can be added, and the spacer arm itself must have a terminal group suitable for conjugation. It follows that a group (not required for functional integrity) suitable for addition of the spacer arm (or for direct conjugation) must be present on the hapten analyte itself. If not, a suitable relative or metabolite of the analyte must be used or an appropriate group must first be added by derivatization, or by *de novo* synthesis. The most common conjugation procedures link enzymes to free carboxylic acid groups on the hapten or hapten-spacer arm derivative.

A wide variety of common steroids and other haptens derivatized by the addition of potential bridging groups are available commercially (Steraloids; Sigma). Provided that there is just one relevant active group on the hapten, such derivatives are often not difficult to prepare 'in house' by standard chemical procedures; otherwise the cooperation of a skilled synthetic chemist may be essential. A range of haptens, including estriol, estradiol-17β, digoxin, theophyline, triiodothyronine and thyroxine, with bridging groups and active functions already attached are available from Boehringer Mannheim (Section 3.2.2.3).

In an EIA for hapten, the type of spacer group and its site of attachment to the hapten molecule may be the same in the enzyme–hapten conjugate as in the hapten–protein immunogen used to raise the antibody (homology) or they may be different (heterology). Heterology may concern the bridging group and/or the site of attachment, or even the hapten itself (32). Site or bridge heterology decreases the affinity of the antibody for the enzyme–hapten conjugate (which may be much greater than for the analyte) and it was formerly widely claimed that heterology is a necessary precondition for an EIA with a low detection limit. However, most hapten EIA are homologous, and many of these are highly sensitive. Conversely, site-heterology may result in reduced specificity. These considerations apply to all hapten immunoassays for which labels with spacer arms are used (see also Section 3.2.1 of Chapter 3).

The optimum hapten–enzyme ratio in a conjugate for an EIA should be investigated each time by preparing a range of test conjugates starting with different ratios of reactant molarities. Most often, an incorporation ratio of 1:1 is suitable and a higher ratio results in a decrease in sensitivity (33, 34). Determination of the ratio for hapten–horseradish peroxidase conjugates can be by spectral differences if such exist (as they do for steroids such as progesterone), but radioactive hapten may be used as a quantifiable tracer, or an immunoassay may be used to estimate the accessible haptens. The recovery of enzyme activity should be 100%, or near 100%, and there should be negligible nonspecific binding; conjugates not meeting these criteria should normally be rejected for use in high-performance assays.

The most usual coupling procedures for haptens and proteins are the carbodiimide, the mixed anhydride (*Protocol 11*) and the active-ester (*Protocol 12*) procedures. Hetero-bifunctional reagents may also be used (35), as described in *Protocol 13*.

Protocol 11

Mixed anhydride conjugation of progesterone to HRP

Equipment and reagents

- Progesterone 11α-hemisuccinate or 3-CMO derivative (Steraloids)
- HRP type IV (Sigma, P8375)
- DMF anhydrous (Aldrich, 27,054-6)
- N-ethymorpholine (Sigma, E 0252, Aldrich, 10,993-2) diluted to 1:10 in ethyl alcohol
- Isobutyl chloroformate (Aldrich, 17, 798-9) diluted to 1:10 in ethyl alcohol
- Ethyl alcohol, anhydrous (Aldrich, 45,983-6)

- 0.1 M PBS, pH 7.0: 0.1 M sodium phosphate, 0.15 M NaCl, pH 7.0
- Sephadex G-25 (F) column (1.0 cm diameter × 45 cm long) equilibrated with PBS
- Cytochrome *c* from horse heart (Sigma, C 7752)
- BSA, fraction V powder (Sigma, A2153)
- Ice bath on magnetic stirrer
- Glass vials, 5 ml e.g. of Wheaton type (screw-top vials with magnetic stirrer)

Procedure

1. Weigh 10 mg HRP (250 nmol) into a glass vial and dissolve in 0.5 ml deionized water. Add 2 μl double distilled N-ethylmorpholine. Add 485 μl DMF. Mix gently and place on ice bath in readiness for step 6.

2. Activation of progesterone derivative. Place another glass vial containing 4.31 mg of progesterone-11α-hemisuccinate (10 μmol) or 3.88 mg progesterone-3-CMO in an ice bath ($-15\,°C$)

Protocol 11 continued

3. With the aid of a small stirring bar, add 275 μl dimethylformamide while mixing continuously. Add 12.6 μl N-ethylmorpholine in ethanol.

4. Start activation by adding 13 μl of isobutyl chloroformate in ethanol, and mix for a further 2–5 min.

5. To the HRP solution prepared at step 1, add 15 μl of this anhydride-activated progesterone (This will provide 2:1 progesterone to enzyme ratio). Mix occasionally while leaving on ice bath for 1 h.

6. Separate conjugate from excess reactants with the Sephadex G25 column, eluting with PBS, and pool the protein peak fractions.

7. To prepare for storage, add BSA at 1 mg/ml, cytochrome c at 0.5 mg/ml and mix with an equal volume of glycerol. Store at −20 °C.

Protocol 12

Active ester method for conjugation of hapten to enzyme

Equipment and reagents

- EDAC hydrochloride (Sigma E-1769)
- 1,4-Dioxane, anhydrous (Aldrich 29,630-9) or DMF, anhydrous (Aldrich, 27,054-6)
- N-hydroxysuccinimide (Aldrich 13,067-2)
- Ethyl acetate (Riedel de Haën 24233; Aldrich 27,052-0)
- Dichloromethane (Aldrich, 27,099-7)
- Hapten or hapten derivative with one free carboxyl group, e.g. progesterone 11α-hemisuccinate (Steraloids)

- Enzyme of suitable quality, e.g. HRP type IV (Sigma, P8375)
- Wheaton vial with stir bar (Sigma)
- 0.01 M PBS, pH 7.0; 0.01 M sodium phosphate, 0.15 M NaCl, pH 7.0
- 0.1 M PBS, pH 7.0; 0.1 M sodium phosphate, 0.15 M NaCl, pH 7.0
- Sephadex G-25 column as for *Protocol 11* but equilibrated with 0.1 M PBS, pH 7.0
- Magnetic stirrer

A. Procedure

1. Weigh out 2.8 mg EDAC (14.6 μmol), 1.7 mg N-hydroxysuccinimide (14.6 μmol), 4.31 mg progesterone 11α-hemisuccinate (10 μmol) into a Wheaton glass bottle.)

2. Add 500 μl dioxane or dimethyl formamide and stir for 2 h.

3. Dilute the activation mixture with 500 μl deionized water. Add 500 μl ethyl acetate, cap, shake vigorously and allow layers to separate.

4. Take the ethyl acetate layer and place into clean glass vial, add 500 μl deionized water, shake vigorously and allow layers to separate.

5. Transfer the ethyl acetate layer to a clean tube and dry down under nitrogen.

6. Redissolve the activated progesterone ester by adding 200 μl dichloromethane.

Protocol 12 continued

7. To prepare enzyme for conjugation, dissolve 10 mg HRP (250 nmol) in 200 μl 0.01 M PBS, pH 7.0.

8. Transfer the required amount of the activated ester to a clean glass vial (the amount transferred is dependent on the desired molar ratio, e.g. 50 μl for 10:1 ratio of steroid to HRP) and dry down under nitrogen.

9. Add 200 μl HRP solution to the activated progesterone.

10. Mix gently and allow to stand overnight at 4°C.

11. Separate the free from conjugated HRP-progesterone on a Sephadex G-25 column using 0.1 M PBS as elution buffer.

12. To prepare for storage, add BSA at 1 mg/ml, cytochrome *c* at 0.5 mg/ml and mix with an equal volume of glycerol. Store at −20°C.

Protocol 13

Conjugation of hapten containing an amino group to enzyme with a hetero-bifunctional reagent

Equipment and reagents

- Hapten (e.g. peptide) with one available amino group
- Enzyme, e.g. HRP
- SAMSA (Sigma, A1251)
- SMCC (Pierce)
- Anhydrous DMF
- 1 M hydroxylamine-HCl, pH 7.0
- 0.1 M phosphate buffer, pH 6.5
- Phosphate-EDTA: 0.1 M sodium phosphate, 5 mM EDTA, pH 6
- 1 M glycine

- 0.1 M EDTA
- 0.1 M Tris-HCL, pH 7.0
- Sephadex G-25 (F) column (1 cm diameter × 45 cm long; Pharmacia) equilibrated with phosphate-EDTA
- Ultrogel AcA 44 column (1.5 cm diameter × 45 cm) (Biosepra Inc.) equilibrated with phosphate buffer, pH 6.5.
- 0.1 M phosphate buffer, pH 6.5
- Centriprep-10 concentrators (Millipore)

A. Preparation of maleimide-hapten

1. Dissolve the hapten (100 nmol) in a suitable solvent such as dioxane, methanol, ethanol or DMF.

2. Add SMCC (1000 nmol) dissolved in 50 μl DMF and mix.

3. Incubate for 2 h at room temperature.

4. To inactivate excess SMCC, add 20 μl 1 M glycine and incubate for 30 min

B. Preparation of mercaptosuccinylated-enzyme

1. Dissolve 100 nmol enzyme (e.g. 4 mg HRP) in 0.5 ml 0.1 M phosphate buffer, pH 6.5.

Protocol 13 continued

2. Dissolve 0.87 mg (5000 nmol) SAMSA in 0.01 ml DMF, add to enzyme solution and mix.

3. Incubate for 30 min at room temperature with occasional mixing.

4. To cleave the acetylmercaptan bonds and expose the sulfhydryl groups, add 0.02 ml 0.1 M EDTA, 0.1 ml 0.1 M Tris, pH 7.0, and 0.1 ml 1 M hydroxylamine and mix.

5. Incubate for 30 min at 30 °C.

6. Apply the reaction mixture to G-25 column and elute with phosphate-EDTA. Measure absorbance at 280 nm.

7. Pool protein fractions and concentrate (Centriprep concentrators), the fractions containing the mercaptosuccinylated enzyme to 50 nmol.

8. Measure the thiol group content of the activated enzyme as described in *Protocol 9B*

C. Conjugation of activated enzyme with maleimide-hapten

1. Mix the activated maleimide-hapten (100 nmol from Step A above) with 50 nmol of mercaptosuccinylated enzyme in 0.25 ml phosphate-EDTA.

2. Mix the two solutions and incubate at 4 °C for 20 h, or at 30 °C for 1 h.

3. Block remaining thiol groups with 20 λl N-ethylmaleimide.

4. Apply the reaction mixture to Sephadex G-25 column and elute with phosphate buffer, pH 6.5. Adjust the flow rate to 0.3–0.5 ml/min and collect fractions with a volume of about 1.0 ml.

5. Read the absorbance of each fraction at 280 and 403 nm and measure the peroxidase activity of each fraction.

6. Store the Fab'-peroxidase conjugate at 4 °C with 1 g/l thimerosal (**not** azide) as preservative. Block remaining thiol groups with N-ethylmaleimide to prevent reaction with the preservative thimerosal.

3.5 Fluorescence labelling

Many different fluorescent compounds are available for use in fluorescence labelling procedures and it would be impractical to deal with all of them here. A conjugation procedure for fluorescein is included because of its widespread use both as a fluorescent label and as a ligand label. Fluorescein isothiocyanate is the reagent used for coupling fluorescein to amino groups.

The DELFIA system developed by Wallac (Turku, Finland) is the most common implementation of labelling with lanthanide ion chelates and time-resolved fluorescence measurement. The label contains a stable, hydrophilic europium chelate and, on completion of the assay, the europium is released into a lipophilic environment with a β-diketone chelator that forms highly efficient fluorescent chelates. The principal DELFIA labelling reagent is N^1-p(isothio-cyanatobenzyl)-diethylenetriamine-N^1,N^2,N^3,N^3-tetraacetic acid, known as N-1.

Wallac supply N-1 as an Eu-labelling reagent, as part of an Eu-labelling kit and in a Sm-labelling kit. As with FITC, an efficient and mild isothiocyanate reaction occurs to form covalent bonds with free amino groups (36). Lanthanide labelling is a very attractive alternative in many 'research' situations where radio-iodination has commonly been used in the past. As the above labelling kits come with full instructions for use, no protocol for lanthanide labelling is given here.

Protocol 14

Labelling IgG with fluorescein

Equipment and reagents

- FITC, isomer I (M_r 389 Da, Sigma, F4274)
- Carbonate buffer: 0.1 M carbonate–bicarbonate buffer, pH 9.5
- IgG (10 mg/ml in 0.1 M carbonate–bicarbonate buffer, pH 9.5)
- DMSO (Sigma)

- 0.1 M PBS, pH 7.5 containing 0.1% sodium azide
- Sephadex G-50 (M) column (1.0 cm diameter × 45 cm long; Pharmacia) equilibrated with 0.1 M PBS, pH 7.5
- Centriprep-10 concentrators (Millipore)

Method

1. Prepare FITC stock solution at 1 mg/ml in DMSO

2. Add 0.1 ml FITC solution (256 nmol) dropwise to 10 mg antibody solution (67.7 nmol). Mix and leave for 2 h in the dark at room temperature

3. Remove unreacted FITC by means of Sephadex G-50 column, eluting with PBS.

4. Collect the first coloured peak to emerge (this contains the labelled IgG) and concentrate with a Centriprep-10 to the original volume that was applied.

5. Calculate the degree of FITC coupling with IgG as follows. The absorption contributed by FITC at 280 nm (a constant fraction of its absorption at 495 nm) is subtracted from the total absorption at 280 nm, before deriving the protein concentration.

   $$\text{FITC, mg/ml} = 3.3 \times \text{absorbance at 495 nm}$$
   $$\text{IgG, mg/ml} = (\text{absorbance at 280 nm} - 0.35 \times \text{absorbance at 495 nm})/1.4$$
   $$\text{FITC/Protein ratio, mol/mol} = (\text{FITC, mg/ml/IgG, mg/ml}) \times (M_r \text{ IgG}/M_r \text{ FITC})$$

6. Sterile filter through 0.22 μm (Millipore). Store the conjugate in dark at 4°C or in aliquots at −20°. Repeated freezing and thawing should be avoided.

3.6 Biotin coupling

The insertion of biotin into proteins requires a reactive biotin derivative as a labelling reagent. The most common is a hydroxysuccinimide ester (NHS-biotin) which reacts with primary amines to form amide linkages. The reaction occurs via a nucleophilic attack of the amine and is favoured at alkaline pH. NHS-biotin is not soluble in aqueous buffers. To use NHS-biotin in physiological buffers, first dissolve the reagent in a minimal amount of DMSO or DMF before addition to the buffer containing the molecules to be labelled. Avoid buffer components containing amines, such as Tris.

The molar ratio of NHS-biotin to IgG or whatever is being labelled should be adjusted to ensure a suitable substitution ratio. Many large proteins can react with several molecules of biotin without loss of biological activity, and each biotin may bind a molecule of avidin. In addition, avidin and streptavidin are tetravalent and have the strongest known noncovalent biological interaction ($K_a = 10^{15}$/M) between protein and ligand. Optimal protein binding capability can be obtained by using a biotin derivative that has an extended spacer arm which reduces steric hindrance. The NHS-biotin spacer arm is 13.5 Å long, but other spacer arm lengths may be employed, such as EZ-Link™ NHS-LC-biotin with a 22.4 Å arm from Pierce, to enhance binding capability. Exploitation of these factors has been used to allow many molecules of secondary label to associate with each primary immune complex, thereby increasing assay sensitivity (37).

Protocol 15

Biotinylation of IgG

Equipment and reagents

- IgG or other protein to be labelled
- 50 mM sodium bicarbonate buffer, pH 8
- Anhydrous DMF (Aldrich, 27,054-6)
- N-hydroxysuccinimide ester of biotin (Pierce Chemical Company)
- 0.1 M sodium phosphate buffer, pH 7.0
- Sephadex G-25 column (1.0 cm diameter × 45 cm long; Pharmacia) equilibrated with phosphate buffer, pH 7.0

A. Procedure

1. Dissolve 20 mg (133 nmol) IgG in 1 ml 50 mM sodium bicarbonate buffer, pH 8.5, in clean glass test tube.

2. Dissolve 0.3 mg (880 nmol) NHS-biotin in 10 μl DMF and add to the test tube containing the IgG and buffer.

3. Incubate for 2 h on ice, or for 30 min at room temperature.

4. Remove unconjugated biotin, etc., by filtration through Sephadex G-25, eluting with phosphate buffer, pH 7.0.

5. Store the biotinylated protein at 4°C with 0.1% sodium azide as preservative.

4 Label characterization

Two basic properties are relevant to the evaluation of a label, namely immunoreactivity and specific activity. With low immunoreactivity little of the label will bind and with low specific activity, large amounts of the label must bind to be measurable.

With a labelled antigen, immunoreactivity is defined as the fraction of label activity that can be bound by excess antibody, while with labelled antibody increasing concentrations of antigen may be used to estimate its immuno-reactive fraction. In either case, a separation technique with charcoal absorption, second antibody precipitation or solid-phase antibody/antigen is needed. Put simply, a fixed amount of label is incubated with increasing concentrations of the second reactant until equilibrium has been attained, bound label separated and the range of bound activities measured. To analyse the data, bound activity (expressed as a percentage of total label added) is plotted against the concentration of second reactant to give a hyperbolic curve, and the label activity corresponding to the asymptote of the curve estimated by extrapolation. Alternative methods, such as plotting the reciprocals of both parameters, may facilitate estimation of the immunoreactivity, usually expressed as a percentage.

Low immunoreactivity may simply indicate that the preparation used for labelling was impure and, for a labelled polyclonal antibody, could show the presence of considerable nonspecific immunoglobulin. Estimation of the im-munoreactivity of labelled antigens is important if they are to be used to investigate the binding kinetics of antibodies, particularly if absolute estimates of binding parameters are required (38).

The estimation of the specific activity of a label was described for radio-iodinated protein in *Protocol 2* and equivalent methods can be used for many other kinds of labels. As with immunoreactivity, knowledge of its specific activity is important if a label is to be used in kinetic investigations. However, in the characterization of conjugate labels, it is the conjugation ratio, that is usually estimated, and with enzyme conjugates the retention of enzymatic activity is also directly relevant since it affects specific activity.

To estimate a conjugation ratio accurately, the preparation to be studied must be pure, the molar concentration of each component measured, and the ratio calculated. Difficulties arise with components lacking spectral or other properties that facilitate their measurement, or with properties that are com-promised by the presence of the second component. Occasionally, an accurate result may require destruction of the conjugate to overcome such interference. When applied to the characterization of a whole conjugate, an immunoassay (with an alternative label type) can be used to measure the 'accessible concentration' of a component, which may be a hapten.

When a protein is linked to a small molecule (e.g. enzyme–hapten), the conjugation ratio can be determined easily if the hapten has an ultraviolet or visible spectrum that does not overlap with that of the protein carrier. An example is the determination of molar incorporation of progesterone in progesterone–HRP conjugates, where the unconjugated pure hapten and enzyme can be use to establish calibration spectra. The characteristic absorbance of haem at 403 nm has been used for the determination of HRP concentration at 403 nm with molar extinction coefficient of 91 000 $M^{-1}.cm^{-1}$ and progesterone at 241 nm with molar extinction coefficient of 16 600 $M^{-1}.cm^{-1}$. Even if the hapten spectrum overlaps with that of the enzyme, accurate determinations of numbers of hapten molecules per protein can still be made by calculating the differences in absorption, the ratio of the extinction coefficients at the appropriate wavelength can be used to calculate the molar incorporation (see *Protocols 6* and *14*).

As an example, take the following data. A progesterone–HRP conjugate had absorbance readings at 403 nm and 241 nm of 0.423 and 0.216, respectively, while for unconjugated HRP the readings were 0.92 and 0.36. First, calculate the HRP contribution to the total absorbance at 241 nm, which is 0.165 [0.423 × (0.36/0.92)]. Then, calculate the absorbance due to progesterone at 241 nm by subtracting this from the total absorbance (0.216 − 0.165 = 0.051). Then, calculate the concentrations of both progesterone and HRP in the conjugate by dividing the net absorbances at 241 nm and 403 nm by their respective molar extinction coefficients (progesterone = 0.051/16 600 = 3.07 μM; HRP = 0.423/91 000 = 4.65 μM). Finally, the molar incorporation of progesterone (progesterone–HRP, 3.07:4.65) can be estimated to be about 0.66.

A more accurate method may involve the incorporation of radioactively labelled hapten – normally a label which is chemically the same as the hapten with the isotopic atoms (^{14}C, ^{3}H, etc.) substituting for endogenous atoms – in the conjugation procedure. With such a tracer the extent of hapten incorporation into the conjugate can be directly estimated by measuring the specific radioactivity of the conjugate. However, in practice, since radioactive conjugates are generally undesirable, such procedures would usually be used to calibrate a standardized conjugation procedure.

Analysis of the relevant reactive groups on the protein(s) involved can also be used to estimate conjugation ratios. In such a case the decrease in the number of relevant reactive groups, such as sulfhydryl (*Protocol 9*, or *Protocol 11* of Chapter 6) or amine (*Protocol 10* of Chapter 6) is measured chemically in the conjugate and compared with the unconjugated protein(s).

5 Conjugate stabilization

The properties of the labels used in immunoassays are as varied as their components. Highly unstable components are obviously avoided where possible, but the variety of antigens and antibodies used in labels ensures that the stability of labels is also varied. Except for radioisotopes and enzymes, the labelling substances that may be used for research applications (mainly fluorophores) are generally stable. The stabilities and shelf-lives of radiolabels is often almost completely determined by the half-life of the radioisotope used and storage conditions that maximize stabilities are determined by the nature of the labelled compound. When one considers label or conjugate stability it is usually a question of enzyme conjugate stability, and the remainder of this discussion will be concerned with this. However, and as appropriate, all labels and conjugates should be passed through a 0.22 μ pore filter and stored in sterile containers at 2–8 °C or frozen (preferably at −70 °C for longer periods).

Traditionally, enzyme conjugates to be used in immunoassays are stored mixed with one or more substances that are judged to stabilize either the enzyme, the antibody or other component or the linkage. Stabilizing substances commonly used include proteins such as BSA, gelatin, FCS, or casein; sugars such as sucrose, sorbitol or trehalose (39), preservative such as gentamicin sulfate, chlorohexidine or sodium azide (not for HRP), and proteolytic inhibitors. In addition, up to 50% of glycerol is often added.

A typical stabilizing reagent for conjugates containing HRP (40) is as follows: sodium phosphate (0.1 M) buffer, pH 6.5, with 0.15 M sodium chloride, 5% BSA (or 10% FCS), 0.5 mg/ml cytochrome c (Sigma), 0.002% gentamicin sulfate and 0.0035% chlorohexidine (Sigma) or 0.01% methiolate (Sigma), and finally glycerol to 30%.

For conjugates with alkaline phosphates conjugate, a suitable medium may be 0.05 M tris buffer, pH 8.0, with 1 mM $ZnCl_2$, 1 mM $MgCl_2$, 0.1% sodium azide and, finally, 50% glycerol. Avoid using phosphate buffer with alkaline phosphatase as high concentrations of inorganic phosphate act as strong competitive inhibitors of that enzyme.

References

1. Edwards, R. (1997). In *Principles and practice of immunoassay* (eds C. P. Price and D. J. Newman), 2nd edn, p. 325. Macmillan Reference Ltd, London.
2. Gosling, J. P. (1997). In *Principles and practice of immunoassay* (eds C. P. Price and D. J. Newman), 2nd edn, p. 349. Macmillan Reference Ltd, London.
3. Wood, P. and Bernard, G. (1997). In *Principles and practice of immunoassay* (eds C. P. Price and D. J. Newman), 2nd edn, p. 389. Macmillan Reference Ltd, London.
4. Harmer, I. J. and Samuel, D. (1989). *J. Immunol Methods* **122**, 115.
5. Weeks, I. Sturgess, M., Brown, R. C., and Woodhead, J. S. (1986). In *Methods in Enzymology* (eds M. A. DeLuca and W. D. McElroy). Vol. 133, p. 366. Academic Press, San Diego.
6. Weeks, I. (1997). In *Principles and practice of immunoassay* (eds C. P. Price and D. J. Newman), 2nd edn, p. 425. Macmillan Reference Ltd., London.
7. McCapra, F., Watmore, D., Sumun, F, Patel, A., Beheshti, I., Ramakrishnan, K., and Branson, J. (1989). *J. Biolum. Chemilum.* **4**, 51.
8. Rongen, H. A.H., Hoetelmans, R. M.W., Bult, A., and van Bennekom, W. P. (1994). *J. Pharm. Biomed. Anal.* **2**, 433.
9. Gosling, J. P. (1990) *Clin. Chem.* **36**, 1408.
10. Kricka, L. J. (1994) *Clin. Chem.* **40**, 347.
11. Channing Rodgers, R. P. (1984). *Practical immunoassay. The state of the art* (ed. W. R. Butt), p. 253. Marcel Dekker Inc., New York.
12. Hemmilä, I., Holttinen, S., Pettersson, K., and Lövgren, T. (1987). *Clin. Chem.* **33**, 2281.
13. Hemmilä, I., Malminen, O., Mikola, H., and Lövgren, T. (1988). *Clin. Chem.* **34**, 2320.
14. Hashida, S., Nakagawa, K., Yoshitake, S., Imagawa, M., Ishikawa, E., Endo, Y., Ohtaki, S., Ichioka, Y., and Nakajima, K. (1983). *Anal. Lett.* **16**, 31.
15. Kricka, L. J. (1991). *Clin. Chem.* **37**, 1472.
16. Kricka, L. J. (1993). *Clin. Biochem.* **26**, 325.
17. Bronstein, I., Edwards, J., and Voyta, J. C. (1989). *J. Biolum. Chemilum.* **4**, 99
18. Calvo, J. C., Radicella, J. P., and Charreau, E. H. (1983). *J. Biochem.* **212**, 259.
19. Chiang, C. S. (1987). *Clin. Chem.* **33**, 1245.
20. Hashida, S., Imagawa, M., Inoue, S., Ruan, K., and Ishikawa, E. (1984). *J. Appl. Biochem.*, **6**, 56.

21. Kabakoff, D. S. (1980). In *Enzyme-immunoassay* (ed. E. T. Maggio), p. 71. CRC press Inc., Boca Raton.
22. Weston, P. D., Devries, J. A., and Wrigglesworth, R. (1980). *Biochim. Biophys. Acta* **612**, 40.
23. Duncan, R. J.S., Weston, P. D., and Wriggelsworth, R. (1983). *Anal. Biochem.* **132**, 68.
24. Ishikawa, E., Imagawa, M., Hashida, S., Yoshitake, S., Hamaguchi, Y., and Ueno, T. (1983). *J. Immunoassay* **4**, 209.
25. Ishikawa, E. (1987). *Clin. Biochem.* **20**, 375.
26. Tournier, E. J.M., Wallach, J., and Blond, P. (1998). *Anal. Chim. Acta* **361**, 33.
27. Munro, C. and Stabenfeldt (1984). *J. Endocrinol.* **101**, 41.
28. Gendloff, E. H., Casale, W. L., Ram, B. P., Tai, J. H., Pestka, J. J., and Hart, L. P. (1986). *J. Immunol. Methods* **92**, 15.
29. Sauer, M. J., Foulkes, J. A., and Cookson, A. D. (1981). *Steroids* **38**, 45.
30. Welman, J. K., Johnson, S., Langevin, J., and Riester, E. F. (1983). *BioTechniques* Vol. 1, no 1, **Sept/Oct.**, 148.
31. Hames, B. D. and Rickwood, D. (1990). In *Gel electrophoresis of proteins: a practical approach* (eds B. D. Hames and D. Rickwood), IRL Press, Oxford.
32. Colburn, W. A. (1975). *Steroids* **25**, 43.
33. Hosada, H., Takasaki, W., Aihara, S., and Nambara, T. (1985). *Chem. Pharm. Bull.* **33**, 5393.
34. Hosada, H., Tsukamoto, R., and Nambara, T. (1989). *Chem. Pharm. Bull.* **37**, 1834.
35. Hata, N., Miyai, K., Endo, Y., Lijima, Y., Doi, K., Amino, N., and Ichihara, K. (1987). *Clin. Chem.* **33**, 172.
36. Hurn, B. A. and Chantler, S. M. (1980). In *Methods in enzymology* (eds H. van Vunakis and J. J. Langone). Vol. 70, p. 104. Academic Press, San Diego.
37. De Lauzon, S., El Jabri, J., Desfosses, B., and Cittanova, N. (1989). *J. Immunoassay* **10**, 339.
38. Zherdev, A. V., Romanenko, O. G., and Dzantiev, B. B. (1997). *J. Immunoassay* **18**, 67.
39. Nielsen, K. (1995). *J. Immunoassay* **16**, 183.
40. Presentini, R and Terrana, B. (1995). J. Immunoassay 16, 309.

Chapter 5
Solid-phase reagents

Robert S. Matson
Advanced Technology Center, Beckman-Coulter Inc., 4300 North Harbour Boulevard, D-20-A, Fullerton, CA 92834-3100, U.S.A.

1 Introduction

This chapter is concerned with the preparation and use of solid-phase reagents in immunoassay. The merits in using a solid-phase, as well as the various approaches to preparing solid-phase reagents will be addressed. Information on the kinds of supports available will be given. Finally, detailed protocols for various formats (microtitre plates, membranes, beads, tubes) will be provided, along with sources of commercial solid-phase reagents.

The homogenous, or separation-free immunoassay, in which antibody and antigen are free to associate in solution, with direct determination of antibody–antigen complex formation in the solution phase is often regarded as the optimal format. Unfortunately, the direct measurement of complex formation in such assays is insufficiently sensitive and accurate to meet many needs. However, solid phase, heterogeneous or separation immunoassay with one reactant immobilized to a solid support (i.e. bead, membrane or vessel) is highly versatile. It has allowed the development of numerous assay formats that would be impossible if, as in the earliest assays, a separate precipitating or absorptive reagent and a centrifugation step had to be employed. In particular, such assays allow for multiplexing and parallel analysis of large sample sets making them attractive for automation. Solid-phase immunoassay is the basis for a very wide range of accurate and sensitive measurement tools and has made significant contributions to analytical science (1). However, there are certain attributes or features that are desired of an efficient and reliable solid phase reagent or immunosorbent.

1. Preservation of the native structure and biological activity of the immobilized reagent.
2. Stability of the surface attachment bonds such that there is negligible loss of reagent.
3. Inertness that affords little nonspecific binding of interfering substances to the support.

4. Presentation of the reagent (e.g. antibody) binding sites away from the surface to promote rapid and efficient molecular recognition by the incoming reactant (e.g. antigen).

1.1 Liquid phase assay with solid-phase separation

Because binding reactions between agents that are free to diffuse occur more quickly, several new types of assay have been developed in which the initial step involves antibody–antigen association in a liquid phase. Some of these assays have been automated for commercial diagnostic applications. The advantage is both speed and sensitivity as interactions in solution, unrestricted by steric hindrance, result in more efficient binding. With all reactants in the liquid phase, the issue remains of how to discriminate bound from unbound label. In the tradition of classical RIA this is accomplished using a solid-phase reagent to separate one from the other.

These new assays include magnetizable bead-based separation assays, membrane capture assays, as well as centrifugal assays. In one scenario, antibody is biotinylated (biotin-Ab) and the suspension mixed with the solution containing the antigen (**Ag**) and antibody enzyme–conjugate (Ab-enzyme) to give the classic two antibody and antigen sandwich (biotin-Ab–**Ag**–Ab-enzyme), but which is still in solution. After incubation streptavidin-coated magnetizable beads are added, the suspension placed near a magnet and the beads (bead-streptavidin-biotin-Ab–**Ag**–Ab-enzyme) 'pelleted'. The beads can then be separated from the supernatant, washed, resuspended to remove nonspecific biomolecules and the signal developed. This is often referred to as a particle capture assay and may be conducted with a microtitre plate that is then attached to a magnetic base to pellet the magnetizable microspheres. A variation of particle capture assay involves the use of normal latex microspheres. In this case, suction is used to capture the particles onto the 'filter bottoms' of special microtitre plates. Other tests involve centrifuging plates or tubes to pellet larger microspheres; or centrifugal filtration to capture smaller particles on membranes.

1.2 Choice of solid-phase support

1.2.1 Material

The most widely used solid-phase materials are plastics, especially thermoplastics such as polystyrene, polypropylene, polysulfone or polycarbonate which can be moulded into any of an unlimited variety of shapes. Each has distinctive chemical and physical properties that make it useful as a support. However, polystyrene is the most commonly used plastic for manufacture of microtitre plates for ELISA.

Latex particles (microspheres or beads) which are used in agglutination or other capture assays are generally made from polystyrene or styrene copolymerized with divinylbenzene. Polymethyl methacrylate and methcrylate copolymer beads are also used. Most latex particles have a density of ≈ 1.0–1.05 g/ml such that they remain suspended in solution, and may contain certain additives to ensure a neutral buoyancy. Magnetizable (superparamagnetic) latex beads are available for use with magnetic capture. Coloured particles are used in one-step assays and fluorescent dyed latex particles are used for membrane capture assays and in flow cytometry. Because of their higher protein binding capacities nylon, nitrocellulose, cellulose mixed esters, and PVDF membranes are used in membrane-based solid supports.

Most solid-phase assays are based upon the passive adsorption or coating of antibody or antigen onto the support surface. Only recently have covalent attachment methods been developed for plastics; this is due to advances in surface chemistries, improved polymer formulations and improved moulding processes.

1.2.2 Form

In addition to the tubes used in solid-phase RIA and the wells of the 'omni-present' microtitre plates and strips, solid-phase supports may take other forms. For example, microsphere-based immunoassays are common, especially in clinical chemistry applications such as latex agglutination. Here, uniform latex beads or microspheres ranging from 0.1 to 100 μm in particle diameter are used. Larger beads (diameters ranging from several to 100 μm, to one or more millimetres) are available in polystyrene, polycarbonate, polypropylene and nylon.

A wide variety of membrane products are used both as direct and indirect solid-phase supports in immunoassays, for example in blot assays (e.g. Western blotting), in flow-through and lateral-flow disposable devices for home testing, and when used to form the bottoms of special microtitre wells.

2 Approaches to immobilization

The goal in the construction of a high-quality solid-phase reagent for use in immunoassay is to immobilize the ligand (e.g. antibody) to the support without adversely affecting ligand–analyte (e.g. antibody–antigen) binding function. Therefore, understanding the solution properties of the ligand and the molecular interactions it undergoes during the immobilization process is important. While the manufacturers of solid-phase materials promote their products by arguing the simplicity of immobilization, they can furnish only general guidelines to efficient ligand coupling. It is up to the user to adapt their recommendations and to develop a specific protocol for immobilization that best matches the intrinsic properties of the ligand to those of the support. This protocol should not only take into account coupling efficiency but also preservation of antibody (or other ligand) activity in order to obtain a reagent with optimal properties for use in a particular immunoassay (2, 3). In this regard, after selection of the support, and before optimization of the attachment procedure, the choice between covalent coupling methods or noncovalent immobilization processes must be addressed.

2.1 Preparation of ligands for immobilization

As above, the general term 'ligand' will be used frequently in the following sections to denote the molecule to be immobilized or attached. In practice, the great majority of immobilized molecules used in immunoassays are proteins, and are either antibodies or protein antigens. Since antigens have highly diverse properties, most of the specific advice given will apply to antibodies.

Although extensive biochemical characterization of the ligand is not generally required in order to perform immobilization, careful consideration of the buffer system, with respect to both pH and ionic strength, in which the ligand is stable is most important. For example, protein stability is well known to be influenced by alterations in pH that lead to charge neutralization. This can result in denaturation and decreased solubility. Ionic strength can lead to increased (salting in) or decreased (salting out) solubility of a protein, depending upon its native structure. The ligand should be delivered to the support free from aggregation so that efficient and even coupling is not impeded. This can be checked easily by size-exclusion chromatography of the ligand preparation on a fast HPLC system. Estimation of the apparent pI of a protein ligand may be useful in selecting the appropriate activation chemistry to use for immobilization. For example, although amino-ligands will couple to NHS-activated supports over a broad pH range of 3–10, most proteins require a narrow pH between 6.5–8.5 to retain function. Acidic proteins (negatively charged, pI < 6.5) do not couple very well to NHS-active ester supports. This is because a competing hydrolysis reaction, in which the NHS ester is converted to the free carboxyl group, imparts a negative charge to the support and repels the negatively charged protein. Conversely, neutral or basic proteins (pI 6.5–11) when presented in a buffer pH < pI react efficiently with the support because of charge attraction. The addition of salt to the coupling buffer is yet another means to reduce charge interaction with the support. For example, the addition of $CaCl_2$, which has a strong binding affinity for carboxyl groups, has been shown to enhance coupling of acidic proteins while NaCl shows a minimal effect.

Buffer components may interfere with coupling processes. For example, Tris buffers react with most amine-directed activation groups such as NHS or CNBr, while phosphate buffers retard NHS-mediated reactions. Certain metal ion contaminants can also inhibit coupling reactions.

Tip

For all these reasons it is highly recommended that the ligand be transferred into a suitable coupling buffer, prepared with high-purity water, by gel filtration or dialysis just prior to immobilization.

2.2 Covalent attachment

Many immunoassays rely upon physical adsorption or coating of ligand (antibody or antigen) as opposed to covalent attachment to the solid phase. If the immobilization is to be direct and the ligand is available in good supply, and is not easily denatured, then noncovalent coating is a reasonable approach (Section 2.3). However, there are instances in which covalent coupling to the solid phase is desirable. Many proteins are known to undergo denaturation upon adsorption to the hydrophobic surface of polystyrene. Conversely, peptide antigens are not easily adsorbed; and the release of free ligand back into solution during assay is obviously undesirable. Thus, covalent attachment methods are recommended when there is a need for increased sensitivity and robustness from the assay. Robustness is achieved by improvements in the preservation (of activity) and stability (reduction in physical loss) of the ligand, while sensitivity is enhanced by optimal presentation of the ligand.

A problem with some commercially available supports is that they may provide for too great an excess of activated group density. While this generally allows for rapid coupling to occur, if excess groups are not properly blocked then multiple crosslinking to the ligand may take place, causing inactivation. Under rapid coupling conditions, the extent of immobilization is more difficult to control, and although generally not recognized, ligand density is very important to the efficiency of solid-phase reagents. With antibodies, an optimal density should be achieved in order to maximize the antigen binding capacity and lowering the IgG density has been shown to lead to increased antigen binding (2, 3), probably by relieving steric hindrance. However, while it may appear then to be desirable to input antibody in dilute form to avoid excessive coupling this may allow for significant increases in the extent of competing hydrolysis reactions. Under these circumstances it is possible that there will be an increase in the nonspecific adsorption background. There is no easy solution to these problems. The best approach is to try a series of experiments aimed at optimization by empirically determining those coupling conditions that provide for high binding activity at minimal background. One approach would be to first vary the coupling buffer conditions (pH, ionic strength) for the protein at a fixed concentration (e.g. 1 mg/ml) over a reasonably long interval (e.g. overnight, 15–20 h) to assure maximum coupling (this is generally conducted at 4–10 °C to reduce the risk of denaturation); the specific and nonspecific binding activity for the set of conditions should then be determined. The protein concentration (e.g. 0.1–5 mg/ml) and coupling times (e.g. 1, 3, 6, 15, 20 h) using the buffer conditions selected in the first series of experiments should then be varied.

Covalent tethering of antibodies has a distinct advantage if the presentation process results in orientation of the antibody such that its antigen-binding sites are freely accessible. Such nonrandom attachments give an increased population of more fully functional antibodies, in which case much less may be necessary to achieve optimal assay conditions. It has also been recognized that providing a spacer molecule or polymer between the solid phase and the immobilized ligand may improve binding. This usually involves indirect immobilization and the choice of spacer molecule, and its immobilization must also be taken into account (Section 2.4).

In summary, every immobilization strategy should take into account how much ligand to place on the solid-phase and, if feasible and appropriate, how to properly orient it relative to the surface.

2.2.1 Reagents and reaction mechanisms

There are numerous methods available for attaching biomolecules to plastics and other solid-phase materials, some of which are listed in *Table 1*. Those offering general utility have become commercial products. It is recommended that several different attachment methods be tested since not all are optimal or necessarily compatible with any one ligand. It is usually advisable to use reagents in modest molar excess ($\approx$ 2–10-fold) over surface groups that you wish to activate in order to drive the reaction. This is especially important in using bifunctional crosslinking agents which are terminated with reactive groups. The use of excess reagent will reduce the likelihood of crosslinking both ends to the support. Therefore, it is useful to have knowledge of the surface group density in order to prepare coupling reagents. This information is usually available from the manufacturer of the solid support. A limited number of reactive groups and corresponding methods are commonly used to attach antibodies and antigens to a variety of solid phase materials (*Figure 1*). See also Chapters 4 and 6 for discussions and details of many similar reagents and methods as applied to the preparation of labels and immunogens, respectively.

2.2.1.1 NHS

Figure 1A depicts a very popular method for protein coupling, particularly for use with beads. Most proteins couple to NHS-supports with excellent retention

Table 1. General purpose covalent attachment methods

Ligand linkage group	Reactive group on solid-phase[a]
Amino (-NH$_2$)	Aldehydes (B) [b], acyl azides, anhydrides (P) aryl halides, carbonates, carbodiimides, epoxides (B), imidoesters, isothiocyanates, NHS esters (P), CNBr, FMP, sulfonyl chloride, tresyl chloride, tosyl chloride (B)
Thiol (-SH)	Alkyl halides, aziridines, haloacetyls, maleimides (P)
Carboxyl (COOH)	Carbodiimides (M), CDI, diazoalkanes,
Hydroxyl (-OH)	Alkyl halogens, CDI (B), chloroformate, DSC, epoxides, isocyanates
Aldehyde (HC=O)	Hydrazide (B, P), amino (to give Schiff base), Mannich reaction[c]
Photochemically reactive giving free radical (R•)	Aryl azides, benzophenones, diazo compounds, diazirines
Abstractable hydrogen (H)	Diazonium, Mannich reaction[c]

[a] Abbreviations used: NHS, *N*-hydroxysuccinimide; CNBr, cyanogen bromide; FMP, 2-fluor-1-methylpyridinium toluene-4-sulfonate; CDI, 1,1'-carbonyldiimidazole; DSC, *N,N'*-disuccinimidyl carbonate.

[b] Methods involving the above reactive groups that are described in detail in this chapter are designated as follows: B, latex beads; P, polystyrene plates; M, nylon-based membranes.

[c] The Mannich reaction is used to immobilize compounds that do not have accessible functional groups but do possess reactive hydrogens that are easily abstractable. The reaction proceeds with the condensation of an aldehyde with the compound and an amine.

of activity (2). Attachment is best accomplished between pH 6.5–8.5. The NHS ester is susceptible to hydrolysis but activated beads can be stored for at least a year in anhydrous isopropyl alcohol. Once beads have been washed for coupling, the reaction must be started within 30–45 min. Coupling is essentially complete within 1 h after the addition of protein. The original method which involved carbodiimide-mediated NHS coupling has been modified to a two-step process in order to avoid the formation of β-alanine side products that lead to elimination of the ligand from the support (4).

2.2.1.2 Maleic anhydride

Anhydrides are generally quite stable and can be stored dry at room temperature. This method (*Figure 1B*) is particularly useful for activation of microtitre plates (see *Protocol 2*). It is important, however, to maintain an alkaline pH (8–9), since the reaction is reversible under acidic conditions (5).

2.2.1.3 Carbodiimides

Many variations on this method (*Figure 1C*) are well established and offer an easy approach to the immobilization of amino-ligands to carboxylated surfaces. There are several varieties available which will permit either organic solvent-based or water soluble (WSC) derivatizations. The *o*-acylisourea intermediate is rapidly hydrolysed in water (see *Protocols 6* and *7*).

2.2.1.4 Epoxides

Surface activation with epoxides (oxiranes) provides a versatile reagent for the coupling of biomolecules containing free hydroxyl, sulfhydral, or amine groups (*Figure 1D*). Reactivity is in the approximate order: SH > NH$_2$ >> OH. Bifunctional oxiranes (bisoxiranes such as 1,4-butanediol diglycidyl ether) offer the advantage of providing a useful spacer arm that can be used as link to a thiol-, hydroxyl- or amine-modified surface. This leaves a terminal epoxide group which can further react with the biomolecule (6).

2.2.1.5 Carbonyldiimidazole

Reactions are possible either with carboxyl groups to form *N*-acylimidazole or with hydroxyl groups to produce an imidazole carbamate (*Figure 1E*). Subsequent reactions with primary amine-containing ligands lead to either amide- or carbamate-linked biomolecules (7,8).

2.2.1.6 Tosylate

This is a highly reactive compound (*p*-toluenesulfonyl chloride) useful in the conversion of hydroxyl groups on a surface. Tosylate-activated surfaces can then react with amino-ligands to form a very stable carbon–nitrogen bond (*Figure 1F*) (9). An example of immobilization using tosylate chemistry is provided in *Protocol 10*.

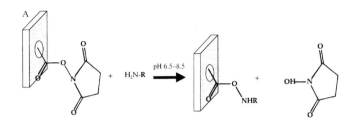

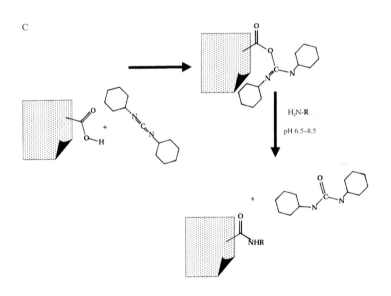

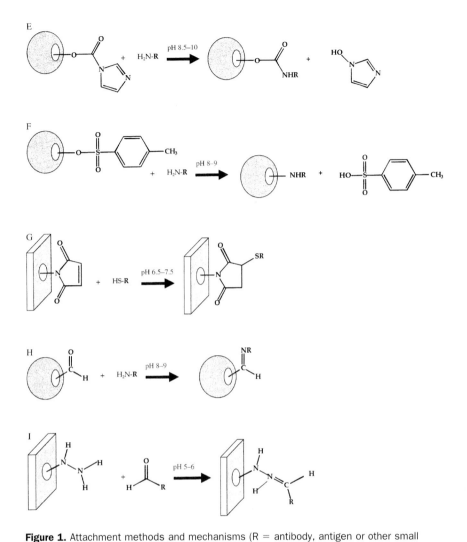

Figure 1. Attachment methods and mechanisms (R = antibody, antigen or other small molecule ligands). A. NHS: the reactive group is eliminated as attachment occurs. B. Maleic anhydride: after substitution the malate group acts as a bridge to the solid phase.
C. Carbodiimides: activation of the carboxylic group, which is to be the site of attachment, is often done just prior to the immobilization reaction and, similar to NHS above, the reactive group is eliminated as attachment occurs (see *Protocols 6* and *7*). D. Epoxides: surfaces activated with epoxides (oxiranes) are versatile and can be used to immobilize molecules containing free hydroxyl, sulfhydral or amine groups. E. CDI: as with NHS-activated surfaces, the reactive group is eliminated as attachment occurs. F. Tosylate: activation of the surface of a solid-phase material with hydroxyl groups and subsequent reaction with amino-ligands leads to the formation of very stable carbon–nitrogen bonds (see *Protocol 10*).
G. Maleimide: this is perhaps the favourite reactive group for linking to free sulfhydrals (see *Protocol 5*). H. Aldehyde: because of the near ubiquity of both amine and aldehyde groups, reactions leading to Schiff base formation are commonly exploited for conjugation and for immobilization (see *Protocol 11*). I. Hydrazide: hydrazides react with aldedyde groups but also with ketone-containing compounds to form hydrazone bonds that, unlike Schiff bases, are quite stable without reduction.

2.2.1.7 Maleimide

Coupling of free sulfhydrals (-SH) is best accomplished using this maleimide (*Figure 1G*). A number of bifunctional maleimide linkers are possible using the Mitsunobu reaction, as described by Walker (10). In *Protocol 3*, a commercially available microtitre plate is used for the immobilization of reduced antibody.

2.2.1.8 Aldehyde

Amines react with aldehyde groups to form a Schiff base (*Figure 1H*). The reaction is reversible, therefore to stabilize the ligand bond it is recommended that the double bond in the Schiff base be reduced. This is usually accomplished by incubation in the presence of sodium cyanoborohydride (see *Protocol 11*).

2.2.1.9 Hydrazide

Aldedyde- and ketone-containing compounds react with hydrazide to form a hydrazone bond similar to that of a Schiff base (*Figure 1I*) but much more stable. It is usually unnecessary to reduce the hydrazone bond, especially if multiple bonds are formed with the ligand (11). This method is particularly attractive for the immobilization of antibodies through vicinal aldehyde groups formed by periodate oxidation of carbohydrate located in the Fc-region of the protein (12). The coupling process leads to site-directed (oriented) coupling of the antibody such that the active antigen binding sites face away from the surface.

2.2.2 Influencing the orientation of attachment

In the construction of the link between ligand and solid-phase material, the finite moment at which the ligand collides with the activated surface may randomly determine the orientation of the ligand to the surface. However, the goal is to sequester the ligand only in such a manner as to preserve its full binding activity, which for an IgG molecule means its ability to bind two molecules of antigen. Most preparations of immobilized antibody, however, exhibit less than one-third of the theoretical antigen-binding efficiency. Published antigen-binding efficiencies for monoclonal antibodies covalently linked to various activated supports include the following: Hopp *et al.* (13) 15–40%, Park *et al.* (14) 11%, Staehelin *et al.* (15) 29%, Bird *et al.* (16) 1–10% and Ohlson *et al.* (17) 28%.

A number of factors contribute to this situation. First, many covalent attachment methods immobilize antibody via free amino residues, the great majority of which are ε-amino groups on lysine residues. Such groups are distributed throughout the protein structure, thereby resulting in coupling that often occurs through residues near a binding site, leading to steric hindrance of antigen binding or altered conformation of the site preventing antigen binding. In the case of monoclonal antibodies especially, the extent to which this occurs can vary from antibody to antibody.

However, attachment of antibodies and antibody fragments can be accomplished in such a manner as to greatly increase the probability that the antigen-binding sites will be directed away from the surface. Accordingly, attachment methods may be categorized as random coupling and oriented coupling pro-

Table 2. Covalent and noncovalent immobilization methods that may give attached antibodies that are favourably orientated

Functional groups and ligands that lead to oriented coupling of antibodies	
Antibody linkage	**Solid-phase functional group**
Oxidized carhohydrate[a] (located on Fc region) (aldo-IgG)	Hydrazide[b] (B,P)[d], Schiff's base
Free sulphydryl of Fab', reduced disulfide linkages	Maleimide (P), Alkyl Halides, aziridines, haloacetyls
Fc-region	Protein A[c], Protein G, antibody against Fc (noncovalent)
Biotin attached site-specifically	Streptavidin (P) (noncovalent)

[a] Preparation of oxidized protein using periodate should be done by titration of the periodate concentration in order to achieve optimal coupling of active protein.

[b] Hydrazone bonds generally do not require reduction, while bonds formed with Schiff bases should be reduced using cyanoborohydride.

[c] Protein A and Protein G have different binding affinities for different immunoglobulin classes and subclasses, and affinity may also depend on species of origin.

[d] Methods involving the above reactive groups that are described in detail in this chapter are designated as follows: B, latex beads; P, polystyrene plates.

cesses (*Tables 1* and *2*). Methods that favour oriented coupling should be considered whenever possible because these may allow the optimal presentation of immobilized antibodies.

Random coupling methods may also be carried out in such a way as to favour certain orientations (*Figure 2*). The key element is optimization. For example, well-established activation processes, such as those based upon CNBr or NHS generally do not normally facilitate oriented coupling. However, it is possible to reduce the degree of randomness associated with the coupling of antibodies via

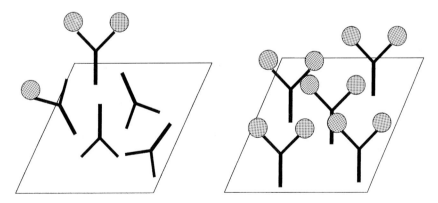

Random coupled antibodies   Oriented coupled antibodies

Figure 2. Antigen (tinted circles) binding to random- versus oriented-coupled antibodies (black Y shapes) on a solid phase. Antibodies may be immobilized on the solid phase by a variety of methods. Noncovalent adsorption or random covalent attachment are generally less effective than oriented attachment in the preparation of immunosorbents with a high level of antigen-binding activity.

such amino-group reactive ester displacement mechanisms. Cuatrecasas and Parikh (18) suggested many years ago on that pH could be manipulated to potentate the reactivity of one type of free amino-group over another, thereby decreasing the randomness of immobilization. In addition, Frost *et al.* (19) demonstrated the influence of protein charge on the immobilization process using NHS activated supports. Taking into consideration the relationship between protein-surface charge repulsion, Matson and Little (2) were able to prepare an anti-tPA monoclonal antibody support that was as efficient as that prepared by an activation process which favoured oriented coupling. It should be noted, however, that extensive optimization (coupling pH, buffer composition and protein concentration) of the NHS-mediated coupling process was required.

2.3 Noncovalent adsorption

The majority of immunosorbent assays are conducted with microwells coated noncovalently with antibody or antigen. This is because proteins easily and passively adsorb onto many surfaces; especially those of the hydrophobic plastics such as polystyrene (Section 3.1). Noncovalent methods are popular because they are generally straightforward, reproducible and simple to perform.

Antibody adsorption to a surface is influenced primarily by protein concentration, incubation time and temperature. The most popular coating buffer is 50 mM bicarbonate, pH 9.6 , but PBS, pH 7.2 or Tris-saline, pH 8.5, are also employed. Coating buffers usually do not contain detergent because these effectively compete with the protein for hydrophobic sites on the surface (Section 2.5.2). The protein concentration is generally held in the range of 1–10 μg/ml. The use of higher input concentrations of protein is not recommended because it results in the formation of unstable secondary adsorption layers, from which weakly associated protein is often released during assay. Thoroughly rinsing the coated plate with wash buffer (three to six times) prior to use is strongly advised. Coating is often conducted by incubating the plate overnight at 4–20 °C in a humidified container. However, this can be greatly accelerated by incubating at 37 °C in a covered water-bath if time is of concern. Examples of coating protocols are provided in *Protocols 1* and *2*.

The protein-surface adsorption process is complex. For most proteins the major driving force in adsorption is hydrophobic interaction. As a general rule, the more hydrophobic the protein the stronger the adsorption to the hydrophobic surface. The magnitude of the effect can be very dramatic, especially at lower input concentrations where protein can be spread over a large surface area, thereby maximizing the interaction with hydrophobic surface groups.

Consequently, when proteins are adsorbed to a surface a series of conformational changes may occur. Such alterations in protein structure can lead to denaturation and, with adsorbed antibodies, reduction in the ability to bind antigen. For example, Friguet *et al.* (20) found that monoclonal antibodies raised against denatured proteins recognized proteins adsorbed to polystyrene but not to these same native proteins held in solution. Schwab and Bosshard (21) found that when native protein antigen (cytochrome *c*) was coated onto several different polystyrene plates new antigenic sites were created. These were recognized by monoclonal antibodies raised against a*po*-cytochrome *c*. Butler *et al.* (22) studied the adsorption of both monoclonal and polyclonal antibodies in detail. They found that less than 3% of the monoclonal antibodies and only 5–10% of the polyclonal antibodies retained the ability to bind antigen when adsorbed to a polystyrene surface.

There is also evidence to suggest that proteins adhere to the surface of plastics in clusters. These clusters may represent the residual functional (e.g. antigen binding) species while the majority of those distributed in monolayers may be fully denatured (22).

2.4 Indirect immobilization

As discussed above, adsorption can have a profound affect on the native structure of an immobilized ligand, but, in addition, binding to ligands is often sterically hindered when they are in direct contact with a surface. Steric hindrance can usually be reduced by the inclusion of a spacer between the surface and the ligand. For example, Peterman *et al.* (23) found that the inclusion of streptavidin as a spacer between the surface and a biotinylated antibody increased antigen-binding activity 160% over direct adsorption of the same antibody. Alternatively, and commonly (e.g. 24), the indirect binding may be through an anti-species Ig antibody that is passively adsorbed to the surface. This antibody is then used to sequester the anti-analyte antibody which can then more efficiently capture antigen. Indirect immobilization by secondary antibody raised against Fc fragments from the primary species, or by Protein A (25), may also lead to more favourable orientation of attachment.

Another bridging approach used is to first lay down a protein–avidin conjugate coating e.g. BSA–streptavidin, to which a biotinylated capture antibody can be immobilized. Since the adsorbed streptavidin (or avidin) generally retains more binding activity than an adsorbed anti-species antibody, the PABC (protein–avidin–biotin-capture) system has become popular, especially for small molecules such as peptides (26) or other antigens (27) which are difficult to immobilize.

An alternative approach is to coat the immunosorbent with a reactive layer. In 'Hydrocoating' (28), free hydroxyl groups in a soluble dextran are first activated with tresyl chloride, which is then coated onto amino-modified polystyrene plates forming a covalent layer. The remaining tresyl groups can be used to immobilize ligands with free amino groups, which then reside in a hydrophilic environment removed from the original surface.

In a related approach, which allows for the preparation of coatings with varied properties, Brillhart and Ngo (29) prepared several hydrazide-activated preparations from aldehyde-dextran formed from soluble dextran by periodate oxidation. Adipic hydrazide was used to produce a hydrophilic hydrazide coating, or a mixture of adipic hydrazide and phenyl hydrazide or napthyleneacetyl hydrazide were used to produce hydrophobic hydazide coatings, all of which

141

had the added advantage of providing for oriented coupling of periodate-oxidized antibodies (3, 12). The various hydrocoatings (hydrophilic, hydrophobic) were then matched to a variety of commercial microtitre plates with different surface properties (Section 3.1) to obtain both an optimal and stable coating for ELISA.

2.5 Treatments after coating

When antibody (or antigen) has been immobilized either by covalent attachment (Section 2.2) or by passive adsorption (Sections 2.3 and 2.4) it is necessary to determine the extent of nonspecific binding (NSB). The sensitivity of the assay will be greatly compromised if NSB is substantial. Sources of NSB include impurities in reagent preparations (e.g. crossreactive species or antigens), proteins or lipids in the samples (or from hands) that bind label or exposed surface areas (unblocked areas) to which assay reagents can directly adsorb. A common source of NSB in serum is the presence of rheumatoid factors or autoantibodies. These can bind to the capture antibody or can be adsorbed at the surface where they can serve as a nonspecific capture antibody.

Minimizing NSB can be addressed in a number of ways. Often, it is sufficient to only use high-quality reagents and labels, and to take steps that will minimize the denaturation of antibody, enzymes or other proteins used in the assay. The use of Fab fragments (which are less 'sticky' and not as susceptible to denaturation) instead of whole antibodies and the inclusion of protein and detergent components in wash and assay buffers may also help. Since rheumatoid autoantibodies react mainly with the Fc region, the use of Fab fragments can also reduce this problem. In other instances it may be necessary to perform a separate blocking step to further reduce NSB.

2.5.1 Protein-blocking agents

Dilute solutions of BSA or gelatin are commonly used as blocking agents for microtitre plates, but they may not always be the best choice. Note that while blocking agents may mask nonspecific sites they may also contribute to new sites. For example, albumin, a common blocking agent, is known to adsorb to basic immunoglobulins.

Vogt *et al.* (30) systematically examined the adsorption of various protein blocking agents to Immulon™ 2 polystyrene microtitre plates (Dynatech) over 20 twofold serial dilutions. These were scored in terms of their inhibition of nonspecific binding measured by the binding of an antibody–peroxidase conjugate to the surface. All proteins were able to block at high concentration (120–3750 μg/well) either by pretreatment or simultaneous with the application of the antibody. The exception was hydrolysed gelatin, which was a poor blocker under any of the conditions studied. Nonfat dry bovine milk, casein and lipoprotein maintained coverage over a 10 000-fold dilution (0.2–1 μg/well), while BSA and hydrolysed gelatin exhibited a rapid drop-off in coverage with dilution.

Using a similar approach, Pratt and Roser (31) compared blocking agents on

MaxiSorp™ polystyrene plates (Nunc). They found that casein was a superior blocking agent to BSA and NBCS in its ability to prevent nonspecific adsorption of a rat immunoglobulin and enzyme conjugates. Fractionation of the casein demonstrated that lower molecular weight species were responsible for the blocking efficiency on the polystyrene surface. Thus, blocking potency was inversely proportional to the protein's molecular weight.

Other issues to consider about proteins as blocking agents include source, stability and immunoreactivity in the form of crossreactivity with antibodies or antigen employed in the assay. When selecting proteins careful attention must be paid to manufacturer's specifications. Not all proteins are prepared in the same manner i.e. the same protein may be manufactured using different purification methods and contain different stabilizing compounds and antimicrobial agents. Many different grades are available and, because these are biological materials, there can be considerable lot-to-lot variation.

Certain proteins used as blocking proteins, such as BSA are also conjugated to haptens to prepare immunogens. It is therefore possible that an anti-hapten antibody may bind to a protein that was added to reduce such 'nonspecific' binding. In such cases control experiments should be included to verify that this is not an issue. Casein derived from milk may contain biotin as an impurity. Blocking proteins may also lead to the introduction of exogenous substances, such as metal ions, lipids or other proteins which may interfere with the assay by inhibiting enzyme or increasing background signal. If fluorescent detection is to be employed, protein blocking agents will also need to be tested for intrinsic fluorescence to avoid adding substantially to the background signal.

2.5.2 Detergents

Detergents can serve two very different purposes in immunoassays. First, they serve to remove nonspecifically bound biomolecules from the surface by disruption of hydrophobic bonds formed between the biomolecule and surface groups. Thus, detergents are included in wash buffers. Generally, these are used in relatively low concentration (0.01–0.1%) in order to avoid potential interference with the assay, such as the inhibition of enzyme activity or the displacement of antibody or antigen coatings from the surface.

Detergent in a blocking buffer may serve to disperse protein aggregates for efficient surface coating but it may itself bind to the surface and serve as a blocking agent. This can be advantageous or deleterious, depending upon the detergent employed. Tween-20, a nonionic detergent, functions to remove nonspecifically adsorbed biomolecules and serves as a blocking agent by covering hydrophobic patches that become exposed by the removal of protein from the surface during repeated wash steps. It also maintains a hydration layer on the surface during processing of the support, protecting surface-bound proteins from denaturation. Conversely, ionic detergents such as SDS or DTAB will impart that charge to the surface upon binding, leading to increased backgrounds due to attraction of oppositely charged biomolecules.

There are also a number of polymers that are useful as blocking agents (32).

Chief among these are polyvinyl alcohols, polyethylene glycols and polyvinyl pyrrolidone. These stable polymers are used to mask out hydrophobic areas and render the surface hydrophilic. They are available in a variety of molecular weight ranges.

3 Solid-phase formats

3.1 Microtitre plates

Polystyrene is by far the most common plastic used in the manufacture of microtitre plates for immunoassay. Plates can be classified according to their binding properties with respect to the noncovalent adsorption of proteins, so that a microtitre plate maybe labelled as low, medium or high binding. There are also ultra-low and tissue-culture grade plates. Polystyrene, a naturally hydrophobic polymer, can be modified by the introduction of carboxyl or amine groups to create mixed hydrophobic–ionic surfaces, or it can be rendered hydrophilic by the grafting of hydrophilic polymers and hydrogels.

The maximal level of surface binding of IgG can be calculated from theoretical constraints (33) based upon the approximate size and shape of the molecule. With all molecules lying down, a monolayer is achieved at 130 ng/cm^2, whereas with all aligned by stacking on end a more densely packed monolayer is achieved at an upper limit of 650 ng/cm^2. The average of these two extremes is about 400 ng/cm^2 and this value is generally taken to represent monolayer coverage. Untreated polystyrene microtitre plates will adsorb 100–200 ng IgG/cm^2 and these are classified as 'Medium Binding' surfaces. Treatment with radiation results in occasional opening or excision of the aromatic polystyrene backbone, which then undergoes oxidation to give carboxyl groups. This imparts a slightly anionic character to the surface that roughly doubles the binding capacity for immunoglobulin to 400–500 ng/cm^2, which is near the theoretical limit. Such plates are considered to possess a 'High Binding' surface. 'Low' or 'Ultra Low Binding' plates are hydrophilic and of neutral charge. These surfaces were developed to permit only very limited protein adsorption and are thought to allow preservation of the native protein. They are used primarily to immobilize antigens or enzymes that are more susceptible to surface denaturation (34). Plates intended for cell culture are not suitable as solid-phase surfaces for immunoassay (34).

Microtitre plates are also not equivalent in performance. Plates will have well-to-well variations in binding that are reported usually in terms of a CV. The average of the high–low well difference from the mean of all wells is often reported. Good-quality plates have a CV in the range 3–5%. For example, a medium-binding plate may have a well-to-well CV = 5% and a high–low well average of ± 15%, while a high-binding plate may have a CV = 3% and a high–low well average of ± 8%.

Another important issue to consider in using microtitre plates are 'edge effects' (see also Section 3.2 of Chapter 7 and Section 3.2.1 of Chapter 8). An edge effect is indicated when there is a significant difference in assay standards readings between the outer wells and the more central wells. This phenomenon is attributed primarily to temperature differences between wells, as outer wells tend to heat up (and cool down) faster than central wells and antibody–antigen binding and enzyme–substrate reaction kinetics are strongly influenced by temperature. Temperature differentials are even more dramatic if several plates are stacked during incubation. Edge effects may be exacerbated if the reporter assay (e.g. peroxidase colorimetric reactions) is light sensitive, as light strikes outer wells of translucent plates with greater intensity. To avoid these problems allow samples, reactant stock solutions and buffers to equilibrate at the desired assay temperature, and pre-equilibrate the microtitre plates. The use of eight-well strips instead of plates is helpful in this regard since heat transfer is much more efficient. Strips also allow flexibility with smaller experiments. Finally, if light-sensitive reactions are to be used, protect the reagents from light, perform the assay in subdued light, and incubate in the dark.

In *Protocol 1* the coating and blocking steps are described in the context of a whole ELISA procedure for measuring an antigen. In the coating step, the capture antibody is presented in PBS, but alternative buffers such as carbonate, pH 9.6, or Tris-saline, pH 8.5, may be considered (Section 2.3). Note that the antibody coating concentration is at the upper end of the recommended range, which is acceptable depending upon the grade of plate. However, it is recommended that a serial dilution series to determine the optimal coating concentration be performed if another manufacturer's plates and grades are to be substituted. A blocking step with a protein-detergent agent is also described, but it should be determined in advance whether or not this step is necessary to reduce NSB. For all the steps of the procedure, it is important to be gentle during dispensing and removal of liquids from the wells; do not fill or rinse wells with a wash bottle or other device that generates a very strong jet of liquid, which might denature molecules by shearing or dislodge coatings from the surface.

As discussed earlier, there are some advantages in using secondary attachment process such as that provided through streptavidin–biotin linkages. *Protocol 2*, after Cordiano *et al.* (27), would be a typical procedure to employ.

An alternative to preparing streptavidin coated plates is to use commercially prepared plates, which have recently become available. The ELISA in *Protocol 3* is based upon such plates.

There are currently only a few commercially available plates with reactive groups for the covalent attachment of biomolecules, but those that are available are adequate for most needs. Therefore, it is now generally unnecessary to undertake harsh chemical treatments of native polystyrene plates (e.g. nitration) in order to achieve covalent immobilization.

In addition to the care needed with standard plates, there are storage and handling issues associated with activated plates and other activated support materials. Pre-activated supports that are susceptible to hydrolysis (e.g. with NHS, tosyl, carbonyldiimidazole groups) must be stored dry or in a compatible, anhydrous solvent. If these are to be stored under refrigeration it is important for the storage container to be re-equilibrated to ambient temperature prior to opening in order to avoid condensation. Make sure not to inadvertently expose the support to various fumes or vapours, such as low molecular weight organic acids, amines, or mercaptoethanol. It is best to handle activated supports with gloves to avoid contamination from hands. If possible, keep the support covered in an air-tight container or in a vacuum desiccator prior to use. If a commercial product is being used, follow the manufacturer's suggestions on storage and handling.

Protocol 1

Coating and blocking steps for a microtitre plate ELISA for antigen

Equipment and reagents

- 96-well microtitre plate (High Binding, Nunc or equivalent)
- PBS: 10 mM sodium phosphate, 150 mM NaCl, pH 7.2
- Blocking buffer: 3% BSA (Sigma), 0.05% Tween 20 in PBS
- Wash buffer: 0.1% BSA, 0.05% Tween 20 in PBS
- Orbital platform shaker

- Capture antibody: goat anti-rabbit IgG (Cappel Laboratories) diluted to 10 μg/ml in PBS
- Antigen: rabbit anti-mouse IgG (Cappel Laboratories)
- Antibody–enzyme conjugate: goat anti-rabbit IgG–alkaline phosphatase (Cappel Laboratories)
- Microtitre plate reader

Method

1. Pipette 100 μl of the capture antibody solution into each well of the plate.
2. Incubate for 20 h at ambient temperature.
3. Carefully remove antibody solution with a pipette and replace with 200 μl wash solution.
4. Gently agitate plate on shaker for 5 min between wash steps. Wash wells of plate twice with wash buffer in this manner.
5. Remove final wash solution and replace with 200 μl blocking buffer. Incubate for 1 h at ambient temperature with gentle agitation.
6. Remove blocking solution and add 100 μl antigen solution. Incubate 1–2 h at ambient temperature.
7. Remove antigen solution (standard, control or unknown) and replace with 200 μl wash buffer. Repeat step 4.
8. Add 100 μl antibody–enzyme conjugate and incubate for 30 min or more until colour development is sufficient.
9. Stop colour reaction by the addition of 1% SDS.
10. Measure the colour intensity in each well with a microtitre plate reader.

Protocol 2

Coating of a polystyrene microtitre plate with streptavidin[a]

Equipment and reagents

- Polystyrene microtitre plate and PBS as in *Protocol 1*
- 10 μg/ml[b] streptavidin (Sigma) in 0.05 M carbonate buffer, pH 9.5
- Wash buffer: PBS containing 0.05% Tween 20, 0.5% Nonidet P40[c], 0.5 mM $CaCl_2$

Method

1. Deliver 50 μl streptavidin solution to each well of the microtitre plate.

2. Incubate overnight at 4°C.

3. Remove the streptavidin solution and replace with 200 μl wash buffer.

4. Rinse each well three times with 200 μl wash buffer.

5. Pipette 200 μl wash buffer into each well and incubate for 30 min at 37°C.

6. Wash each well as in step 4 prior to use.

[a] Method obtained from reference (27), with permission.

[b] The concentration of streptavidin used for coating will depend upon the binding properties of the microtitre plate used. If suitable concentrations are not known it is advisable to perform preliminary binding studies with serially diluted streptavidin. Biotinylated AP or HRP can then be used to assess the coating concentrations obtained.

[c] In the above coating step, Tween 20 is present primarily as a blocking agent, while NP-40 (similar in structure to Triton X-100) is used as a detergent to remove excess or loosely bound streptavidin.

Protocol 3

ELISA with a streptavidin-coated microtitre plate[a]

Equipment and reagents

- Streptavidin coated microtitre plate (Reacti-Bind™, Pierce Chemical Company)
- Tris buffered saline (TBS): 25 mM Tris, 150 mM NaCl, pH 7.6
- Wash buffer: TBS containing 0.1% BSA, 0.05% Tween 20
- Antigen: serially diluted with wash buffer
- Biotinylated capture antibody: 10 μg/ml in wash buffer
- Second antibody–enyzme conjugate: diluted with wash buffer
- Enzyme substrate solution and plate reader

Protocol 3 continued

Method

1. Pipette 100 μl biotinylated capture antibody into each well and incubate for 2 h at ambient temperature.

2. Remove antibody solution from the wells and replace with 200 μl of wash buffer.

3. Rinse each well three times with 200 μl wash buffer.

4. Pipette 100 μl of each serial dilution of antigen into wells.

5. Incubate the microtitre plate for 30 min at ambient temperature.

6. Remove antigen solution from wells and repeat step 3.

7. Pipette 100 μl volumes of enzyme conjugate into each well.

8. Incubate for 30 min at ambient temperature.

9. Remove enzyme solution and repeat step 3.

10. Add substrate for colour development

[a] Method obtained from Pierce Chemical Company, with permission.

An example of the use of an activated microtitre plate is provided in *Protocol 4*, in which a commercially available activated polystyrene plate is used to immobilize a ligand with one or more amino groups. In this case, the reactive group is maleic anhydride which reacts at neutral or basic pH. It is particularly useful for the immobilization of small molecules such as peptides that are not easily absorbed onto polystyrene surfaces. One precaution, however, is to avoid acidic conditions during the application, as hydrolysis occurs at low pH (35). Note that attachment may be random or oriented depending on the number and location(s) of the amine group(s) within the ligand.

Protocol 4

Covalent attachment of a peptide (or biotin) to a maleic anhydride plate[a]

Equipment and materials

- Maleic anhydride activated microtitre plate (Reacti-Bind™, Pierce Chemical Company)

- PBS, blocking and wash buffers from *Protocol 1*

- Peptide stock solution for serial dilution, e.g. 18 μg/ml (10 μM) or, if in short supply, 1.8 μg/ml (1 μM) of a ≈ 1800 Da, 15-residue peptide in PBS

or

- BAPA (328.48 Da, Pierce Chemical company) stock solution for serial dilution, e.g. 3.28 μg/ml (10 μM) in PBS

Protocol 4 continued

Method

1. Pipette 100 μl of 1 to 1/1000 dilutions of peptide or BAPA in PBS into the wells of the plate to establish a sufficient coating concentration[b].

2. Incubate for 1 h at ambient temperature.

3. Carefully remove solution using a pipettor and replace with 200 μl blocking buffer.

4. Incubate the microtitre plate for 1 h at ambient temperature.

5. Remove solution and replace with 200 μl wash buffer.

6. Rinse each well three times with 200 μl wash buffer.

7. Proceed to use plate for intended assay.

[a] Method obtained from Pierce Chemical Company, with permission.

[b] Serial dilutions of BAPA gave an OD of 1.0 with a streptavidin–HRP conjugate at a BAPA concentration of 61 nM (20 ng/ml, 2 ng/well), while a 15 amino acid peptide gave the same adequate optical density reading at 67 nM (12 ng/well).

Maleic anhydride plates may be used to immobilize larger biomolecules such as antibodies or streptavidin. It is also possible to convert this group into additional reactive functional groups such as hydrazide for the oriented coupling of periodate-oxidized antibodies.

Fab' fragments and other proteins with free sulfhydryl groups can be immobilized on maleimide-activated surfaces and this may be more or less site-specific, depending on the number and locations of the groups. If the sulfhydryl groups are participating in disulfide linkages in the protein, they are first reduced with a gentle reducing agent such as DTT. The protein is then maintained in the reduced state by incorporating trace amounts of DTT into the buffers. EDTA is also added to chelate any oxidizing metals that might be present. In addition, it may be appropriate to add sulfhydryl groups by means of a suitable reagent (*Table 4.2*).

Protocol 5

Coupling of a reduced antibody to a maleimide activated microtitre plate[a]

Equipment and reagents

- Maleimide-activated microtitre plate (Corning Costar)
- DTT (Sigma)
- PBS: 10 mM sodium phosphate (6.85 mM monobasic, 3.15 mM dibasic) containing 150 mM NaCl, pH 6.5
- Coupling buffer: 1 mM EDTA, 0.1 μM DTT in PBS
- Blocking buffer: 0.2% nonfat dry milk in coupling buffer
- [b]Thiol-ligand: DTT-reduced antibody (1-100 μg/ml) in coupling buffer

Protocol 5 continued

Method

1. Pipette 100 μl reduced antibody solution into the wells of the microtitre plate.

2. Incubate for 1 h at ambient temperature.

3. Decant off the solution and rinse wells three times with wash buffer.

4. Pipette 200 μl blocking buffer and incubate for 30 min at ambient temperature.

5. Decant off the solution but do not rinse the microtitre plate.

6. Proceed to perform immunoassay[c].

[a] Method obtained from Corning Costar, with permission.

[b] Proteins lacking available sulfhydryls can be modified through free amino groups with Traut's reagent – prepare by diluting protein (1–10 μg/ml) in 15 mM Traut's reagent (2-iminothiolane; Sigma) containing 50 mM Tris, 150 mM NaCl, 1 mM EDTA, pH 7.6. Incubate 1 h, ambient temperature and use directly in step 1.

[c] It is recommended by the manufacturer to use subsequent reagents for the immunoassay supplemented with 10% fetal bovine serum to reduce NSB.

3.2 Tubes

The coated tube ELISA is well known but has largely been displaced by the microtitre plate. Protein ligands may be passively adsorbed to polypropylene or polystyrene tubes by following procedures similar to those described for plates (*Protocols 2* and *3*). The kinds of tubes used (e.g. 10 mm × 75 mm) are usually much larger than microtitre wells. They provide more surface area for binding. This is accomplished through efficient mixing by means of a circular rotator with the rotor held in a near-horizontal position.

Howell *et al.* (36) compared untreated polystyrene with glutaraldehyde-activated plastic and glass and they found the covalent attachment process to be more suitable. The glutaraldehyde-activated polystyrene tubes were prepared by incubation with 0.1% glutaraldehyde in 0.1 M sodium carbonate buffer, pH 9 for 3 h at 56°C followed by distilled water rinses. Another protocol described by Tijssen (37) involves pretreatment of polystyrene tubes with glutaraldehyde under acidic conditions. This is followed by a shift to pH 8–9.5 in the presence of the antibody to promote attachment while avoiding unwanted prepolymerization of glutaraldehyde that can take place under basic conditions.

3.3 Membranes

Most membranes that are used for immunoassay are derived from nylon 6,6 which is poly(iminoadipoyliminohexamethylene) or -[-NH-$(CH_2)_6$-CO-$(CH_2)_4$-CO-]- that is cast onto an inert matrix such as a nonwoven polyester. Nylons are mechanically and chemically resilient hydrophilic polymers. They can be chemically modified to include surface carboxyl or amino groups, thereby imparting negative, positive or amphoteric charges. Nylon membranes are also easily wettable which is of great advantage when 'spotting down' (coating) reagents or during washing. Another attractive feature is that only small amounts of antibody or antigen need to be used for spotting. Solutions are easily wicked into the membrane to provide a small concentrated spot. Finally, membranes can be housed in a variety of flow-through devices such as vacuum blots or microplates that allow the application of large sample volumes. These formats can be used automated. One disadvantage of nylon membranes is their rather high level of intrinsic fluorescence, which limits the range of applications for which they can be used.

An alternative to the use of microtitre plates for ELISA is to employ arrays of dots on membranes, and, if carefully organized with the right equipment, this can be very efficient and may be economical with reagents in quantitative or semiquantitative assays. Either covalent (*Protocols 6* and *7*) or noncovalent (*Protocol 8*) immobilization methods can be used. For preliminary spot tests to evaluate various signal development reagents, or when only a few samples need to be analysed, membranes can be used in free form (*Protocol 8*, Method A). If the immunoassay conditions need to be varied in optimization studies, or if many samples are to be analysed, the membrane can be assembled and processed in a vacuum dot–blot apparatus (*Protocol 8*, Method B). In *Protocol 6* a nylon membrane with carboxyl groups is activated with carbodiimide (*Figure 1c*). In *Protocol 7* a capture antibody is covalently attached to the membrane, residual activation groups capped (quenched) with ethanolamine and the membrane blocked with casein. The activation procedure is best accomplished using the free membrane in a bulk process. However, untreated membrane could have been cut in advance to the fit a vacuum blot apparatus and then assembled after processing to perform the protein coupling protocol and the immunoassay.

Protocol 6

Preparation of a carbodiimide-activated membrane[a]

Equipment and reagents

- Biodyne® C membrane (Nylon 6,6 functionalized with carboxyl groups, Pall Corporation)
- Methylene chloride (Aldrich)
- 10% (v/v) DCCD (Sigma): in methylene chloride
- Shaker
- Plastic or glass container with lid

Method

1. Cut membrane to desired size.
2. Submerge membrane in DCCD[b] solution, seal container and incubate for 30 min at ambient temperature with gentle agitation.
3. Decant DCCD solution and rinse membrane in methylene chloride.
4. Wash membrane with methylene chloride at least three times with 5 min agitation before decanting.

5. Air-dry membrane for 2 min then store in a vacuum desiccator. Short-term storage at ambient temperature (e.g. 1–3 h) is acceptable. Prolonged storage should be at 4°C under desiccation.

[a] Method obtained from Pall Corporation, with permission.

[b] Safety precautions: DCCD and methylene chloride are toxic; the latter is also flammable. The method should be conducted in a properly vented fume hood. Wear appropriate solvent resistant gloves, safety goggles and a lab coat.

Protocol 7

Coupling of antibody to DCCD activated membrane[a]

Equipment and reagents

- DCCD membrane prepared in *Protocol 6*
- Coupling buffer: 50 mM sodium bicarbonate buffer, pH 8.0
- PBS: 40 mM sodium phosphate (dibasic), 8 mM sodium phosphate (monobasic), 150 mM NaCl, pH 7.2
- Antibody[b]: 1 mg/ml in coupling buffer

- Quenching buffer: 0.1 M ethanolamine, pH 8–9
- Blocking buffer: 0.5% casein (BDH Biochemicals Ltd) in PBS
- Wash buffer: 0.1% Triton X-100 (Bio-Rad Laboratories) in PBS
- Orbital platform shaker

Method

1. Place dry activated membrane in a flat bottomed plastic or glass dish[c].
2. Carefully spot down 1 μl antibody solution onto the surface using a micropipettor.
3. Incubate for 1 h. All procedures are performed at ambient temperature.
4. Apply sufficient quenching buffer to thoroughly soak membrane and to allow it to float.
5. Incubate for 1 h with gentle agitation using an orbital platform shaker.
6. Decant and replace with blocking buffer.
7. Incubate for 1 h.
8. Decant and replace with wash buffer.
9. Rinse membrane three times with wash buffer with 5 min of agitation between rinses.
10. Store membrane in wash buffer at 4°C until ready for use.

[a] Method obtained from Pall Corporation, with permission.

[b] Other proteins or amino-ligands may be covalently coupled at similar input concentrations.

[c] Membrane may also be cut in advance to be used in a vacuum dot blot apparatus as described in *Protocol 8*, Method B.

Protocol 8

Immunodot–blot ELISA with antibody adsorbed to a membrane[a]

Equipment and reagents

- Biodyne® A or B nylon 6,6 membrane (Pall Corporation)
- Antibody, antigen and conjugate as in *Protocol 1*
- PBS, blocking, and wash buffers from *Protocol 7*
- Tris substrate buffer: 0.1 M Tris, 0.1 M NaCl, 50 mM MgCl$_2$, pH 8.5

- Nitro blue tetazolium (NBT, Sigma): 75 mg/ml in 70% (v/v) dimethylformamide
- 5-Bromo-4-chloro-3-indolyl Phosphate (BCIP, Sigma): 50 mg/ml in DMF
- Orbital platform shaker for Method A
- Vacuum Dot Blot Apparatus (Bio-Rad Laboratories) for Method B

Method A (with free membrane)

1. While wearing gloves[b], cut a 10 × 10 cm square of membrane. Cut into 1 cm strips for testing. Subdivide these into 1 cm segments by lines drawn with a pencil and number each strip for identification. Perform all procedures at ambient temperature.

2. Serial dilute the capture antibody (goat anti-rabbit IgG) in PBS to give concentrations equivalent to 10 ng/μl, 100 ng/μl and 1 μg/μl.

3. Place the membrane strips on a nonadsorbent surface. Pipette onto the surface 1 μl volumes containing the capture antibody to give spots in the centre of each square on the membrane strips.

4. Air dry the membrane strips for 5 min.

5. Place the membrane strips in a Petri dish and cover with blocking buffer and gently agitate for 30 min

6. Air-dry the membrane strips for 30 min.

7. Dilute antigen (rabbit anti-mouse IgG) to 1 μg/ml and 100 ng/ml in PBS. Place membrane strips in Petri dishes containing 10 ml of each dilution of antigen. Gently shake the membranes for 30 min.

8. Decant, replace with 10 ml wash solution and gently agitate the strips for 5 min. Wash twice in the same manner.

9. Replace the final wash solution with 10 ml PBS. Gently agitate the strips for an additional 1 min and decant.

10. Dilute the antibody-conjugate (goat anti-rabbit IgG-alkaline phosphatase) 1:100 (v/v) in PBS. Apply 10 ml of the conjugate solution to the membrane strips and gently agitate on the orbital shaker for 60 min.

11. Repeat step 8.

12. Wash twice with deionized water, gently agitating for 1 min between rinses.

Protocol 8 continued

13. Immediately before use, prepare enzyme substrate solution by mixing 33 μl NBT and 25 μl BCIP into 7.5 ml Tris substrate buffer.

14. Decant the rinse water and replace with 7.5 ml substrate solution. Gently agitate for 5 min.

15. Decant and add 10 ml deionized water. Gently agitate for 2 min.

16. Remove the membrane strips from the Petri dishes and blot the strips between paper towels. While protecting from light, air-dry the strips on a fresh paper towel for 30 min, or longer if necessary.

17. Analyse the results by measuring the spot colour intensities with a reflectometer or scanning densitometer[c].

Method B (using a vacuum dot blot apparatus)

1. Cut the membrane to the desired size to fit the apparatus (e.g. 9 × 12 cm).

2. Wet the sized membrane by first floating on top of a solution of PBS, then fully submerge.

3. Place the wet membrane in the vacuum dot blot apparatus and assemble properly such that the membrane is sealed to prevent cross-talk (diffusion) between wells.

4. Pipette 10–100 μl of serially diluted capture antibody into wells. Load empty wells used for negative controls with an equivalent volume of PBS.

5. Allow the wells to stand for 30 min, then apply a vacuum to the apparatus to remove the solutions in the wells.

6. Load each well with 100 μl blocking buffer. Allow to stand for 30 min, then vacuum and rinse each well with 100 μl PBS while still under vacuum.

7. Load each well with 100 μl of antigen sample and allow to stand 1 h, then vacuum and rinse with wash buffer.

8. Release the vacuum and load each well with 100 μl PBS. Apply a vacuum to remove the buffer. Repeat the rinse step once more.

9. Load each well with 100 μl antibody enzyme conjugate and allow to stand 1 h, then vacuum and rinse in PBS.

10. Load each well with 100 μl deionized water and vacuum-rinse the wells.

11. Load each well with 100 μl of the enzyme substrate solution. Incubate 5 min then vacuum to remove solution. With the vacuum still on, rinse each well twice with 100 μl deionized water.

12. Disassemble the apparatus and allow the membrane to air-dry at ambient temperature. Read the results using an appropriate densitometer or scanner.

[a] Method obtained from Pall Corporation, with permission.

[b] Gloves should be worn at all times during this procedure to avoid contamination of the membrane by fingerprints.

[c] There are various kinds of scanners available for detection of colorimetric precipitating substrates such as NBT/BCIP.

3.4 Microspheres

The use of small uniform latex particles (microspheres) in the IVD (*in vitro* diagnostic) industry is widespread, especially for immunodiagnostic applications. They offer advantages over other solid phases (e.g. microtitre plates) in sensitivity (higher binding capacity, the attribute of small uniform particle size and high surface area–volume ratios) and ease of use (provided by the ability to maintain stable colloidal suspensions).

Microspheres are used for protein immobilization either by passive adsorption or covalent attachment to the surface. They are available in a wide range of particle diameters from 0.02–1000 μm (20 nm–1 mm). However, immunoassays generally employ microspheres at 1 μm. As a general guide, bead sizes used are: 0.01–0.3 μm for turbidimetric immunoassays, 0.3–0.9 μm for particle-capture ELISA, 0.1–0.4 μm for strip tests, > 0.8 μm for solid-phase immuno-assays and 0.2–0.9 μm latex agglutination. Suspensions of these are stable up to 0.25 M electrolyte (total monovalent ion concentration).

3.4.1 Protein adsorption

Latex particles prepared from pure polystyrene are hydrophobic. They are commonly used for protein (e.g. antibody or antigen) coating by passive adsorption. Most polystyrene microspheres contain sulfate groups covalently attached to the surface. Sulfated latex microspheres ($pK_{sulfate} < 2$) are stable under moderately acidic conditions. Their presence serves to stabilize the suspension and prevent aggregation. During processing a number of these sulfate groups are hydrolysed to give hydroxyl groups. Adsorbed surfactant used as a stabilizing agent during polymerization may also be present on the beads. They can be cleaned to remove surfactant but then are more prone to aggregation (38). For this reason, they are generally used as supplied from the manufacturer.

Protocol 9 describes a typical process for preparing passively adsorbed im-munosorbents based upon microspheres. At first inspection it may appear to be a simple mixing experiment, however, there is an important underlying strategy based upon estimating the microsphere–protein ratio required to reach mono-layer saturation. For estimations of monolayer coverage the following equation may be used:

$$S = \frac{6}{\rho D} \times C$$

where S = amount of protein (mg protein/g solid) necessary for monolayer satura-tion, $6/\rho D$ = surface area/mass (m^2/g) for microspheres of diameter D (μm) and density ρ (g/cm^3), and C = microsphere protein binding capacity (mg protein/m^2).

For 1 μm polystyrene beads with a density of 1.05 g/cm^3 and a protein binding capacity of 2.5 mg protein/m^2 to be coated with bovine IgG, then

$$S = (6/[1.05 \times 1]) \times 2.5 = 14.3 \text{ mg IgG per gram of beads.}$$

In practice, a protein concentration of 3–10-fold above monolayer saturation (S) is used to achieve an optimal spatial orientation (presentation) and to minimize nonspecific binding (inertness).

Protocol 9

Adsorption of antibody to uncoated polystyrene microspheres[a]

Equipment and reagents

- Microspheres: uncoated polystyrene beads, 1 μm diameter, 10% solids (Bangs Laboratories)
- Antibody: prepared in adsorption buffer at ≈ 0.5-1.5 mg/ml
- Adsorption buffer: 50 mM sodium bicarbonate–carbonate,150 mM NaCl, pH 9.5

- Blocking buffer: 10 mM PBS, 0.1% Tween 20, pH 7.2
- Rotator (end-over-end) or rocking platform
- Centrifuge[b]: 1 μm beads pellet at 1200 **g** for 15 min in a standard benchtop centrifuge

Method

1. Dilute microspheres to ≈ 1% solids (10 mg/ml) with adsorption buffer.

2. Add 1 ml microsphere suspension to 1 ml antibody solution[c].

3. Gently mix using an end-over-end rotator or rocking platform for 2 h at ambient temperature.

4. Incubate overnight at 4°C with continuous mixing.

5. Centrifuge, remove supernatant, and resuspend the microsphere pellet in blocking buffer.

6. Mix at ambient temperature for 1 h, then centrifuge and remove supernatant.

7. Resuspend pellet at 10% solids in fresh blocking buffer and store at 4°C until ready for use.

[a] Method obtained from Bangs Laboratories with permission.

[b] Centrifuge particles 0.5-0.8 μm at 2200 **g** for 15 min.; 0.3-0.5 μm at 9300 **g** for 15 min.

[c] Gentle mixing of the bead suspension into the protein solution is more efficient and coating more uniform than attempting to resuspend the bead pellet using the protein solution.

3.4.2 Covalent coupling

There are situations in which covalent tethering of antibody (or antigen) to beads is preferred. First, not all proteins form coatings that remain stable upon storage or under assay conditions without crosslinking them to the surface. Second, proper presentation of the ligand on the surface is best achieved using covalent linking methods that direct spatial orientation.

Both amino- and carboxyl-modified latex beads are useful surfaces for the covalent attachment of proteins using the reactive groups and reagents described in Section 2.2.1 and in *Table 5.1*. For example, carboxyl groups can be directly activated with a carbodiimide , which in turn will react with amino-ligands (e.g. proteins such as antibodies, streptavidin, amino-biotin) or with a bifunctional spacer arm (e.g. aminocaproic acid to extend the carboxyl group away from the surface, or hexanediamine to create a terminal amino linker). Amino groups can be converted to terminal epoxide groups using a bisoxirane such as 1,4 butanediol diglycidyl ether, or reacted with glutaraldehyde to prepare beads with surface aldehyde groups. Selection of the coupling method to use is determined by the intrinsic properties of the protein to be immobilized (pH stability, hydrophobicity and availability of free amino or thiol amino acid residues) and the bead's surface properties. Some properties relevant to covalent coupling or surface derivatization of carboxy and amino latex beads are described below.

Carboxyl-modified latex beads are stabilized by the negatively charged carboxyl anions ($pK \approx 5$), but, because the charge is lost at low pH they spontaneously aggregate and are not suitable for use under such conditions. However, carboxyl latex is well suited for the covalent attachment of biomolecules and is available in a variety of derivatives. These include styrene/acrylic acid–COOH, styrene/malic acid–(COOH)$_2$, or styrene/aminocaproic acid–COOH, which have different reactivities with respect to the covalent attachment of biomolecules. It is advisable to screen several types and select those that give the best retention of ligand-binding activity (39).

Amino-modified latex beads can be produced by a number of synthetic routes. Polymerization with amino-styrene results in surface amines pendant to aromatic rings, while other methods introduce amine groups into the aliphatic (polyethylene) backbone. Since aromatic amines are electron resonance stabilized they tend to be less reactive than the aliphatic amines (32).

Most covalent attachment methods lead to the attachment of antibodies or antigens through the protein's free amino groups. The linkage between the solid support and the protein is usually an amide peptide bond (i.e. support–CO–NH–protein). For example, surface carboxyl groups activated with carbodiimide, NHS, maleic anhydride or CDI result in the formation of amide bonds to proteins. Under acidic conditions (pH 3–4), as in the case of maleic anhydride, the protein is cleaved from the support. If this is an issue, there are covalent coupling chemistries that can result in the more stable alkyl amine (support–CH–NH–protein) linkage. Below are two examples.

In *Protocol 10*, a tosyl-activated solid phase is used to couple antibody. Tosylates are derived from conversion of the support's free hydroxyl groups (support–C–O–tosyl). Reaction with an amino-ligand (e.g. antibody) leads to the formation of a stable alkyl amine bond. In *Protocol 11*, protein coupling to an aldehyde activated support occurs by Schiff base (support–C=NH–protein). This is an unstable bond and must be converted to the more stable alkyl amine linkage using a reducing agent such as cyanoborohydride.

Protocol 10

Coupling of an antibody to tosyl-activated beads[a]

Equipment and reagents

- Tosyl-modifed Microspheres ($\approx$ 10% w/v, Bangs Laboratories)
- Coupling buffer: 0.1 M sodium borate, pH 8.5
- Quenching-blocking buffer: 30-40 mM ethanolamine, 1% BSA

- Amino-ligand[b]: 1 mg/ml antibody in coupling buffer
- Storage buffer: 10 mM PBS, 0.1% Tween 20, pH 7.4
- Vortex mixer
- Rotator or angled platform shaker

Method

1. Wash 1 ml (100 mg/ml) beads twice in 10 ml coupling buffer. Use a microcentrifuge to pellet and resuspend the beads between wash steps.

2. Resuspend the pellet in 5 ml coupling buffer by vortexing to ensure that complete suspension has occurred.

3. Mix 5 ml amino-ligand solution with 5 ml bead suspension.

4. Incubate at ambient temperature for 16–24 h with continuous mixing using a rotator.

5. Centrifuge beads then wash-resuspend pellet in quenching buffer. Repeat process once more.

6. Resuspend pellet with 10 ml quench buffer and mix gently using a rotator for 30 min.

7. Centrifuge beads then wash-resuspend pellet twice in storage buffer.

8. Resuspend pellet in 5 ml storage buffer and store at 4°C until needed.

[a] Method obtained from Bangs Laboratories, with permission.

[b] Other ligands that contain free primary amino groups include other proteins, peptides and small molecules.

Protocol 11

Coupling of an antibody to aldehyde-modified beads[a]

Equipment and reagents

- Aldehyde-modified microspheres ($\approx$ 10% w/v, Bangs Laboratories)
- Sodium cyanoborohydride (Aldrich)

- Ligand solution, other buffers and equipment as in *Protocol 10*

Protocol 11 continued

Method

1. Wash 1 ml (100 mg/ml) of beads twice in 10 ml coupling buffer. Use a micro-centrifuge to pellet and resuspend the beads between wash steps.

2. Resuspend the pellet in 5 ml of coupling buffer by vortexing to ensure that complete suspension has occurred.

3. Mix 5 ml of amino-ligand solution with 5 ml bead suspension.

4. Incubate at ambient temperature for 2–4 h with continuous mixing using a rotator.

5. Centrifuge beads then wash-resuspend pellet in 10% sodium cyanoborohydride solution. Repeat process once.

6. Resuspend pellet with 10 ml 10% sodium cyanoborohydride solution and mix gently by means of a rotator for 30 min.

7. Centrifuge beads then wash-resuspend pellet in quenching buffer. Repeat process once.

8. Resuspend pellet with 10 ml quench buffer and mix gently using a rotator for 30 min.

9. Centrifuge beads then wash-resuspend pellet twice in storage buffer.

10. Resuspend pellet in 5 ml storage buffer and store at 4 °C until needed.

[a] Method obtained from Bangs Laboratories, with permission.

3.4.3 General advice

Unlike other solid phases, with latex particles one must also take into account the stability of the particle solution, as colloidal suspensions must be maintained for the coupling methods to work. If spacer arms are to be added make sure to dilute (e.g. < 1% solids) the bead suspension prior to coupling in order to avoid crosslinking neighbouring beads to one another. Prior to performing any reactions it is advisable to remove surface-bound surfactants or other water-soluble polymers that may interfere with subsequent additions of functional groups. However, this should not be done if the process leads to irreversible aggregation of the beads. Once the bead has been functionalized it may possess a new set of surface properties. The use of an inert, nonionic detergent (e.g. Tween 20, Triton X-100) to back-coat the bead prior to ligand coupling can serve to stabilize the suspension and at the same time mask nonspecific sites.

Particles also have to be processed differently from other solid supports. One needs to be able to dilute, concentrate and clean microspheres while retaining the ability to maintain stable bead suspensions. Dilution into deionized water is possible for charged beads containing bound surfactant and ions. However, for dilute suspensions (< 1% solids) the addition of surfactant to about 0.1% (w/v) is highly recommended. Particle concentration may be accomplished by centrifugation (see footnotes in *Protocol 9*) for aqueous suspensions and by rotary evaporation under vacuum (with warming to 40–50 °C) for particles in organic solvent. Larger beads (> 5 μm) can also be recovered from solution and rinsed using a vacuum filtration apparatus. Cleaning and buffer exchanges for small particles can be accomplished by centrifuge–decant or dialysis methods. When performing dialysis select a dialysis membrane or hollow fibre system with the largest pore size rating available that will still retain beads. Completely replace external water or buffer supply frequently (at least three changes) to ensure efficient removal of water soluble surfactants and buffer salts.

4 Handling and storage

4.1 Surface denaturation

Biomolecules removed from their natural environment are subject to denaturation. Many enzymes and other proteins are susceptible to denaturation by sonication, vortexing or other rigorous mixing procedures. The drying of proteins on a surface can also lead to irreversible conformational changes (40). Denaturation of proteins at interfaces is to be regarded as a serious problem. Drying may also take place, causing even more denaturation. The use of Tween 20 and PBS which maintain a hydration sphere of ordered water molecules around the protein may minimize denaturation.

4.2 Microtitre wells and tubes

Microtitre plates and tubes are highly electrostatic and will attract lint and other dust particles to their surface. This can lead to nonuniform attachments by the physical blocking of sites. Oils from hands, vacuum pumps or other laboratory equipment can form hydrophobic films on the exposed surface, preventing the direct attachment of proteins or other reagents. Plastics are also damaged by UV radiation in the presence of air, causing discolouring, cracking and surface oxidation. They should be stored in their original packaging, away from sunlight, and not be removed from it until immediately before use.

For the extended storage of 'ready for use' microtitre plate immunosorbents (i.e. with attached proteins) it is advisable to fill wells with a stabilizing agent that will maintain protein hydration. Agents used for this purpose include sucrose, glycerol, casein or BSA. They may be used separately or in combination. A nonionic detergent capable of maintaining hydration, such as Tween 20, is often included as well. The addition of an antimicrobial such as sodium azide (0.1%) is recommended if plates are to be stored wet. For dry storage, use PBS as the storage buffer since it also maintains protein hydration. Do not use carbonate–bicarbonate or other volatile buffer systems because these have little protective effect upon drying. Plates should be stored at 4 °C and not frozen.

Just prior to use, the plates need to be returned to ambient temperature. If the plates were stored dry with buffer salts or other stabilizing agents the wells need to be filled with deionized water in order to reconstitute the solution. Use a volume of water that returns the solution to its original concentration prior to drying. Let the plates stand for $\approx$ 30 min, then rinse three to six times in assay buffer before use. For plates stored in an aqueous buffer, bring to ambient conditions and remove storage buffer. Rinse in assay buffer as just described.

4.3 Membranes

Nonactivated membranes are very stable and can be stored dry at ambient temperature in their original packaging. They can be quite electrostatic and should be placed in a clean environment, preferably in subdued light. If the packaging has been opened place them between sheet liners (normally supplied with the product) and store in a sealed container or plastic pouch. Avoid the use of plastic bags that may contain antistatic or slip agents and plastic containers made of polystyrene that may contain injection-mould release agents. These substances can become adsorbed to the membranes surface and present a serious source of contamination. A good storage medium for membranes is KaPak™ (KaPak Corp.) polyester sealing bags. Always handle membranes with clean cotton gloves to avoid contamination.

4.4 Microspheres

Store latex microspheres at 4°C in tightly sealed containers to avoid evaporation. Guard against freezing because this will cause aggregation that is often permanent. For efficient passive adsorption of proteins to latex particles the concentration of bead solids should be kept in the range of 0.5–1% (w/v). This is to avoid aggregation which can occur by protein bridging to neighbouring particles. Nonspecific adsorption can be minimized by the use of nonionic detergents such as Tween 20 which hydrate the surface and reduce the effective hydrophobicity of the particle.

If charged particles are to be used, certain conditions should be avoided to reduce the likelihood of inadvertent aggregation. For negatively charged particles (e.g. carboxyl, sulfate) do not use buffers that contain divalent cations such as Ca^{+2} or Mg^{+2}. In the case of positively charged latex (e.g. with amino groups) do not use phosphate, citrate or sulfate-based buffers. Maintain protein concentrations in the range of 20–200 μg/ml in the latex suspension. Wash the particles at least three times in the buffer used for adsorption, then block residual hydrophobic sites with a blocking agent such as casein + Tween 20 ($\approx$ 0.5 mg/ml).

5 Sourcing of reagents

The decision as whether to purchase from a commercial source or to prepare the immunosorbent in the laboratory should be based upon need, availability, costs and safety issues.

1. Need: if the immunoassay is based upon a unique ligand or capture antibody then there is little choice but to prepare the immunosorbent. However, manufacturers are now offering solid phases with Protein A, streptavidin and various secondary antibodies. It may be possible, in some instances, to modify

the immunoassay format to utilize these new products. Another important issue is quality. Manufacturers must provide quality certification with their product, which may be of great benefit to the user concerned with lot-to-lot variation.

2. Availability: solid phases may not be available that match a particular immunoassay's specification for sensitivity. It may be necessary to further modify the surface to meet such performance requirements using, for example, coupling methods that are not commercially available.

3. Costs: Untreated solid phases are relatively inexpensive compared with activated or precoated forms. Passive adsorption coating will work well in most cases but requires the use of more ligand. If the ligand itself is expensive, then covalent attachment is recommended because chemical coupling methods generally consume much less ligand. The purchase of chemical reagents in bulk that are used in covalent coupling protocols can be expensive. However, because only small quantities are required (for e.g. per plate well) the actual cost per assay is generally low. The cost of commercially prepared solid phases includes manufacturing labour, QA/QC and sales, distribution and marketing burdens, all of which must be passed onto the customer.

4. Safety issues: certain coupling methods require a great deal of skill in the proper handling of toxic and flammable or potentially explosive chemicals. Procedures involving chloromethylation, hydrazines, and *p*-toluene sulfonyl chloride are best performed by experienced chemists. Otherwise, it is recommended that these supports be purchased from a reliable commercial source.

References

1. Ekins, R. and Chu, F. (1997). *J. Int. Fed. Clin. Chem.* **9**, 100.
2. Matson, R. S. and Little, M. C. (1988). *J. Chromatog.* **458**, 67.
3. Schramm, W. and Paek S.-H. (1992). *Anal. Biochem.* **205**, 47.
4. Wilchek, M. and Miron, T. (1987). *Biochemistry* **26**, 2155.
5. Endo, N., Umemoto, N., Dato, Y., Takeda, Y., and Hara, T. (1987). *J. Immunol. Methods* **104**, 253.
6. Sundberg, L. and Porath, J. (1974). *J. Chromatog.* **90**, 87.
7. Bethell, G. S., Ayers, J. S., Hancock, W. S., and Hearn, M. T. (1979). *J. Biol. Chem.* **254**, 2572.
8. Hearn, M. T. W., Harris, E. L., Bethell, G. S., Hancock, W. S., and Ayers, J. A. (1981). *J. Chromatog.* **218**, 509.
9. Mosbach, K. H. and Nilsson, K. G. I. (1983). US Patent **4,415**, 665.
10. Walker, M. A. (1994). *Tetrahed. Lett.* **35**, 665.
11. O'Shannessy, D. J. and Wilchek, M. (1990). *Anal. Biochem.* **191**, 1.
12. Little, M. C., Siebert, C. J., and Matson, R. S. (1988). *BioChromatog.* **3**, 156.
13. Hopp, T. P., Prickett, K. S., Price, V. L., Libby, R. T., March, C. J., Cerretti, D. P., Urdal, D L., and Conlon, P. J. (1988). *Biotechnology* **6**, 1204.
14. Park, H. S., Jung, M. Y., Oh, M. S., Koh, J. H., Kim, H. S., and Hyun, H. H. (1987). *Korean Biochem. J.* **20**, 336.

15. Staehelin, T., Hobbs, D. S., Kung, H., Lai C.-Y., and Pestka, S. (1981). *J. Biol. Chem.* **256**, 9750.
16. Bird, P., Lowe, J., Stokes, R. P., Bird, A. G., Ling, N. R., and Jefferis, R. (1984). *J. Immunol. Methods* **71**, 97.
17. Ohlson, S., Lundblad, A., and Zopf, D. (1988). *Anal. Biochem.* **169**, 204.
18. Cuatrecasas, P. and Parikh, I. (1972). *Biochemistry* **11**, 2291.
19. Frost, R. G., Monthony, J. F., Engelhorn, S. G., and Siebert, C. J. (1981). *Biochem. Biophys. Acta* **670**, 163.
20. Friguet, B., Djavadi-Ohaniance, L., and Goldberg, M. E. (1984). *Mol. Immunol.* **21**, 673.
21. Schwab, C. and Bosshard, H. R. (1992). *J. Immunol. Methods* **147**, 125.
22. Butler, J. E., Ni, L., Nessler, R., Joshi, K. S., Suter, M., Rosenber, B., Chang, J., Brown, W. R., and Cantareo, L. A. (1992). *J. Immunol. Methods* **150**, 77.
23. Peterman, J. H., Tarcha, P. J., Chu, V. P., and Butler, J. E. (1988). *J. Immunol. Methods* **111**, 271.
24. Kakabakos, S. E., Evangelatos, G. P., and Ithakissios, D. S. (1990). *Clin. Chem.* **36**, 497.
25. Schramm, W., Yang, T., and Midgley, A. R. (1987). *Clin. Chem.* **33**, 1331.
26. Ivanov, V. S., Suvorova, Z. K., Tchikin, L. D., Kozhich, A. T., and Ivanov, V. T. (1992). *J. Immunol. Methods* **153**, 229.
27. Cordiano, I., Steffan, A., Randi, M. L., Pradella, P., Girolami, A., and Fabris, F. (1995). *J. Immunol. Methods* **178**, 121.
28. Gregorius, K., Mouritsen, S., and Elsner, H. I. (1995). *J. Immunol. Methods*, **181**, 65.
29. Brillhard, K. L. and Ngo, T. T. (1991). *J. Immunol. Methods* **144**, 19.
30. Vogt, R. F., Phillips, D. L., Henderson, L. O., Whitfield, W., and Spierto, F. W. (1987). *J. Immunol. Methods* **101**, 43.
31. Pratt, R. P. and Roser, B. (1997). *NUNC product bulletin*, No. 7: Comparison of Blocking Agents for ELISA.
32. Bangs Laboratories (1998). *Technical note*, No. 22: Carboxylate-modified Microspheres.
33. Esser, P. (1997). *NUNC product bulletin*, No. 6: Principles in Adsorption to Polystyrene.
34. Corning Costar (1995). *ELISA techniques bulletin*, No. 1: Immobilization Principles-Selecting the Surface.
35. Hermanson, G. T. (1996). *Bioconjugate techniques*, p. 137. Academic Press, San Diego.
36. Howell, E. E., Nasser, J., and Schray, K. J. (1981). *J. Immunoassay* **2**, 205.
37. Tijssen, P. (1985). *Practice and theory of enzyme immunoassays*, p. 297. Elsevier, Amsterdam.
38. Interfacial Dynamics (1994). *How to handle latexes, product guide*.
39. Seradyn (1988). *Microparticle immunoassay techniques*.
40. Ansari, A. A., Hittikudur, N. S., Joshi, S. R. and Medeira, M. A. (1985). *J. Immunol. Methods* **84**, 117.

163

Chapter 6
Standards and immunogens

M. Q. Chaudhry
MAFF Central Science Laboratory, Sand Hutton, York YO41 1LZ, UK

1 Introduction

Standards are preparations of analyte that are used for calibration, that is, in an assay 'unknown' samples are compared with them to estimate concentrations of analyte in the samples. While for hapten immunoassays standards are chemically quite different from the corresponding immunogens, for immunoassays that measure naturally immunogenic antigens the same purified preparation may be used as both standard and immunogen. However, the criteria for a good standard may be quite different from those for a good immunogen. Standards are considered in Section 6.

An immunogen is a substance capable of eliciting an immune response. In contrast, an antigen can be anything that is specifically recognized by components of the adaptive immune system, whether it is immunogenic or not. Thus, not all antigens are immunogenic (and, for those that are, their immunogenicity varies considerably), but all immunogens are essentially antigenic. Substances that are both antigenic and immunogenic include whole cells, viruses, and macromolecules (proteins, complex polysaccharides or lipids, polynucleotides), but antigenic determinants (epitopes), i.e. the portions of antigens complementary to combining site of antibodies, are of limited molecular size. Smaller non-immunogenic molecules that can be made immunogenic by coupling to a carrier macromolecule are called haptens. Thus, haptens are bound specifically by antibodies produced in response to an immunogen that contained the hapten as part of its structure (see Section 4).

1.1 Criteria for a good immunogen

1.1.1 Requirements for immunogenicity

In the first stage of a primary immune response, an immunogenic antigen is specifically recognized by antibodies acting as receptors on the surfaces of B lymphocytes, leading to the selected stimulation of a few B cell clones. In parallel, the antigen may be nonspecifically phagocytosed by antigen-processing cells, partly degraded, and antigen fragments displayed on the cell surfaces, bound to MHC class-II proteins. Then, helper T-cells with appropriately specific surface receptors bind to the displayed antigen fragments, stimulating them to secrete cytokines, which, in turn, further promote the proliferation and differentiation of the selected B lymphocytes into antibody-producing cells. Therefore, to elicit a strong immune response, an immunogen must:

1. Have an epitope that can be recognized by a B-cell antibody, and
2. Be degradable, and
3 Have a site which can simultaneously bind to class-II protein and T-cell receptor.

Proteins and other macromolecules usually contain a large and indefinable number of antigenic determinants but only some of these are immunogenic. Failure to evoke an adequate immune response may be because of similarities to host 'antigens', since the B and T cells with receptors specific for host molecules are removed during development of self-tolerance. Thus, despite their huge number, there is a theoretical limitation to the antigen-binding sites available in B-cell antibodies, T-cell receptors, and class-II proteins in any one animal (1, 2).

1.1.2 Natural immunogens

While raising antibodies to natural immunogens is relatively straightforward, their complexity, heterogeneity and fragility must be taken into account. Antigens of interest may be present in complex matrices in specific physiological environments that must be disrupted during their isolation. Such disruption can lead to spontaneous physical and chemical changes in complex biomolecules, which may be degraded by proteolysis, or react with other components and lose native form. Such changes may affect the immunogenicity of antigens, and the specificity of the antibodies elicited. Similarly, some haptens may also become inadvertently chemically modified, affecting the immunogenicity of their conjugates with carrier proteins.

Although, peptides with a molecular mass of less than 2000 Da are generally of poor immunogens, some exceptions have been reported; for example, a decapeptide-amide (1275 Da) has been used to raise antibodies reactive to leucosuppressin-like peptides from the central nervous system of cockroach (3). In my own laboratory, antibodies to a synthetic peptide of around 1420 Da representing an allatostatin from the tobacco hornworm *Manduca sexta* have been successfully raised (J. N. Banks, unpublished data).

To summarize, when purifying and handling immunogens, do not use prolonged procedures for isolation of peptides and add inhibitors of proteolytic enzymes if necessary. Use sterile laboratory ware and mild conditions for handling and storage of all immunogens. Avoid chemical modification of susceptible haptens by the use of pure reagents, by excluding oxygen and by careful manipulation.

1.1.3 Haptens and carriers

With hapten–carrier molecule conjugates as immunogens, antibodies have been raised to a wide range of otherwise non-immunogenic substances, including

166

small-molecule compounds such as pharmaceuticals, hormones, toxins, pesticides, etc. (4–6). The immunogenicity of a hapten-carrier and the specificity of the antibodies generated are influenced by the orientations of the haptens relative to carrier, the length of any spacer residue, the substitution ratio, the nature of the carrier, and the conjugation method used. As with steroids and other haptens, studies on peptide conjugates prepared to give different orientations with respect to the carrier molecule, indicate that amino acid residues specific for antibody recognition are generally located near the terminal opposite to the one used for coupling (7).

For the same reasons that are relevant to the preparation of labels (Chapter 4) and solid phase reagents (Chapter 5), the presence of a reactive group in a hapten facilitates chemical conjugation with carrier protein for immunogen synthesis. Haptens without a suitable reactive group may be derivatized to introduce one, or a metabolite with an appropriately located group may be used. Depending on what is required, derivatization may be highly complex and require the skill of a synthetic chemist or may be quite readily accomplished with the aid of a bifunctional reagent (see below and Chapters 4 and 5). The use of metabolites is common with small molecules such as steroids, e.g. the most common immunogen for progesterone contains 11α-hydroxyprogesterone.

Alternatively, haptens 'without' reactive groups may be nonspecifically linked to carrier protein by photo-activation of arylazide-containing linkers, or by formaldehyde condensation (see Section 4.2.4). Such nonspecific methods often result in heterogeneous hapten–carrier conjugates, i.e. a hapten is linked to carrier molecules in more than one orientation. While this may make selection of a monoclonal antibody-producing clone more difficult, and may need another conjugate for screening, the polyclonal antibodies raised are generally more reactive owing to recognition of the hapten in different orientations.

The aqueous solubility of haptens also facilitates coupling with proteins, since conjugation reactions do not work efficiently unless haptens and proteins are dissolved in the same solvent. Most proteins can tolerate some degree of organic solvents, but high solvent ratios usually lead to protein precipitation. To avoid this problem, haptens with little or no aqueous solubility may be dissolved in an organic solvent, and added to the protein solution in appropriate aliquots. The conjugation of hydrophobic haptens to proteins in this way can lead to precipitation of the resulting conjugate, especially if the ratio of hapten to carrier molecules is relatively high. This, however, does not present any problem in immunizations, as insoluble conjugates can be used as immunogens. It has been found that insoluble materials are usually more immunogenic than the soluble ones, because they are more readily engulfed and processed by the antigen-processing cells.

1.2 Animal welfare

Special care also must be taken to avoid injecting anything that may be harmful to the health of the animals, such as pathogens or toxins. Where possible, the

167

use of intact viral particles or microbial cells in immunizations should be avoided and purified antigen preparations or, if appropriate, peptide–carrier conjugates used instead. Preparations containing viral proteins should be treated with nuclease enzymes (RNAase, DNAase) to eliminate the possibility of infectivity. Immunogens with harmful biological activity, such as peptide toxins, must be denatured, partly fragmented or crosslinked to a carrier before use in immunizations (see also Chapter 2).

2 Purification of immunogens

Ideally, a preparation used in immunizations should contain only pure immunogen, and the use of high-purity immunogens may be essential for some applications that require high-affinity, immunogen-specific polyclonal antibodies, such as affinity chromatography and immunohistochemistry. Some impurities may be highly immunogenic, and even in trace amounts could lead to a poly-clonal antiserum with reduced specificity, or decrease the probability of finding a clone secreting a suitable, specific monoclonal antibody. However, for many applications, anti-carrier or anti-contaminant antibodies can be removed by selective precipitation or by immunoaffinity chromatography prior to the use of polyclonal antisera and, with monoclonal antibodies, the extra effort required to screen more clones may be worthwhile.

A wide range of techniques is available for the purification of proteins, pep-tides and other immunogens from any given source (*Table 1*). The design of the purification scheme and choice of each individual method will depend on the physical and chemical properties of the substance to be purified and on its abundance in the particular source. The first stage of a successful approach to purification involves gathering as much information as possible on its chemical nature (peptide, protein, lipoprotein, glycoprotein etc) and physical properties (molecular weight, solubility, hydrophobicity, pI, stability etc). Based on this information, an appropriate purification scheme can be designed. It would be

Table 1. Purification methods commonly used for proteins

Purification method	Separation based on	Protein denatured
Salt fractionation	Changes in salt concentration and pH	No
Electrophoresis		
Nondenaturing gel	Molecular size and charge	No
SDS-PAGE	Molecular size	Yes
Isoelectric focusing	Isoelectric point	No
Chromatography[a]		
Gel filtration	Molecular size	No
Ion exchange	Overall ionic charge	No
Hydrophobic interaction	Hydrophobic interaction	No
Bio-specific affinity	Natural binding site	No

[a] Low- or high-pressure systems (e.g. column, capillary, FPLC, HPLC).

outside the scope of this chapter to discuss the different available techniques and strategies in detail, as suitable manuals with such information are readily available in the *Practical Approach Series* (8–12).

A useful approach to immunizing small animals when only impure antigen is available, is to separate the mixture by PAGE or SDS–PAGE and use the desired 'band' from the gel to elute the antigen in a suitable buffer (see section 3.1 of Chapter 2). The meltable synthetic gel matrix OligoPrep (National Diagnostics) offers a convenient way of isolating protein antigens. The matrix containing the desired band can be solubilized at 60°C. Once melted, the matrix does not re-gel, and can be directly mixed with an adjuvant and used for antibody production.

3 Synthetic and recombinant immunogens

The use of synthetic and recombinant immunogens offers some unparalleled benefits, such as the potential for developing subunit vaccines (13). The potential usefulness to the developer of an immunoassay, however, is dependent on the context in which the assay is being developed. In general, unless such immunogens are of proven efficacy and are commercially available, or unless they can be prepared and used in the context of a much broader programme of research and development (in vaccine development, for example), they may be prohibitively expensive to design, prepare and validate.

3.1 Synthetic peptide immunogens

Developments in peptide synthesis have made it feasible to prepare immunogens containing synthetic peptides that will induce antibodies that bind to proteins containing the same sequences. Thus, if the gene sequence for a protein is known, or if part of the protein has been sequenced (e.g. the *N*-terminal region), it is possible to synthesize an immunogen and to raise antibodies that will bind to that protein, without the need to isolate the native protein itself. However, since only a relatively small subset of partial peptide sequences are capable of representing a sufficiently large portion of potential epitopes ('continuous epitopes'), the choice of a suitable sequence can be very difficult. Many computer-aided methods have been developed to identify sequences with certain 'promising' characteristics, such as hydrophobicity, surface accessibility, secondary structure, etc. (14). Peptides representing the *N*- and/or *C*-terminal segments are often worthy of investigation.

The main advantages of immunogens containing synthetic peptides are their potential purity and, provided that sufficient sequence and structural information is already available on the antigen or its close relatives, the convenience of being able to avoid what may be an arduous purification procedure. The main disadvantage is that, compared with anti-native antibodies, anti-peptide antibodies generally bind with lower affinity to the native protein than antibodies raised against the protein itself. In addition, antibodies raised to very small peptides are generally more crossreactive because smaller peptides are more likely to match randomly with sequences in other proteins.

Unless the synthetic peptide is large enough to be immunogenic, which is uncommon, it must be coupled to a carrier molecule to give an immunogen and then anti-carrier antibodies will be found in polyclonal antisera. This can be prevented by use of a peptide–peptide copolymer as immunogen, without conjugation to a carrier (15, 16), or the immunogen may be prepared with a non-immunogenic carrier, such as modified gelatin or polysaccharides.

The production of anti-carrier antibodies can also be avoided by using a totally synthetic carrier, such as polylysine to give MAPs. A MAP carrier is an immunogenically inert molecule of radially branching lysine residues with α- and ε-amino groups for either synthesis of peptide antigens or subsequent linking of multiple copies of classic solid-phase preformed peptides (17–19). The resulting MAP has a high ratio of peptide antigen, and is generally more immunogenic than the monomeric peptides attached to a carrier protein. The MAP system has been further developed to reduce structural ambiguity (20) and to give a built-in lipophilic adjuvant (21). MAP constructs are also used as antigens for the specific detection of anti-pathogen antibodies. A companion volume *Peptide Antigens: a Practical Approach* (22) is a comprehensive source of information and methods on this subject.

3.2 Recombinant peptide immunogens

Recombinant DNA techniques have made possible the use of polypeptides expressed by cloned genes as immunogens. The use of viral expression vectors, with the exposure of the polypeptide on the virion surface (23), has further boosted the pace of designing effective recombinant immunogens.

Similar to synthetic peptide immunogens, recombinant immunogens have limitations with respect to the availability of preliminary information and the requirement of expertise and resources. In addition, preparations of recombinant proteins must be purified to remove all expression vector proteins and may contain a substantial proportion of improperly folded, denatured or incompletely glycosylated immunogen.

4 Conjugation of haptens and carriers

There are several approaches to chemically linking peptides and other haptens with carrier molecules (22, 24, 25) and most of these are very similar to those used to prepare labels (Chapter 4) and solid-phase reagents (Chapter 5). Consult these chapters for further discussion, protocols that may have useful supplementary information, and explanatory diagrams.

The reactive groups in peptide haptens that are commonly targeted for crosslinking include: primary amines in lysine residues and terminal amino groups, carboxylate groups in aspartic and glutamic acid residues and terminal carboxylic acids, and sulfhydryl group in cysteine side-chains. The same reactive groups are commonly found on nonpeptide haptens and on their derivatives used for conjugation. Crosslinking to hapten can also be carried out nonspecifically, such as by photo-activation of arylazide-containing cross-linkers (Pierce Chemical Company).

For the preparation of label conjugates (Section 3.4 of Chapter 4), a spacer group between the hapten and the carrier is often necessary to allow immunological recognition of the hapten. In immunoassays (e.g. EIA) for haptens that have conjugate labels, the hapten–spacer–enzyme conjugate may be exactly equivalent to hapten–spacer–carrier immunogen (homology) or it may be different (heterology). Small peptides are preferably coupled through the terminal amino acid on the opposite end from which antibodies are desired, and for other haptens the site of linkage may be crucial to the specificity of the antibodies generated and must be chosen carefully.

The reactive groups present in carriers that are used for coupling are most commonly primary amines but sulfhydryls, carbonyls and carboxyls may also be used.

4.1 Materials and reagents

4.1.1 Carriers

The most commonly used carriers are proteins, such as BSA, keyhole limpet haemocyanin, chicken egg albumin, and thyroglobulin. A positively charged form of BSA (cationized-BSA or cBSA, Pierce Chemical Company), with carboxylic acids converted to aminoethylamide groups, is claimed to be more immunogenic than the native form. Because of its net positive charge, cBSA should have a greater affinity for the negatively charged cell surface membrane of the antigen-presenting cells, which leads to efficient uptake, antigen processing and stimulation of helper T-cell (26). Other carriers used for conjugating small peptide haptens include inactivated toxins, such as tetanus toxoid (24), and hepatitis B core antigen (27). Nonprotein carriers include polylysines (MAP), dextrans modified either with oxirane (28), aldehyde, or hydrazide groups (Pierce Chemical Company), amino-modified polysaccharides such as polysaccharine (Bionostics Inc.), nucleic acids, and some resins.

4.1.2 Crosslinking reagents

A wide variety of crosslinking reagents with a choice of reactive groups is commercially available. Homo-bifunctional crosslinkers have two identical reactive ends, whereas hetero-bifunctional linkers have different reactive ends. The suitability of a crosslinking reagent depends on the types of reactive groups in the hapten and carrier molecules. Other factors that must be taken into consideration include the solubility of the hapten, the carrier and the final conjugate, and the effectiveness of the residual linker as a 'spacer' between the hapten and the carrier.

For small-molecule haptens, provision of an appropriate-length spacer is essential to increase exposure, and to provide additional molecular structure for recognition by the immune system. The optimal length of spacer for different hapten–carrier combinations can only be established empirically, and commonly it is about four to six atoms long. When a crosslinking reagent would not by itself separate the linked molecules sufficiently, the hapten is usually derivatized by the addition of a 'bridging group' such a hemisuccinate. This is discussed at greater length in Chapter 4.

The poor solubility of some crosslinkers in aqueous buffers can be overcome by dissolving in a water-miscible organic solvent, such as acetonitrile, ethanol, methanol, DMF or DMSO. The solvent of choice for crosslinking water-insoluble haptens to proteins is DMSO, because it dissolves both polar and nonpolar compounds. The solubility of some haptens in aqueous buffers may similarly be increased by adding appropriate proportion of a water-miscible solvent (e.g. up to 40% DMF or DMSO).

4.2 Methods

4.2.1 Conjugation through carboxyl groups

The commonly used methods to link carboxyl groups in a hapten or carrier to amine groups involve activation by carbodiimides, isobutylchloroformate or cabonyldiimidazole. The carbodiimides react with carboxyl groups to form an unstable O-acetylisourea intermediate, which reacts with amines to form amide bonds. The most commonly used carbodiimide is 1-ethyl-3-(3-dimethylamino-propyl)carbodiimide (EDAC), which does not produce a spacer between the two molecules. The optimum pH for EDAC coupling is between 4.5 and 5. Addition of NHS or sulfo-NHS improves the stability of the intermediate and enhances the yield (29). Excess of EDAC could lead to precipitation of carrier proteins due to intra- or inter-molecular crosslinking. Similar crosslinking could take place between hapten molecules that contain both amino and carboxyl groups, and therefore simultaneous activation and coupling of such haptens is carried out in the presence of carrier protein. Typical coupling reactions with EDAC are described in *Protocol 1*.

Protocol 1

Carbodiimide method

Reagents

- 20 mM hapten solution in a suitable buffer (e.g. 20 mg of a 1000 Da hapten in 1 ml 0.1 M MES buffer, pH 4.7, or in PBS, pH 7.4; for haptens insoluble in water, add up to 40% of a suitable organic solvent such as DMF, DMSO, ethanol or methanol to the buffer before attempting dissolution)

- 1 M EDAC, dissolve 20 mg in 100 μl distilled water
- 0.5 M sulfo-NHS, dissolve 10 mg in 100 μl water (or DMSO for the less soluble NHS)
- 150 μM carrier protein (e.g. 10 mg/ml BSA, 67 000 Da) in the same buffer used for hapten

Protocol 1 continued

A. For haptens that do not contain any amino groups

1. Add 100 μl each of EDAC and NHS (or sulfo-NHS) to 1 ml (20 000 nmol) of hapten solution at a final concentration of 0.1 M and 5 mM, respectively.

2. React at room temperature for 15–20 min.

3. Add up to 450 μl activated hapten (7500 nmol) per ml of protein solution (150 nmol) (i.e. up to 50 × molar excess of activated hapten).

4. Allow to react at room temperature for 2 h.

5. Purify conjugate by gel filtration or dialysis.

B. For haptens that contain both amino and carboxyl groups

1. Mix up to 375 μl (7500 nmol) of hapten in 1 ml (150 nmol) of protein solution (i.e. up to 50 × molar excess of hapten).

2. Add EDAC at a final concentration of 50–100 mM (69–138 μl), and NHS (or sulfo-NHS) at 5 mM (14 μl). Add EDAC in small aliquots and appropriate proportion to avoid protein precipitation.

3. Allow to react at room temperature for 2 h. The reaction can be quenched by addition of excess glycine.

4. Purify conjugate by gel filtration or dialysis.

Carbonyldiimidazole (CDI) reacts with carboxylic acids to form an *N*-acylimidazole intermediate, which reacts with amine groups to form amide bonds without any spacer (*Protocol 2*). CDI also reacts with hydroxyl groups to form imidazolyl carbamate. In this case, reaction with amines introduces a one-carbon spacer between the linked molecules. Owing to rapid hydrolysis of CDI in aqueous media, activation of carboxyl- or hydroxyl-containing haptens is carried out in anhydrous organic solvents. Following CDI-activation, a hapten can be conjugated to carrier protein in a 'non-amine-containing' aqueous buffer of pH between 8 and 10.

The carboxyl groups on hapten molecules can also be activated and coupled

Protocol 2

Carbonydiimazole method

Reagents

- 200 mM stock solution of CDI, dissolve 32 mg in 1 ml of an anhydrous solvent, such as acetone, DMF or DMSO

- 20 mM solution of hydroxyl- or carboxyl-containing hapten in the same solvent (e.g. 10 mg of a hapten of molecular weight 500 in 1 ml of solvent)

- 150 μM carrier protein (e.g. 10 mg/ml BSA, 67 000 Da) in sodium carbonate buffer pH 9.6

Protocol 2 continued

Method

1. Mix equimolar (20 µmol) amounts of CDI (100 µl) and hapten (1 ml) solutions.

2. Incubate at room temperature for 1 h.

3. Add up to 50 × molar excess of CDI-activated hapten (up to 412 µl) dropwise to 1 ml (150 nmol) of protein solution while gently stirring.

4. Allow to react at room temperature for at least 4 h.

5. Purify conjugate by gel filtration or dialysis.

to carrier proteins by a direct and simple method with isobutylchloroformate (*Protocol 3*). The reaction results in conversion of carboxyl groups to acid anhydrides, which react readily with protein amine groups to form amide bonds.

Protocol 3

Isobutylchloroformate (mixed anhydride) method

Reagents

*   150 µM carrier protein (e.g. 10 mg/ml BSA, 67 000 Da) in sodium carbonate buffer pH 9.6. If hapten is not soluble in water, add up to 40% DMF to protein solution before adding the activated hapten

*   20 mM solution of hapten in DMF (e.g. 10 mg of a hapten of molecular weight 500 in 1 ml of DMF)

Method

1. Keep hapten solution cold on ice-ethanol, and add 3 µl triethylamine and 4 µl isobutylchloroformate to 1 ml hapten solution.

2. Mix and allow the reaction to proceed for 10 min.

3. Add up to 50 × molar excess of activated hapten to protein solution (i.e. up to 378 µl of activated hapten per ml of BSA solution) while gently stirring.

4. Allow the reaction to proceed at room temperature for at least 4 h.

5. Purify conjugate by gel filtration or dialysis.

4.2.2 Conjugation through amino groups

Amine groups in haptens, carrier proteins, or both, can be modified for conjugation. A number of homo- and hetero-bifunctional cross linkers with different spacer lengths and amine-reactive end(s) are commercially available (Pierce Chemical Company). The groups reactive to primary or secondary amines include NHS esters, sulfonyl chlorides or imidoesters.

Protocol 4

NHS and sulfo-NHS

Reagents

- 15 μM carrier protein (e.g. 1 mg/ml BSA, 67 000 Da) in PBS pH 7.4
- 10 mM stock solution of hapten (e.g. 10 mg of a 1000 Da hapten) in 1 ml of PBS pH 7.4, or in DMSO
- 20 mM stock solution of EDC, 4 mg in 1 ml water
- 50 mM stock solution of sulfo-NHS, 10 mg in 1 ml water (or if NHS, in DMSO)

Method

1. Add EDC and sulfo-NHS to protein solution at a final concentration of 2 and 5 mM, respectively (i.e. 110 μl of each stock solution per ml of protein solution).

2. React at room temperature for 15–20 min.

3. Purify the activated protein by gel filtration quickly to avoid hydrolysis. Sephadex-25 desalting columns, such as HiTrap (Amersham Pharmacia Biotech), can be used for quick removal of excess linker from the activated protein.

4. Add up to 50 × molar excess of hapten to the activated protein solution, e.g. up to 75 μl (750 nmol) of hapten per ml (15 nmol) of activated BSA solution). Add up to 40% DMSO if the hapten is not soluble in water.

5. Mix and react for at least 2 h at room temperature.

5. Purify conjugate by gel filtration or dialysis.

Imidoesters are acylating agents that react specifically with primary amines at alkaline pH (8–10) to form amidine bonds (*Protocol 5*). The commonly used homo-bifunctional imidoesters for cross linking two amine-containing compounds include DMA, DMP, DMS, and DTBP (Pierce Chemical Company).

Protocol 5

Imidoesters (DMA, DMP, DMS, DTBP)

Reagents

- 200 mM stock solution of the imidoester linker, dissolve 30 mg in 1 ml of an organic solvent (e.g. DMF, DMSO)
- 20 mM solution of the amine-containing hapten (e.g. 10 mg of a 500 Da hapten) in 1 ml 0.1 M sodium borate, pH 8.2 containing 0.2 M triethanolamine
- 30 μM carrier protein (e.g. 2 mg/ml BSA, 67,000 Da) in a buffer which does not contain amines (e.g. 0.1 M sodium borate, pH 8.2).

Protocol 5 continued

Method

1. Mix equimolar amounts (20 μmol) of the linker and the hapten (i.e. 100 μl linker to 1 ml hapten solution) and allow to react at room temperature for 1 h.

2. Add up to 50 × molar excess of the activated hapten to protein solution, e.g. up to 75 μl (1500 nmol) hapten to 1 ml (30 nmol) protein.

3. Allow to react at room temperature on a gentle shaker for at least 4 h (preferably overnight).

4. Purify conjugate by gel filtration or dialysis

The amine groups in two compounds can be coupled using homo-bifunctional reagents such as acid anhydrides (e.g. succinic anhydride), diacid chlorides (e.g. succinyl chloride), or dialdehydes (e.g. gluteraldehyde). By appropriate selection of the reagent, a desired-length spacer can also be provided between the hapten and the carrier molecules. Because of the rapid hydrolysis of acid anhydrides and acid chlorides in aqueous media, activation of amine-containing compounds is carried out in anhydrous solvents, such as acetone or DMSO. The hapten and linker are first reacted in equimolar amounts for about 30 min. The activated hapten is then added, in appropriate molar excess, to the protein solution in a non-amine-containing buffer (pH 8–9). A typical coupling method for conjugating an amine containing hapten and protein using gluteraldehyde is given in *Protocol 6*.

Protocol 6

Gluteraldehyde method

Reagents

- 10% stock solution of gluteraldehyde in a non-amine solvent (e.g. acetone, ethanol, methanol, DMSO)

- 20 mM stock solution of hapten in PBS pH 7.4, or DMSO (e.g. 10 mg of a 500 Da hapten in 1 ml of buffer)

- 30 μM carrier protein (e.g. 2 mg/ml BSA, 67 000 Da) in a buffer which does not contain amines (e.g. sodium carbonate buffer pH 8.5)

Method

1. Add up to 50 × molar excess of hapten to protein solution (i.e. up to 75 μl (1500 nmol) of hapten per ml (30 nmol) of BSA solution). Add up to 40% DMSO if hapten is not soluble in water.

2. Add gluteraldehyde to achieve 0.2–1% final concentration (i.e. 22–110 μl/ml of protein solution) avoiding protein precipitation.

3. Place the reactants on a gentle shaker, and react at 4 °C for at least 2 h.

4. Purify conjugate by gel filtration or dialysis.

4.2.3 Conjugation through sulfhydryl groups

Sulfhydryl groups in hapten or carrier molecules can be selectively targeted to produce conjugates which may be cleavable under controlled conditions. If free sulfhydryl groups are not present on the hapten or the carrier molecules, they can be generated by reduction of disulphide bonds (S–S) with dithiothreitol (DTT) or tris-(2-carboxyethyl)phosphine (TCEP). New sulfhydryl groups can also be introduced (e.g. by thiolating amine groups), if disulphide bonds are not available, or if reduction causes changes in protein conformation. This can be achieved with SPDP followed by reduction with DDT, or by SATA or SATP, followed by removal of acetyl group with 50 mM hydroxylamine (24). The thiolation of amine groups can also be carried out directly using 2-aminothiolane, or introduced by modifying EDC-activated carboxylic acid groups with cystamine, followed by reduction of the disulphide with DTT.

A number of homo- and hetero-bifunctional linkers reactive to sulfhydryl groups are commercially available (Pierce Chemical Company). The most commonly used ones are the hetero-bifunctional linkers reactive to both amine and sulfhydryl groups. The coupling is first carried out with carrier protein through the amine-reactive end of the linker, followed by reaction with the sulfhydryl containing peptide or other haptens.

The sulfhydryl-reactive functional groups include maleimides, haloacetyls alkyl halides, and pyridyl disulphides. Maleimides have specific reactivity to sulfhydryl groups in a pH range 6.5–7.5 and produce thioether linkage which is stable under physiological conditions. Haloacetyls (such as iodoacetyl) also react with sulfhydryl groups at physiological pH to form a stable thioether linkage. Pyridyl disulphides react with sulfhydryl groups to form a cleavable disulfide bond at pH 4–5. A typical coupling procedure is given in *Protocol 7* for hetero-bifunctional crosslinkers which contain one end reactive to amines (e.g. NHS-ester) and the other reactive to sulfhydryl groups (e.g. maleimide, haloacetyl, or pyridyl disulfide):

Protocol 7

Cross linkers with sulfhydryl reactive groups

Reagents

- 150 μM carrier protein (e.g. 10 mg/ml BSA, 67 000 Da) in PBS pH 7.4
- 20 mM stock solution of the linker, dissolve 20 μmol in 1 ml of the same buffer, or in DMSO
- 20 mM stock solution of hapten in PBS pH 7.4, or DMSO (e.g. 10 mg of a 500 Da hapten in 1 ml buffer)

Method

1. Add up to 375 μl (7500 nmol) of the linker to 1 ml (150 nmol) of protein solution (i.e. 50 × molar excess of the linker), mix and incubate at room temperature for at least 2 h.

Protocol 7 continued

2. Quickly remove the unincorporated linker by gel filtration using a Sephadex-25 desalting column (such as HiTrap, Amersham Pharmacia Biotech).

3. Add the sulfhydryl-containing hapten in 10–20 × molar excess to the activated protein solution (75–150 μl/ml of protein).

4. Incubate for at least another 4–6 h (or preferably overnight).

5. Purify conjugate by gel filtration or dialysis.

4.2.4 Conjugation with other crosslinkers

Haptens without any reactive functional group can be linked to carrier molecules through nonselective coupling. The presence of certain groups on hapten molecules (e.g. electron-donating groups on aromatic rings, ketones, esters or phenols) makes some carbon atoms 'active', and hydrogens at these positions replaceable to form new bonds when condensed with formaldehyde and an amine (Mannich reaction), or when reacted with a photoreactive linker. A number of hetero-bifunctional crosslinkers are commercially available which contain one end that is reactive to a specific group, such as amine or sulfhydryl, and an arylazide (e.g. phenyl azide) group on the other end which can be activated by short-wave UV light to react nonspecifically with haptens. On photolysis, the arylazides form very reactive nitrene intermediates which react nonselectively with molecules in close proximity to form bonds involving active hydrogens. There is also some evidence to suggest that the photolysed intermediates react preferentially with nucleophilic groups, especially amines (24). In our laboratory, we have successfully used sulfo-HSAB, an amine- and photo-reactive bifunctional linker (Pierce Chemical Company) to produce immunogens for a number of small-molecule compounds. Another example of a photoreactive crosslinker is APG (Pierce Chemical Company) which has one end that is selectively reactive to the guanidium side-chain of arginine. These cross-linkers are first reacted with selective groups of carrier protein under dark room conditions to avoid degradation of the phenylazide group. After removal of the unconjugated linker, activation of the phenylazide end is carried out under short-wave UV light to link to the desired hapten. A typical coupling scheme using sulfo-HSAB or APG is given in *Protocol 8*.

The hydrogen atoms at 'active' carbon positions in a hapten molecule can also be replaced in nonselective conjugation to carrier molecules by reagents such as diazonium compounds or formaldehyde. The latter reaction, termed 'Mannich condensation', is a convenient way of producing conjugates of haptens without an easily-reactive functional group by condensation of active hydrogens with primary or secondary amines of a carrier molecule (*Protocol 9*). The nonselective nature of this reaction may lead to extensive inter- and intra-molecular cross-linking in proteins, which can be minimized by using the cationized form of the carrier protein (e.g. cationized BSA, Pierce Chemical Company).

Protocol 8

Hetero-bifunctional crosslinkers with the photoreactive phenylazide group

Reagents

- 30 μM carrier protein (e.g. 2 mg/ml BSA, 67 000 Da) in PBS pH 7.4
- 2 mg/ml stock solution of the photoreactive linker (e.g. sulfo-HSAB or APG) in PBS (avoid exposing to light)
- 20 mM stock solution of hapten in PBS pH 7.4, or DMSO (e.g. 10 mg of a 500 Da hapten in 1 ml of buffer)

Method

1. Under dark room conditions, add 20–50 molar excess of the linker to protein solution (up to 150 μl APG, or 275 μl sulfo-HSAB/ml of protein solution), mix and incubate for 1–2 h at room temperature.

2. Under dark room conditions, remove the unreacted linker by gel-filtration (e.g. D-Salt column, Pierce, or PD10 column, Amersham Pharmacia Biotech).

3. Add 50–100 × molar excess of hapten to the linker-activated protein solution and mix.

4. Expose the reactants to short wave UV light (265–275 nm) for 10 min.

5. Purify conjugate by gel filtration or dialysis.

Protocol 9

Mannich condensation

Reagents

- 10 mg/ml cationized BSA (Pierce Chemical Company) in 0.1 M MES, 0.15 M NaCl, pH 4.7 (coupling buffer)
- 37% formaldehyde solution in water
- 10 mg/ml hapten which contains active hydrogen in coupling buffer, or in ethanol if hapten is insoluble in water

Method

1. Mix 200 μl each of protein and hapten solutions and add 50 μl of 37% formaldehyde solution.

2. Allow to react at 37–57 °C for 2–24 h.

3. Remove unincorporated hapten and formaldehyde by gel filtration or dialysis.

4.3 Characterization of hapten immunogens

In general, the effects of a conjugation procedure can be empirically assessed by means of nondenaturing agarose gel electrophoresis. A change in the rate of migration of a conjugate band, in comparison with the carrier band, or a change in the direction of migration due to a change in the overall charge will indicate success in the procedure, provided, of course, that such changes correspond to those expected (30). However, the standardization of hapten–carrier conjugates requires a more accurate estimation of the ratio of conjugation. For relatively large 'hapten' molecules and/or when the incorporation ratio is sufficiently large, this can be roughly estimated by resolution of relative sizes of the conjugate and unconjugated carrier by SDS-PAGE. Spectral differences in the absorption of UV or visible light by a hapten compared with the carrier, can also be used to estimate the ratio of conjugation (Chapter 4).

Another method widely used for conjugates prepared through protein amine groups, involves assay of the total number of free amine groups. The molar ratio of conjugation would be equal to the difference in free amine groups in the unconjugated carrier and the conjugate. Such estimations, however, are not suitable for peptides or other haptens containing additional amine groups. A method for determining free amine groups (adapted from references 31 and 32) is given in *Protocol 10*.

Protocol 10

Determination of conjugation ratio by estimation of free amine groups

Reagents

- 0.2 M sodium hydroxide, 0.8 g in 100 ml distilled water
- 7.2 mg/ml TNBS (2, 4, 6-trinitrobenzenesulphonic acid) in water
- 2 mg/ml solutions of unconjugated protein, and purified conjugate in 0.1 M sodium acetate, pH 4.7

Method

1. Pipette out 200 µl of protein and conjugate solutions (in triplicate) in separate test tubes or disposable cuvettes. Use similar amount of 0.1 M sodium acetate buffer in a separate cuvette to be used as blank.
2. Add 200 µl of 0.1 M sodium borate buffer pH 9.5 to each cuvette and mix.
3. Add 50 µl of 0.2 M sodium hydroxide to each cuvette and mix.
4. Add 50 µl TNBS solution to each cuvette, mix, and incubate at room temperature for 2–16 h.
5. Add 2.5 ml of distilled water to each tube, and read absorbance at 367 nm.
6. The difference in absorbance obtained with conjugate and unconjugated protein can be used to calculate the ratio of conjugation ($\varepsilon_{367\,nm} = 1.1 \times 10^4\,M^{-1}.cm^{-1}$).

For conjugates prepared via the sulfhydryl groups, determination of the remaining number of free sulfhydryl groups can provide an estimate of the conjugation ratio (see also *Protocol 9* of Chapter 4). The following method (adapted from ref. 24) can be used to determine the number of free sulfhydryl groups in a protein. The molar ratio of conjugation would be equal to the difference in free sulfhydryl groups in the unconjugated carrier and the conjugate.

Protocol 11

Determination of conjugation ratio by estimation of free sulfhydryl groups

Reagents

- 4 mg/ml stock solution of Ellman's reagent (5,5'-dithiobis-(2-nitrobenzoic acid)), in 0.1 M sodium phosphate pH 8
- 2 mM (3.5 mg/ml) cysteine standard and 1:1 dilutions down to 0.125 mM in 0.1 M sodium phosphate pH 8

- 1–10 mg/ml carrier protein (unconjugated) in 0.1 M sodium phosphate pH 8
- 1–10 mg/ml purified conjugate in 0.1 M sodium phosphate pH 8

Method

1. Pipette out 10–100 μl of protein and purified conjugate in separate wells of a microtitre plate (in triplicate). Set aside separate wells for use as blank.

2. Add 0.1 M sodium phosphate pH 8 to make up the total volume to 210 μl in each well.

3. Add 20 μl of Ellman's reagent to each well.

4. Incubate at room temperature for 15 min, and measure absorbance at 410 nm using a microplate reader.

5. The difference in absorbance obtained with conjugate and unconjugated protein can be used to calculate the ratio of conjugation ($\varepsilon_{412 \text{ nm}} = 1.36 \times 10^4 \text{ M}^{-1}.\text{cm}^{-1}$). More accurate quantification can be achieved from the linear range of a standard line obtained with cysteine standards.

A method described by Tsao *et al.* (33) for estimation of the ratio of synthetic peptides coupled to carrier proteins is based on amino acid analysis, and uses a marker amino acid, α-aminobutyric acid, included in the sequence during peptide synthesis. The amino acid analysis of an hydrolysate of the conjugate may be used to estimate coupling ratio of peptide to carrier protein. Provided that it was absent from the carrier molecule, any natural amino acid could just as easily be used as a marker.

Other more powerful techniques that have been used to characterize conjugates include MALDI and LC-ESI. These techniques have been compared by Adamczyk *et al.* (34), who showed that while SDS–PAGE was more useful in detecting protein crosslinking, MALDI–MS and LC-ESI–MS gave comparable qualitative results.

There is no optimum ratio to which a hapten may be conjugated to a carrier. For good antibody titre, a ratio of between eight and 25 molecules of hapten per carrier molecule is considered adequate, although conjugates with a hapten ratio of as low as two have also been successfully used (35). The only real test of immunogen quality, however, is a demonstration that it is capable of easily inducing antibodies with the desired characteristics.

5 Storage of immunogens

Being commonly and largely proteinaceous in nature, the storage of immunogens should be done with the care devoted to proteins in general. Long-term storage above 0°C can lead to deterioration due to microbial contamination; handling of samples in sterile containers, filtering through microfilters, and adding a suitable preservative such as 0.05% sodium azide prior to storage, should minimize this risk. However, a better temperature for the storage of pure or semi-pure immunogen preparations is −20°C in an appropriate buffer containing up to 50% ethylene glycol or glycerol. Some conjugate stabilizers, which contain buffered antifreeze for use at −20°C (such as SuperFreeze, Pierce Chemical Company) are available.

With impure immunogen preparations, the presence of certain contaminants, such as proteases, can lead to deterioration unless special precautions are taken. Addition of a suitable protease inhibitor can ensure protection of immunogens during isolation and storage, and may also enhance immunogenicity by inhibiting certain proteases in serum and in the lysosomal/endosomal compartment of cells (36, 37). The most commonly used inhibitors are metal chelators, such as EDTA or EGTA at a concentration of 5–10 mM. Addition of a serine protease inhibitor, e.g. PMSF at a concentration of 50–100 μM, and a cysteine protease inhibitor, e.g. leupeptin hemisulfate, at a concentration of 10–100 μM may also provide protection against proteolysis during handling and storage of immunogen preparations. Protease inhibitor 'cocktails' are also available from Calbiochem (see also Section 5 of Chapter 4).

6 Standards

Standards are essential for the calibration of assays. In its crudest form (often entirely appropriate when a new analyte is in question) a standard may be just a designated serum sample, batch of culture broth or tissue extract to which other samples are compared. Preferably, standards contain precisely and accurately known amounts of pure, homogenous analyte and are also available in a matrix that perfectly suits the assay and the samples to be assayed. Apart from their use for standard curves, standards are also needed for the preparation or authentication of control samples, and for assay development, optimization and validation. In many fundamental and essential respects, an assay can only be as good as its standards.

Standards fall broadly into two groups, those that can be exactly defined chemically (organic compounds, synthetic peptides and nucleic acids), and those that cannot be so defined (proteins, especially large glycoproteins and complex carbohydrates). Certified reference standards are normally available for all common analytes in the first group, while the second group can be further split into the well-studied (analytes of major clinical importance) and relatively poorly studied analytes. Reference standards for some of the well-studied complex analytes may also be available; for example, WHO standards have been used in comparing performance of different assays, and in the validation of working standards of a variety of analytes, including vaccines (38–40), hormones (41–44), growth factors (45, 46), cytokines (REFS) and cancer markers (47) (48, 49).

The best methods to be used for the preparation and validation of good quality standard for a new analyte would be dependent on its availability in reasonable quantity, on its chemical and biological properties, and on how well these are understood. For chemically definable compounds, a high-resolution chromatographic method, perhaps coupled to mass spectrometry, would be the method of choice to establish concentration and purity. For biologically active proteins, one must start by empirical standardization in terms of units of biological activity per mg of protein. 'Biological activity' would be measured by an *in vivo* or *in vitro* bioassay, perhaps that used to discover the new analyte and a suitable assay would be used to determine the total concentration of proteins. The amount of protein is determined from a standard line obtained with known amounts of a protein (e.g. BSA). The most commonly used protein assays include Coomassie blue (50), bicinchoninic acid (51) and Lowry (52) (an improved Lowry assay is available from the Pierce Chemical Company). These assays are very sensitive and can be used to determine accurately protein concentrations down to few μg/ml. More accurate quantification of reference standard preparations of proteins can be achieved by amino acid analysis (53).

Many efforts have been made to achieve uniform standardization for immunologicals world-wide to avoid discrepancies in results obtained by tests carried out at different laboratories. The WHO has published guidelines for preparation and characterization of International Standards (IS) and other reference reagents for biological substances (54). The developments in standardization of biological substances have been reviewed (55–57), and preparation of ISs for various immunologicals has been published (58–61). Many immunological standards may be obtained from the NIBSC for use in calibration of other working standards (56).

References

1. Arnon, R. and Geiger, B. (1977). In *Immunochemistry: an advanced textbook* (eds L. E. Glynn and M. W. Steward), p. 307. Wiley-Interscience, New York.

2. Weir, D. M., Herzenberg, L. A., Blackwell, C., and Herzenberg, L. A. (eds) (1986). *Handbook of experimental immunology, vol. 1: immunochemistry.* Blackwell Scientific Publications, Oxford.

3. Meola, S. M., Wright, M. S., Holman, G. M., and Thompson, J. M. (1991). *Neurochem. Res.* **16**, 543.

4. Sherry, J. P. (1992). *Crit. Rev. Anal. Chem.* **23**, 217.

5. Nelson, J. O., Karu, A. E. and Wong, R. B. (ed.) (1995). *ACS Symposium Series*, **586**. American Chemical Society, Washington DC.

6. Skerritt, J. H.; Lee, N. (1996). In *ACS Symposium Series*, **621** (ed. R. C. Beier and L. H. Stanker), p. 124, American Chemical Society, Washington DC.

7. Schaaper, W. M. M., Lankhof, H., Puijk, W. C., and Meloen, R. H. (1989). *Molec. Immunol.* **26**, 81.

8. Hames, B. D. and Rickwood, D. (ed.) (1984). *Gel electrophoresis of proteins: a practical approach.* IRL Press, Oxford.

9. Harris, E. L.V. and Angal, S. (eds) (1989). *Protein purification methods: a practical approach.* IRL Press, Oxford.

10. Harris, E. L.V. and Angal, S. (eds) (1990). *Protein purification applications: a practical approach.* IRL Press, Oxford.

11. Lim, C. K. (ed.) (1986). *HPLC of small-molecules: a practical approach.* IRL Press, Oxford.

12. Oliver, R. W. A. (ed.) (1989). *HPLC of macromolecules a practical approach.* IRL Press, Oxford.

13. Ertl-Hildegund, C. J. and Xiang, Z. (1996). *J. Immunol.* **156**, 3579.

14. Pellequer, J.-L., Westhof, E., and van Regenmortel, M. H. V. (1994). In *Peptide antigens: a practical approach* (ed. G. B. Wisdom), p. 7. IRL Press, Oxford.

15. Jolivet, M., Lise, L., Gras-Masse, H., Tartar, A., Audibert, F., and Chedid, L. (1990). *Vaccine* **8**, 35.

16. James, M. A., Montenegro-James, S. and Fajfar-Whetstone, C. (1993). *Parasitol. Res.* **79**, 501.

17. Posnett, D. N., McGrath, H., and Tam, J. P. (1988). *J. Biol. Chem.* **263**, 1719.

18. Tam, J. P. (1988). *Proc. Natl. Acad. Sci. USA* **85**, 5409.

19. Herrera, M. A., De-Plata, C., Gonzalez, J. M., Corradin, G., and Herrera, S. (1994). *Mem. Inst. Oswaldo Cruz Rio de Janeiro* **89**, 71.

20. Lu, Y-A., Clavijo, P., Galantino, M., Shen, Z-Y., Liu, W., and Tam, J. P. (1991). *Molec. Immunol.* **28**, 623.

21. Huang, W., Nardelli, B., and Tam, J. P. (1994). *Molec. Immunol.* **31**, 1191.

22. Wisdom, G. B. (ed.) (1994). *Peptide antigens: a practical approach.* IRL Press, Oxford.

23. Minenkova, O. O., Il'ichev, A. A., Kishchenko, G. P., Il'icheva, T. N., Khripin, Y. L., Oreshkova, S. F., and Petrenko, V. A. (1993). *Mol. Biol. (Moscow)* **27**, 561.

24. Hermanson, G. T. (1996). *Bioconjugate Techniques.* Academic Press, San Diego.

25. Aslam, M. and Dent, A. (1997). *Bioconjugation.* Macmillan, London.

26. Apple, R. J., Domen, P. L., Muckerheide, A., and Michael, J. G. (1988). *J. Immunol.*, **140**, 3290.

27. Loktev, V. B., Ilyichev, A. A., Eroshkin, A. M., Karpenko, L. I., Pokrovsky, A. G., Pereboev, A. V., Svyatchenko, V. A., Ignat'ev, G. M., Smolina, M. I., Melamed, N. V., Lebedeva, C. D., and Sandakhchiev, L. S. (1996). *J. Biotechnol.* **44**, 129.

28. Bocher, M., Giersch, T., and Schmid, R. D. (1992). *J. Immunol. Methods* **151**, 1.

29. Staros, J. V., Wright, R. W., and Swingle, D. M. (1986). *Anal. Biochem.* **156**, 220.

30. Kamps-Holtzapple, C., Carlin, R. J., Sheffield, C., Kubena, L., Stanker, L. and Deloach, J. R. (1993). *J. Immunol. Methods* **164**, 245.

31. Habeeb, A. F. S. A. (1966). *Analyt. Biochem.*, **14**, 328.

32. Plapp, B. V., Moore, S., and Stein, W. H. (1971). *J. Biol. Chem.* **246**, 939.

33. Tsao, J., Lin, X., Lackaldn, H., Tous, G., Wu, Y., and Stein, S. (1991), *Anal. Biochem.* **197**, 137.
34. Adamczyk, M., Gebler, J. C., and Mattingly, P. G. (1996). *Bioconjug. Chem.* **7**, 475.
35. Erlanger, B. F. (1980). In *Methods in Enzymology* (eds J. J. Langone and H. V. Vunakis), Vol 70, p. 85. Academic Press, San Diego.
36. Falo, L. D., Colarusso L. J., Benacerraf, B., and Rock, K. L. (1992). *Proc. Natl. Acad. Sci. USA* **89**, 8347.
37. Vidard, L., Rock, K. L., and Benacerraf, B. (1991). *J. Immunol.* **147**, 1786.
38. Diaz, A. M. O., Miller, R. A., Cortes, M. A., Dellepiane, N., Elberger, D., Fabrega, F., Miceli, G., Mendoza, G., and Obarrio, M. E. (1990). *Biologicals* **18**, 281.
39. Lyng, J., Bentzon, M. W., Ferguson, M., and Fitzgerald, E. A. (1992). *Biologicals* **20**, 301.
40. Lin, C. P., Chen, T-L., Yang, R-I., Chen, C-J., and Hsieh, J-T. (1993). *J. Food Drug Anal.* **1**, 3.
41. Bristow, A. F. Gaines-Das, R. Jeffcoate, S. L., and Schulster, D. (1995). *Growth Regul.* **5**, 133.
42. Robbins, D. C., Andersen, L., Bowsher, R., Chance, R., Dinesen, B., Frank, B., Gingerich, R., Goldstein, D., Widemeyer, H-M., Haffner, S., Hales, C. N., Jarett, L., Polonsky, K., Porte, D., Skyler, J., Webb, G., and Gallagher, K. (1996). *Diabetes* **45**, 242.
43. Rose, M. P. (1998). *Clin. Chim. Acta* **273**, 103.
44. Rose, M. P. and Gaines-Das, R. E. (1998). *J. Endocrinol.* **158**, 97.
45. Pestka, S. and Meager, A. (1997). *J. Interferon Cytokine Res.* **17**, S9.
46. Krakauer, T. (1998). *J. Immunol. Methods* **219**, 161.
47. Robinson, C. J. (1998). *Fresenius J. Anal. Chem.* **360**, 476.
48. Meager, A. and Das, R. E.G. (1994). *J. Immunol. Methods* **170**, 1.
49. Brawer, M. K., Bankson, D. D., Haver, V. M., and Petteway, J. C. (1997). *Prostate* **30**, 269.
50. Bradford, M. M. (1976). *Anal. Biochem.* **72**, 248.
51. Smith, P. K., Krohn, R. I., Hermanson, G. T., Mallia, A. K., Gartner, F. H., Provenzano, M. D., Fujimoto, E. K., Goeke, N. M., Olson, B. J., and Klenk, D. C. (1985). *Anal. Biochem.* **150**, 76.
52. Lowry, O. H., Rosenborough, N. I., Farr, A. L., and Randall, R. J. (1951). *J. Biol. Chem.* **193**, 265.
53. Sittampalam, G. S., Ellis, R. M., Miner, D. J., Rickard, E. C., and Clodfelter, D. K. (1988), *J. Assoc. Off. Anal. Chem.* **71**, 833.
54. World Health Organisation (1990). *WHO technical report series 800.* World Health Organisation, Geneva.
55. Jeffcoate, S. L. (1992). In *Developments in biological standardization, vol. 74. Biological product freeze-drying and formulation; symposium* (eds J. C. May and F. Brown), p. 195. S. Karger Ag, New York.
56. Thorpe, R. (1998). *J. Immunol. Methods* **216**, 93.
57. Saldanha, J. (1998). *Biologicals* **26**, 115.
58. Anonymous (1998). *Revue Scientifique et Technique Office International des Epizooties.* **17**, 600.
59. Castle, P. (1998). *Rev. Sci. Techn. Off. Int. Epizoot.* **17**, 585.
60. Wright, P. F. (1998). *Rev. Sci. Techn. Off. Int. Epizoot.* **17**, 527.
61. Wright, P. F., Tounkara, K., Lelenta, M. and Jeggo, M. H. (1997). *Rev. Sci. Techn. Off. Int. Epizoot.* **16**, 824.

Chapter 7
Optimization

Eric Ezan and Jacques Grassi

CEA, Service de Pharmacologie et d'Immunologie, CE-Saclay 91191 Gif-sur-Yvette, France

1 Introduction

The ultimate goal of immunoassay optimization is to satisfy previously determined criteria of accuracy and precision along with the achievement of adequate sensitivity and practicability. All of these four basic characteristics must be kept in mind at all three stages of assay development:

1. Choice of assay format and reagents,

2. Setting assay conditions (optimization),

3. Validation, including application to biological samples.

Assay practicability and precision are mainly determined by technological components such as assay format, the method used to separate bound and free forms, and whether or not analyte is extracted from the sample before being analysed. Assay sensitivity is largely determined by reagent characteristics (tracer specific activity and antibody affinity) and by assay conditions (reagent concentrations, time and temperature of incubation). Finally, accuracy relies on antibody specificity, calibration, and on sample matrix interference being eliminated.

In this chapter we focus on the optimization of sensitivity by the study of the influence of reagent concentrations and general assay conditions on the lower limit of detection, and on the optimization of accuracy by the study of factors that interfere with the specific immunological reactions.

2 Sensitivity

2.1 Estimators of sensitivity

For a given assay and set of reagents, the optimization of assay sensitivity is a compromise (or balance) between the ratios of reagent concentrations and the errors associated with signal measurement. In competitive assays, the lower the concentrations of antibody and tracer, the better the sensitivity (i.e. the lower the detection limit), since the analyte 'competes' more effectively when reagent concentrations are low. However, low reagent concentrations give low signals with high variability. In noncompetitive (reagent excess) assays, increased labelled antibody concentration facilitates analyte detection but may also contribute to high nonspecific binding and signal variability.

Sensitivity may be defined as the limit of detection or quantification, or may be estimated from the slope of the dose–response curve or from a precision profile. A well-accepted estimator is the lower limit of detection (LLD) which is defined as the smallest concentration of antigen giving a signal that can be distinguished from that obtained in the absence of antigen (1). The LLD has a precise statistical meaning and corresponds to the concentration which gives a signal (S_{LLD}) such that:

$$S_{LLD} = S_0 + ts \sqrt{\frac{1}{n_0} + \frac{1}{n}} \qquad [1]$$

in a noncompetitive assay, or

$$S_{LLD} = S_0 - ts \sqrt{\frac{1}{n} + \frac{1}{n}} \qquad [2]$$

in a competitive assay, where S_0 is the signal obtained in absence of antigen, t is the t-value in the Student's t-test at the 95% confidence level, s is the standard deviation of the signal S_0, n_0 is the number of replicates used for the antigen at the zero concentration, and n is the number of replicates used for the standards or samples.

Since immunoassays are usually performed in two or three replicates, the LLD is often estimated as the concentration that gives a signal $S_0 + 3$ s (noncompetitive assays) or S_0–3 s (noncompetitive assay).

Equations [1] and [2] indicate that, for a given assay, the factors limiting the LLD are the experimental errors that determine the standard deviation of the signal response. These errors are due to variance in signal measurement and reagent manipulation (pipetting, separation of bound and free antigen, washing steps) and can be evaluated in *total* by the estimation of the coefficient of variation (CV) of the signal as measured in the assay, S_0:

$$CV(\%) = \frac{s}{S_0} \times 100 \qquad [3]$$

Errors in reagent distribution are due to the variability of pipetting and usually produce a CV of 1-3%. Errors in signal estimation *alone* depend on the intensity and the nature of the signal and on the quality of the instrument used to record it. In the case of radiotracers, the CV of the count rate is inversely proportional to the number of counts collected (N) and is predicted by the relation:

$$CV_{counts}(\%) = 2\frac{\sqrt{N}}{N} \times 100 \qquad [4]$$

The variability of signal measurement of a radioactive tracer can therefore be compared to that of an enzymatic tracer (*Table 1*). With both signals, the lower

Table 1. Comparison variability in signal measurement for radioactive and enzymatic tracers

Radioactive tracer			Enzymatic tracer		
Moles (10^{-18})	Counts (d.p.m.)[a]	CV (%)[b]	Moles (10^{-18})	Absorbance	CV (%)[c]
20	100	20	20	0.015	3.4
50	250	12	50	0.037	1.1
100	500	9	100	0.075	0.8
200	1000	6.3	200	0.15	0.3
1000	5000	2.8	1000	0.75	0.15
2000	20 000	1.4	2000	1.5	0.15
20 000	100 000	0.6	2670	2	0.6

[a] Based on an iodine-125 label with a specific activity of 2000 Ci/mole

[b] From Equation [4].

[c] Obtained experimentally by colorimetric measurements of alkaline phosphatase in a volume of 0.2 ml (Spectrophotometer Multiskan RC, Labsystems, Eragny, France).

the magnitude of the measurement, the greater the uncertainty. In this example, for the same amount of label measured, the ^{125}I-radioactive signal is less precise than the enzymatic signal provided by alkaline phosphatase and measured colorimetrically. This is also true for other enzymes with even higher specific activities, such as horseradish peroxidase, β-galactosidase or acetylcholinesterase. Therefore, the contribution of measurement error is dependent on both the nature of the label and the intensity of the signal.

With competitive RIA the limit of detection is sometimes estimated by the IC_{90}, the concentration of standard at which the initial binding is decreased by 10%. This is reasonable since the magnitude of the S_0 is usually in the range of 2000–40 000 d.p.m. and leads to a total error (due to both measurement and reagent manipulation) of 3–4%. For noncompetitive IRMA the magnitude of the S_0 corresponds to the nonspecific binding and may vary according to several parameters such as time of measurement, concentration of labelled antibody and the level of nonspecific binding.

Tip

LLD is very sensitive to minor fluctuations in the value of standard deviation and can fluctuate between assays. This requires that the calculations be repeated over a number of different days to establish stability.

Recently, we used a commercial noncompetitive ('sandwich') immunoassay for salmon calcitonin for a pharmacokinetic study in humans. We found that the signal obtained for the zero standard was lower than those for samples not containing the antigen, i.e. obtained before salmon calcitonin administration. These false-positive results indicated that sample interference was present and that the LLD provided by the manufacturer had no meaning in the context of our particular samples.

> ## Tip
>
> Matrix effects caused by the between subject variability in sample components are sources of potential interference and, if not eliminated (which is preferable), should also be taken in account when the LLD is being estimated.

Because of these, and other limitations, the LLD is not a good estimator of assay sensitivity in many assays. Therefore, it is also necessary to estimate immunoassay sensitivity by a limit of quantification that is assessed by measuring assay precision and accuracy. A method for estimating such a limit is described in to *Protocol 1*.

Protocol 1

Estimating the limit of quantification of a competitive immunoassay

Equipment and reagents

- All that is required to perform the assay being optimized
- At least five quality controls samples prepared by spiking analyte-free sample (assay buffer, plasma, serum or tissue extract) with known amounts of analyte at concentrations covering the whole range of assay standards. For example, for a competitive assay the concentrations could be those that give readings at around 10, 20, 30, 50, 70 and 85% of the zero reading, with an additional concentration at tenfold the mid-range of the standard curve. (Analyte-free plasma can be prepared as described in *Protocol 4*.)

Method

1. Test the repeatability by assaying each sample at least fivefold in duplicate, on the same day and in the same run. Estimate from the five mean results obtained for each sample the CV of repeatability.

2. Test the reproducibility and the accuracy by assaying each sample in duplicate on five different days. Estimate from the five mean results obtained for each sample the CV of reproducibility.

3. Estimate the accuracy at each sample concentration by dividing the mean of all the results obtained by the concentration of added analyte and multiplying by 100.

4. Estimate the assay limit of quantification by plotting the accuracy, the CV of re-

Protocol 1 continued

peatability, and the CV of reproducibility against analyte concentration and inter-polating the lowest analyte concentration at acceptable accuracy and variability of repeatability and reproducibility is obtained. Typical values of 85–115% in accuracy and 15–20% in CV of repeatability and reproducibility may be acceptable. (The limits of what is acceptable will depend on the degree of confidence required for the assay.) This is illustrated by the example in *Table 2*.

Table 2. Estimating the limit of quantification of a competitive immunoassay

	Concentration of analyte (pg/ml)					
	10	**20[a]**	**40**	**100**	**400**	**1000**
CV of repeatability (%)	21	**14**	11	7	11	12
CV of reproducibility (%)	26	**19**	8	14	9	18
Accuracy (%)	84	**90**	107	101	93	110

[a] Bold values indicate the column for lowest concentration of analyte that provides CVs of repeatability and reproducibility less than 20% and accuracy in the range of 85–115%.

2.2 Optimization of reagent concentrations

Since antigen–antibody complex formation can be modelled easily by means of equations derived from the law of mass action, various authors have proposed mathematical approaches to immunoassay optimization (2–4). These consider several variables such as antigen and antibody concentrations, the specific activity of the tracer, the equilibrium affinity association constant of the antibody (K_a), errors in signal measurement and nonspecific binding. However, such methods are not often used by immunoanalysts because of a number of fundamental limitations. They are complex and require sophisticated com-putational facilities, they do not easily take into account common features of assays such as that the reactions are often not allowed to reach equilibrium, and information on assay parameters such as specific activity or antibody affinity may not be available. However, if such modelling studies do not always accurately reflect reality, they are useful and can provide a theoretical basis for the experi-mental selection of critical parameters to be studied for each assay format.

2.2.1 Competitive assays

Once the technological parameters (antibody and tracer, assay format, mode of reagent separation etc.) have been selected, the experimental approach to the optimization of the LLD may be commenced by comparing standard curves obtained with different reagent concentrations (*Protocol 2*).

The results of a typical optimization experiment for an enzyme immuno-assay of a peptide are shown in *Table 3*. The assay was performed on microtitre plates coated with a mouse monoclonal antibody specific for rabbit IgG. The tracer consisted of the peptide coupled to acetylcholinesterase and a polyclonal rabbit antiserum was used. The results show that, as expected, total binding was proportional to antibody and tracer concentrations and the ratio of nonspecific binding to total binding was increased as the tracer concentration was raised. The best sensitivity index meeting the predetermined criteria is that in the shaded box (*Table 3B*) and the pair of antibody and tracer concentrations giving this value would thereby have been selected. Alternatively, since an even lower tracer concentration could have met the criteria and given an even lower index, the experiment could have been repeated with adjusted ranges of reagent concentrations.

Protocol 2

Optimization of reagent concentrations for a competitive assay

Equipment and reagents

- All that is required to perform the assay being optimized

Method

1. Establish a standard curve at an antibody dilution (Ab_{ref}) and a tracer concentration ($Tracer_{ref}$) which, combined, give an acceptable level of tracer binding (for example 5000 d.p.m. using a radioactive tracer or 1.00 absorbance units in 1 h for an enzymatic tracer). Interpolate a concentration of analyte (C) that displaces between 20 and 40% of the tracer bound at zero standard.

2. Prepare antibody solutions 4 and 16 times more and less concentrated than Ab_{ref}.

3. Prepare tracer solutions 2.5 and 10 times more and less concentrated than $Tracer_{ref}$.

4. Incubate in duplicate each combination of tracer and antibody dilutions in the absence of analyte, and in the presence of the analyte at concentration C. By omitting antibody (and analyte), estimate nonspecific binding at each tracer concentration.

5. For each tracer and antibody combination, measure the signal in the absence of analyte (B_0), the signal obtained in presence of the analyte (B), and a 'sensitivity index' which is the ratio between the two (B/B_0).

6. Select the acceptable tracer and antibody concentration according to the following criteria:

   - total binding should be at a level that minimizes errors in measurements (e.g. > 0.4, see *Table 1*)

   - nonspecific binding should be < 5% of the total binding, as it has been shown that lower levels have in many cases only a small influence on the limit of detection (3).

7. From these selected 'pairs' of tracer and antibody concentrations identify the optimal one which provides the minimal 'sensitivity index'.

8. If needed, repeat steps 1–7 with different antibody and/or tracer.

Table 3. Experimental optimization of a competitive enzyme immunoassay. Bold values indicate optimal binding (absorbance values for total binding $\geqslant$ 0.4 absorbance unit) and underlined values indicate optimal ratios of nonspecific binding (below 5% of total binding)

Concentration of tracer (nM)	Inverse antibody dilution ($\times 10^{-3}$)					
	10	**40**	**160**	**640**	**2560**	**NSB**[b]
	A. Total and nonspecific binding					
5	**2.298**[a]	**1.593**	**1.328**	**1.16**	**0.833**	0.471
2	**1.962**	**1.426**	**1.215**	**0.733**	**0.402**	0.193
0.4	**<u>1.528</u>**[c]	**0.915**	**0.816**	**0.544**	**0.225**	0.052
0.1	**<u>0.703</u>**	**<u>0.646</u>**	**<u>0.436</u>**	0.202	0.088	0.019
	B. Sensitivity indices (B/B_0) at 1 ng analyte per ml					
5	**1.01**	**0.98**	**1.02**	**0.99**	0.95	
2	**0.98**	**1.00**	**0.97**	**0.81**	0.96	
0.4	**<u>0.92</u>**	**0.87**	**0.82**	**0.70**	0.56	
0.1	**<u>0.75</u>**	**<u>0.72</u>**	**<u>0.68</u>**[d]	0.65	0.48	

[a] Optical absorbance units after a 1-h incubation of bound tracer with the substrate values $\geqslant$ 0.4 in bold.

[b] Nonspecific binding obtained in absence of the antibody.

[c] Values for which absorbance $\geqslant$ 0.4 *and* NSB < 5%.

[d] This has lowest 'sensitivity index' for conditions satisfying the criteria of optimal binding and optimal nonspecific binding

2.2.2 Noncompetitive assays

Noncompetitive immunoassays can be experimentally optimized by means of a scheme similar to that of *Protocol 2*. However, compared with competitive assays, the number of parameters to be tested may be larger and the importance of reducing nonspecific binding is so great that preliminary studies with this as an objective should be carried out. These may be concerned with:

- the chemical nature of the solid phase (Sections 1.2 and 3 of Chapter 5),
- the nature of the incubation buffer, and
- the nature of washing steps (buffer, number and procedure),
- the nature and quantity of blocking proteins for nonspecific adsorption sites (Section 2.5 of Chapter 5).

However, the above variables may also affect the antibody–antigen interactions, and other preliminary (or subsequent) optimization experiments should be used to check that the conditions chosen also suit the assay as a whole. The main parameters to be tested in the optimization protocol should include:

- the coating concentration of the capture antibody,
- the concentration of tracer antibody,
- simultaneous, as opposed to sequential, addition of antigen and tracer antibody (one- or two-step procedures) and
- swapping the roles of the pair of antibodies being tested and alternate pairs of antibodies.

Finally, the criteria used for the selection of suitable or optimal parameters are the percentage of nonspecific binding (as low as possible and preferably below 0.1%), and the 'sensitivity index' i.e. the ratio between the signal of a known antigen concentration and the signal for the nonspecific binding (as high as possible).

A potential phenomenon that also should be taken in consideration, is the 'high-dose hook effect', i.e. a decrease in signal at high concentrations of analyte. This mainly occurs in one step-assays (antigen and tracer antibody are added to the capture antibody simultaneously as opposed to sequentially) when the antigen saturates both capture and label antibodies. Obviously, this causes higher concentration samples to generate signals appropriate to lower concentration samples and, when it occurs, must be treated seriously.

Therefore, for all assays, once the general assays parameters have been set (see also Section 2.3), an experiment should be done to give a standard curve with a range of standard concentrations covering at least four orders of magnitude, such as 1 pg to 10 ng. Clearly, the levels and range chosen should be relevant to the purpose to which the assay is to be applied. If a hook effect is observed with a one-step assay it may be necessary to shift to a two step procedure. However, the effect arises most often when true reagent excess has not been achieved and higher purity antibodies or higher quality solid-phase and tracer reagents may cure it. In some two-step assays, hook effects caused by steric hindrance or by the removal of antigen bound to low-affinity sites also occur.

Statistical approaches can be used if the number of parameters to study is large. This is not unlikely as x variables tested at n levels require the exploration of x^n conditions. This may be solved by the fractional factorial design of optimization, whereby the effect that a given variable has on the observed response of a process can be evaluated. The value of this approach has been demonstrated for the optimization of the detection of monoclonal antibodies to the nicotinic acetylcholine receptor (5).

2.3 Optimization of physicochemical parameters

Antibody–antigen interactions occur because of molecular forces including van de Waal's interactions, hydrophobic interactions, hydrogen bonding and electrostatic forces, all of which are affected by temperature and pH.

The contributions of enthalpy and entropy in the binding of binding proteins or antibodies to ligands such as steroids or peptides have been studied (6). It was shown, for example, that steroid binding to transport protein was more favourable at 37°C than at 4°C, whereas binding to antibody was not affected by temperature. Experimental methods for determining the thermodynamic parameters of antigen–antibody reactions have also been proposed (7).

As with the mathematical modelling of the optimization of the LLD, the modelling of environmental influences on the different forces participating in the recognition of antigen by antibody is very complex, and an empirical approach to determining an optimal assay condition such as temperature is required (*Protocol 3*).

However, independently of its effects on the specific immunological reaction, increasing temperature may lead to deterioration of analyte or of reagents, or to sample matrix components having deleterious effects. Some antigens such as peptides or proteins are particularly susceptible to the action of proteases and, although antigen–antibody affinity is sometimes better at 20 or 37 °C, it may be preferable to optimize an assay at 4 °C in order to avoid *in vitro* analyte metabolism during the immunological reaction. The binding of many low molecular weight antigens to other plasma components can also be activated at high temperature.

Protocol 3

Optimization of assay incubation time and temperature

Equipment and reagents

- All that is required to perform the assay being optimized

Method

1. Investigate antigen stability, and the potential effects of sample matrix components, experimentally or by a literature survey. In cases when potential difficulties are identified, limit the investigation to lower temperatures and/or consider the introduction of a preliminary sample extraction step.

2. Choose a range of temperatures and incubation times. With a competitive assay, include incubation procedures where addition of the tracer is delayed after pre-incubation of the analyte and the antibody. With a noncompetitive assay include one- and two-step incubations.

3. Run a standard curve at each combination of conditions, and measure the IC_{50}, (i.e. the concentration of antigen displacing 50% of the initial tracer binding, or giving about 50% of maximum binding for a noncompetitive assay) for each curve.

4. Select the time, temperature and procedure providing the best IC_{50}.

This protocol is illustrated by an example for a competitive immunoassay for a peptide (*Table 4*). The final incubation time chosen often represents a compromise between the IC_{50} and the 'optimal' length of the assay. In this example, a total incubation time of 24 h at 20 °C without delayed addition of the trace was chosen because the desired IC_{50} was as near 40 pg/ml as possible, the analyte was stable at 20 °C and a longer incubation was impracticable.

A similar approach may be undertaken for optimizing the pH of the assay buffer and reagents (incubation pH). Although the optimal pH for antigen–antibody affinity varies between 5 and 8.5, if the assay is to be performed without extraction it is usually recommendable in practice to choose a pH close to that of the sample matrix.

Table 4. Effect of time and temperature on sensitivity of an enzyme immunoassay

Temperature (°C)	Time of total incubation (h)	Time of pre-incubation[a] (h)	Total signal[b] (mAU)	IC_{50} (pg/ml)
4	24	0	180	160
4	48	0	300	105
4	72	0	410	95
4	48	24	150	65
4	72	48	140	70
22	24	0	530	60
22	48	0	830	50
22	72	0	1020	45
22	48	24	430	30
22	72	48	440	25

[a]Time of preincubation of analyte and antibody before addition of the tracer.

[b]Absorbance unit after 3 h of incubation of the enzymatic tracer with the substrate.

3 Accuracy

3.1 Factors affecting accuracy

Accuracy expresses the closeness between the true value and the observed value. A difficulty arises in assessing accuracy when the true value is not a priori known. Alternative biological or physicochemical methods for measuring the analyte, if available, can be used provided that they have satisfied the basic criteria of validation and cover the same range of concentrations. As an alternative, and for some analytes, existing immunoassays allow comparisons with the method in development. However, the literature is rich in examples of the absence of correlation between immunoassays for various types of analytes, such as steroids (8), drugs (9–11), cancer markers (12), cytokines (13) or gonadotrophins (14). When the true value is not known, the best one can do is to identify and eliminate, in so far as this can be done (and shown to be done), all factors which may lead to assay inaccuracy.

Accuracy may be affected by systematic errors that can occur at various levels and their possible existence should be taken into consideration at each level (i.e. preparation of calibrators, manipulation of the samples, sample matrix effects and technological variability).

We find that the preparation of the calibrators used for standard curves is an important potential source of assay bias. Hapten primary standards are usually obtained in liquid solution, or are prepared in-house at a concentration of, say, 100 µg/ml. They are then diluted 10^5–10^8-fold to obtain concentrations in the ng/ml to pg/ml range. For many proteins, and hydrophobic compounds in particular, nonspecific binding to vessels and to pipette tips can be important areas of loss.

As an example, during the recent development of a RIA for a hydrophobic peptide, we found that sequential dilutions of the standard in a phosphate buffer introduced a 50% loss of peptide at each dilution step. This was subsequently reduced to 5% by the addition of protein (0.5% BSA) to the buffer and completely prevented by the simultaneous addition of detergent (0.5% Tween-20 or Triton X-100). See also Section 6 of Chapter 6.

> ## Tip
>
> Only reliable and recently calibrated pipettes and dilutors must be used for the preparation of calibrators, and the integrity of the solutions of analyte should be tested at all dilution steps.

The most diverse and erratic causes of inaccuracy are factors present in the samples being analysed that disturb the antigen–antibody reactions. Such interference has been divided into that caused by exogenous factors and that caused by endogenous factors. Typically, exogenous factors correspond to substances added to the sample (anticoagulant, separating gels, etc.) or arise owing to poor conditions of storage (instability of the analyte, nonspecific binding to vessels, etc.). Endogenous factors are those present in the biological samples and include crossreacting substances, binding proteins, heterophilic antibodies, auto-antibodies against the analyte, rheumatoid factors or plasma lipids and salts. This interference, whether endogenous or exogenous, may affect any of the participating partners in an immunological binding reaction, or the equilibrium between the partners, or the detection of the assay endpoint (*Figure 1*).

In general, the identification and evaluation of interference is a difficult task since it is often highly variable between samples. Some sources of interference recur regularly and deserve special attention since they are perhaps the main source of assay inaccuracy. These are discussed in the subsequent sections.

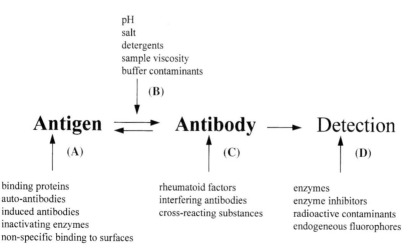

Figure 1. Immunoassay interference affecting the antigen (A), the antigen-antibody equilibrium (B), the antibody (C) or the detection of the label (D).

Immunoassay quality control and standardization are concerned with all factors affecting accuracy and precision. Efforts to make improvements in the immunoassays used in clinical diagnoses have led to the implementation of rigorous laboratory quality control procedures and external quality assessment schemes (13, 14), which are discussed in Chapter 10.

3.2 Technological variables

Any of a wide range of technological variables may be responsible for in-accuracy, but many of these will be specific to the assay format in question. Therefore, the assay developer must be constantly on the look out for such problems and should design experiments to test accuracy whenever a type or source of inaccuracy is suspected or possible.

In any assay that involves the analysis of large batches of samples, positional effects are always possible. For example, 'edge effects' are a common potential source of problems in immunoassays performed on 96-wells microtitre plates. They are tested for by running the same sample in all wells of a plate and, if an edge effect is present, the magnitude of the signal will vary along the rows and columns of the plate to give an overall pattern that is not random. A typical severe example is shown *Figure 2*, where a pronounced 'column effect' that stretches systematically across the whole plate is evident. The importance of such problems is very often underestimated and *all* assays should be carefully checked for positional and edge effects by tests like that of *Figure 2* and by including quality control samples at various positions in the batch of unknown samples or on the microtitre plate.

Any one (or any combination) of a range of phenomena may be at the origin of edge and positional effects. Common causes include:

* uneven induction of static electricity during plate manipulation;
* uneven temperature across plate during incubations steps;
* slow additions of samples or reagents combined with short incubations;

	1	2	3	4	5	6	7	8	9	10	11	12
A	456	464	475	483	491	499	515	523	531	539	547	555
B	458	461	488	496	490	501	509	517	531	539	547	555
C	465	473	481	489	497	505	521	529	528	555	533	572
D	485	493	499	499	498	506	514	521	529	556	561	534
E	487	495	492	496	494	485	493	501	509	525	528	541
F	488	496	492	498	491	498	506	500	504	512	519	551
G	476	484	492	475	493	491	499	507	500	512	533	563
H	477	485	493	495	496	499	498	508	512	519	550	559

Figure 2. Variability across a microtitre plate for a competitive enzyme immunoassay for a peptide. The microtitre wells were indirectly coated (via an anti-rabbit IgG mouse monoclonal antibody) with a rabbit IgG specific for the peptide, and each well was exposed to fixed concentrations of the peptide and the peptide coupled to an enzyme. The 'cells' of the table have been shaded to emphasize the pattern of variability of absorbance $\times$ 1000: no shading < 500, light shading 500–530 and dark shading > 530.

- additions of samples and reagents in different orders and at widely different rates;
- instability of a reagent during distribution
- uneven plate shaking;
- problems of technological standardization (malfunctioning plate washer or plate reader).

In many cases, we have found that avoiding plates having to warm up or cool down during the overall assay protocol has been effective. This can be done by adjusting the temperatures for reagent distribution and the temperatures of incubations or, most simply, by running the entire assay at room temperature. The omission of plate shaking during the incubation and enzyme assay steps was also beneficial in some instances. For problems linked to static electricity, the use of a static discharge pad has been shown to be effective (15).

3.3 Crossreactive compounds

The degree of interference by a crossreactant is dependent on three factors: antibody specificity, assay format and sample preparation.

Antibody specificity is estimated by cross-reactivity measurement, i.e. to which extent an analogue compound may be recognized in the assay. For competitive immunoassays, the traditional procedure for calculating crossreactivity is the 50% displacement method which consists of comparing the dose of analyte and substances tested necessary to displace 50% of bound tracer (16). However, and since crossreactant 'standard' curves may not be parallel to that of analyte, different schemes have been proposed for evaluating crossreactivity. Miller and Valdes (17) reviewed five different methods proposed in the literature and suggested building an 'interferometer' in which the bias is calculated for all combinations of analyte and crossreacting substances.

Whatever the method employed, the crossreactivity should always be carefully examined in a biological context, since compounds which are only slightly recognized by the antibodies will significantly affect assay accuracy if they are present in samples at high concentration. For example, it has been demonstrated that phosphodiesterase inhibitors commonly used in the investigation of cyclic AMP-mediated signal transduction, although recognized to only a low extent by cAMP antibodies, were responsible for an apparent accumulation of cyclic AMP in culture supernatant (18). In this case, the effect of the interference was eliminated by using culture medium, treated exactly like experimental samples, as matrix for preparation of the standard curve and dilution of the samples.

Another example concerns opiates such as morphine or hydromorphine which are extensively metabolised in humans to give hydroxyl and glucuronide derivatives. Although these compounds crossreact only to a few per cent, their concentrations in samples are about 500-fold higher than the parent drug. Therefore, a 'direct' assay procedure was found to be not specific enough and a selective extraction step was included in the assay (19). Unexpected interference from crossreacting substances is also found in therapeutic drug monitoring when multi-medication of patients is done with closely related drugs (20).

These examples emphasize that there is no common solution for all immuno-assays since each situation has its own complexity owing to the pattern of anti-body specificity and the concentrations of analogous endogenous compounds or metabolites present in the samples. However, in many cases modulation of assay specificity is possible and numerous specific assays have been developed with insufficiently specific antibodies. Among solutions that can be adapted to many situations, we may cite selective extraction (21–25), chromatography by HPLC or affinity (26–30), sample transformation (20, 31), immune exclusion (32, 33), coupling to mass spectrometry (34), or modulation of assay temperature or pH (25, 35, 36).

Antibody and assay specificity is also discussed in the context of raising and choosing antibodies in Chapters 2 and 3 and in relation to assay validation in Chapter 8.

3.3 Plasma-binding proteins

Both endogenous compounds and drugs in plasma may be bound to a greater or lesser extent (but often highly variably from patient to patient) to other plasma proteins such albumin, lipoproteins or α-1-acid glycoprotein. This may significantly interfere with the accuracy of an assay, especially if the analyte in its bound form is not recognized by an assay antibody. In the interest of user convenience, most immunoassay kits do not have a preliminary solvent extraction step or other procedure to remove such interference. Rather, an attempt is made to minimize such effects, often by means of standard solutions prepared in a matrix that 'mimics' average sample composition. However, since plasma protein concentrations vary from one subject to another, and even during the day in the same subject, the reference plasma used for standards preparation (for example, pooled drug-free plasma from medical centres) cannot be representative of all samples. This may lead to false results, especially when the sample is not diluted in the reference plasma prior analysis.

Therefore, the incidence of these types of interference needs to be quantified, for example by means of a procedure such as that in *Protocol 4*. By this approach, the variability of tracer binding to the antibody in the presence of different analyte-free plasma samples is estimated, and then this variability is tested by examining how accuracy and variability are affected when the same set of plasma samples are spiked with a known concentration of analyte.

In planning and executing *Protocol 4*, it is important that the panel of samples used be as representative as possible of the samples to be routinely assayed. If it was necessary to use charcoal-treated samples, it should also be kept in mind that this is a very crude procedure that removes most low molecular weight molecules and much more, so that the value of the exercise is greatly reduced. Finally, while the overall degree of variability is important, the incidence of any interference detected and the magnitudes of the effects with individual samples may also be of great importance.

Protocol 4

Estimating the incidence of plasma components that interfere in a direct competitive immunoassay

Equipment and reagents

- All that is required to perform the assay being investigated
- Obtain 5 ml plasma samples from 20–30 different subjects that do not contain the analyte to be tested. For assays of endogenous hormones, etc., if representative samples cannot be obtained directly (e.g. male samples for some female reproductive hormones), they may be prepared as described below. For a drug assay, samples from patients not receiving the drug are suitable.

Preparation of analyte-free plasma samples

1. Add 50 mg of activated charcoal (Norit-A or Norit-GSX charcoal, Aldrich) to 1 ml of plasma.

2. Incubate for 20 h at 20 °C with continuous mixing.

3. Centrifuge 20 min at 20 000.

4. Decant carefully the supernatant and store at −20 °C. Residual charcoal may be eliminated from the supernatant by filtration through a 0.22 or 0.45 μm Millipore filter.

Sample screening

1. To each of the analyte-free plasma samples in duplicate, add tracer and antibody exactly as for the assay in normal operation, and continue until the endpoints have been read.

2. Estimate the variability of the duplicate means. The CV should be less than 10%.

3. Spike a 1 ml aliquot of each sample to give a concentration that corresponds to two- to three-fold the LLD of the assay.

4. Also assay in duplicate each of the spiked samples with standards diluted with the buffer or plasma pool being evaluated.

5. Calculate the mean[a] recovery for each spiked sample and estimate the between sample variability[b].

[a] Also, examine the degree to which any interference detected correlates with high and low readings detected in the initial survey of effects on tracer–antibody binding (Step 1). A high degree of correlation would indicate that the same factors are involved.

[b] The mean recovery should be 100 ± 15% and the variability should be within the normal intra-assay coefficient of variability for the assay in question (i.e. 5–10%).

As an example, we recently assessed the extent and consequences of the variability of a matrix effect on the accuracy of an in-house immunoassay for nomegestrol acetate, an artificial progesterone agonist (25, 37). Twenty-five plasma samples from different subjects were tested. As above, each sample was assessed for the presence of interfering factors, but with a standard curve made with the usual standard reference plasma. We measured the recovery for each sample twice: after spiking with a concentration corresponding to the central part of the standard curve (which did not require pre-dilution), and at a high concentration which required at least a tenfold dilution with reference plasma (*Table 5*).

Table 5. Recovery[a] (%) of analyte added to drug-free plasma from different subjects

Subject	Low analyte concentration[b]	High analyte concentration[c]
1	75	74
2	97	90
3	91	109
4	140	138
5	46	59
6	55	107
7	129	109
8	182	147
9	87	95
10	81	75
11	89	85
12	215	135
13	52	97
14	39	101
15	47	116
16	66	131
17	98	99
18	65	105
19	68	117
20	71	101
21	86	81
22	98	94
23	51	102
24	196	114
25	89	88
Mean (%)	92.5	102.8
CV(%)	50.4	20.3

[a] Recovery is expressed as the ratio of measured concentration/expected concentration.

[b] Undiluted before assay.

[c] Diluted tenfold before assay.

For the low concentrations, although the mean accuracy was close to 100% (92.5%), the variability was enormous (50.4%). Interestingly, a good inverse correlation was found when recovery for low concentration samples was plotted against the percentage of tracer–antibody binding (not shown) in drug-free plasma. For the high concentrations of analyte the variability in the recovery was lower (20.4%) due to the effect of the dilution and no correlation was found.

To check whether this variability was common to other immunoassays, we measured variability in tracer–antibody binding for 13 different drugs measured in our laboratory. Tests were performed in plasma free of analyte and the results show that inter-subject variability was in the range 3–27% (37).

Therefore, the presence and incidence of such effects should be assessed for all analytes, especially if the assay is to be performed without a preliminary extraction step. If the use of *Protocol 4* indicates the existence of a problem, alternative solutions should be tested (some of which have drawbacks):

1. Improve the sensitivity of the assay by choosing another antibody or tracer or by optimizing more thoroughly the assay conditions (Section 2.2)

2. Reduce the interference by pre-diluting the samples. Disadvantage: a much lower LLD may be needed.

3. For each subject, assay samples with a standard curve prepared in analyte-free plasma from the same subject. Disadvantage: this makes the assay cumbersome and can only be applied to drug assay, where it is possible to obtain reliably representative plasma.

4. Use specific inhibitors of the binding of the analyte to plasma protein (25, 38–40). Disadvantage: this approach is generally used in steroids immuno-assays but has not proven wholly satisfactory. For other analytes it also may be difficult to find any inhibitors.

5. Develop an extraction procedure to remove nonspecific plasma components. Disadvantages: assay complexity and time are increased and accurate correction for analyte lost during extraction is necessary.

3.4 Anti-Ig antibodies

3.4.1. Origins

Following the development of sandwich (or immunometric) assays, problems due to the presence in test samples of anti-immunoglobulin (anti-Ig) antibodies became apparent. Anti-Ig antibodies interfere with assays by forming complexes with the reagent antibodies obtained from experimental animals. This phenomenon is complex and affects all types of immunoassays (41–43) and the culprits are variously referred to as 'heterophilic antibodies', 'polyspecific antibodies', human anti-mouse antibodies (HAMA) or 'rheumatoid factors'.

The diversity of mechanisms producing anti-Ig antibodies and the general nature of certain anti-Ig antibodies (food-derived anti-Ig, anti-idiotypes) suggest that anti-Ig antibodies may be present in all blood samples. Their effects on assay accuracy will depend on the kind of antibodies used in the assay.

3.4.2. Mechanisms of interference

Different types of interference may arise, depending on the kind of assay used, according to the nature and concentration of the heterophilic antibodies (*Figure 3*).

When the interference results in overestimation of the antigen concentration, we speak of 'positive interference' and, correspondingly, underestimation is said to be caused by 'negative interference'. In the positive interference observed in two-site immunometric assays, the anti-Ig antibodies often simultaneously recognize the capture antibody (immobilized on the solid phase) and the tracer antibody, and form a 'bridge' between the two, thus mimicking the role of analyte. Positive interference is the best known and most frequently described effect of anti-Ig in the literature.

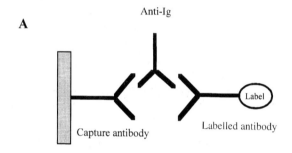

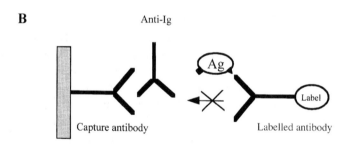

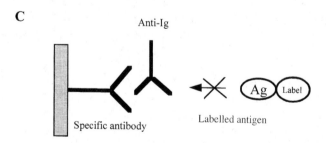

Figure 3. Mechanism of positive (A) and negative (B) interference observed with noncompetitive immunoassays and positive interference (C) observed with competitive immunoassays.

Although less frequent, negative interference is also seen in two-site immuno-metric assays (41, 44, 45). This is notably the case when the anti-Ig antibodies recognize either the capture antibody or the tracer antibody and when they are directed against the idiotope, preventing antigen binding by steric hindrance.

The interference potentially generated by anti-Ig antibodies in competitive assays is often overlooked, even by assay kit manufacturers, but it can be just as conspicuous. Competitive assays essentially suffer from positive interference, when anti-Ig bind to the specific antibody and prevent binding to tracer by steric hindrance.

3.4.3. Demonstrating interference

We have been confronted by the problems posed by anti-Ig antibodies in our development of assays for interleukins (ILs) in plasma and synovial fluid from patients with rheumatoid diseases. These assays involve the use of a pair of mouse monoclonal antibodies, one immobilized on a solid phase (96-well microtitre plate), the other labelled with acetylcholinesterase (Fab'-AChE conjugates) (44, 45). We used the assays to seek evidence for variations in IL1α concentration in relation to their supposed role in the aetiology of rheumatoid diseases. Initial measurements revealed much higher average levels in disease-affected individuals than in normal individuals. In order to demonstrate the specificity of the assay, we developed several procedures to show the degree to which immunoreactivity was due to false-positive responses. One procedure that provided satisfactory results was to fractionate positive samples through a molecular sieve (open columns or HPLC) and measure the immunoreactivity of each fraction. The system was calibrated with the analyte and the elution times (molecular weights) of all 'active' components were determined. This allowed immunoreactive fractions to be related to antigen, IgG and/or IgM.

3.4.4. Overcoming interference

Approaches to the elimination the interference by anti-Ig, whether IgG or IgM, include the following.

3.4.4.1 Choice of antibodies

The severity and incidence of interference can be modulated through the choice of capture antibody and tracer antibody, as illustrated by the results recorded with a large number of different 'assays', each with a different pair of anti-IL1α monoclonal antibodies (*Table 5*). With each 'assay' solid-phase immobilization of the tracer antibody was measured in 88 plasma samples and, since we had demonstrated the absence of IL1α in all of these samples by molecular sieve chromatography, all sample readings for which signal was twice the nonspecific binding were considered to be false positive.

Although pairs of antibodies that bind to identical or overlapping epitopes (homologous or noncomplementary antibodies) are theoretically unable to detect IL1α, such pairs gave as many false-positive results as complementary pairs. This confirms that for all pairs the 'positive' results were due to anti-Ig

Table 6. Frequency of false-positive interference as a function of the antibody pairs used[a].

Group	Capture antibody	Subclass	False-positive (%) tracer α29	False-positive (%) tracer α176
A	α29	IgG1	**72**	22
	α184	IgG1	<u>64</u>	13
	α230	IgG1	<u>32</u>	13
	α25	IgG1	<u>30</u>	22
	α100	IgG2	<u>30</u>	16
B	α185	IgG1	30	<u>18</u>
	α18	IgG1	36	<u>27</u>
	α2159	IgG1	33	<u>22</u>
	α153	IgG1	32	<u>58</u>
	α176	IgG2	30	**100**
	α50	IgG2	26	<u>58</u>
C	α101	IgG1	35	15

[a] Eighty-eight human 'normal' plasma samples were tested and it was assumed that the test samples contained no ILs, as demonstrated by a molecular-sieve chromatography experiment. Measurements were made using a one-step protocol (simultaneous addition of plasma and tracer, immunological reaction: 18 h, 4°C), with Fab'–AChE conjugates and without addition of nonimmune mouse immunoglobulins to the assay medium. We tested 24 pairs of antibodies using 12 different capture antibodies and two tracer antibodies (α29 and α176). To understand the significance of these results it should be realised that the anti-IL1α antibodies fall into three 'complementarity groups' (A, B and C). Antibodies of a given group recognize identical or over-lapping epitopes and therefore cannot bind simultaneously to IL1α. Conversely, their binding is compatible with that of the antibodies of the two other groups. Antibody pairs comprising a capture antibody and a tracer antibody of the same complementarity group (underlined) are by definition unable to detect IL1α. Most pairs comprise two different antibodies (heterologous pairs). Two pairs comprise the same antibody as capture antibody and tracer antibody (homologous pairs, indicated in bold type).

antibodies and not IL1α. Interference was not significantly lower with pairs of antibodies from different subclasses (IgG1/IgG2). It is striking that the greatest interference is noted with pairs of homologous antibodies (72 and 100% for antibodies α29 and α176, respectively). As already suggested (41), the use of homologous pairs provides a good way of characterizing the particular susceptibility of an antibody to anti-Ig.

These tests were done with antibodies raised in the same mouse strain. Some of the pairs tested were even raised in a single mouse. Clearly, the observed variations are not related to the allotype of these antibodies. Furthermore, in these experiments Fab' conjugates were used as tracer and most anti-allotype antibodies would not be detected. It can therefore be concluded that the observed variations are due to anti-isotype or anti-idiotype antibodies.

We finally chose the pair α185 as capture antibody and α29 as tracer antibody because they gave a much lower LLD than other less susceptible combinations. Therefore, we needed to find additional ways to further reduce this interference.

Interference occurs with polyclonal antibodies as well as with monoclonal antibodies, and depends on the species used to raise the antibodies employed in the assay. For a 'normal' population, we found anti-Ig antibodies directed against numerous species, with a marked predominance of anti-bovine immuno-globulins and to a lesser degree anti-rabbit immunoglobulins. At present, it is not possible to state whether this between-species polyspecificity reflects a varied diet or rather the polyspecific nature of certain types of anti-Ig antibody.

3.4.4.2 Selective extraction of the antigen

A highly effective way of abolishing interference is to purify the test sample partly or completely, e.g. by selective precipitation, thereby separating the molecules to be assayed from the anti-Ig antibodies (46). However, while effective, this approach may render an assay considerably more labour-intensive.

3.4.4.3 Blocking with neutralizing antibodies

The most common approach to reducing or abolishing interference from anti-Ig antibodies is the addition of excess nonspecific immunoglobulins. The questions remaining are, which type of anti-Ig antibody should be used and at what concentration? Numerous studies have shown that interference from anti-Ig antibodies can be effectively abolished (or at least greatly reduced) by antibodies of the same species as those used in the assay (generally with mouse or rabbit antibodies). There are, however, several reports of greater efficacy with Ig of other species, notably bovine Ig. Clearly, the effect of the nonspecific Ig will depend both on the samples studied (i.e. on the nature of the anti-Ig) and on the characteristics of the assay antibodies. In our IL1α assay, which was used to study individuals affected by rheumatoid diseases, we found that mouse monoclonal antibody of the same subclass as those of the assay was the most effective in neutralizing interference (45). In general, however, it seems preferable to use polyclonal antibodies prepared from normal serum because they would normally be much cheaper and should, theoretically, be better able to neutralize any of a variety of anti-idiotype anti-Ig antibodies.

An Ig concentration ≥ 50 μg/ml seems to be genuinely effective. Irrespective of the approach adopted, it should be remembered that low-level interference may remain unaffected; we have found that the remaining problematic samples usually contain anti-Ig IgM antibodies (45).

3.4.4.4 Addition of reducing agents

Interference from anti-Ig IgM antibodies are the most difficult to abolish and we found that inclusion in the assay of a strong reducing agent able to depolymerize IgM facilitates their neutralization. We thus showed that addition of 0.01 M dithiothreitol very markedly reduced interference due to anti-Ig antibodies (45). This approach has proved useful in our IL assays, but cannot, however, be generally applied since this agent may considerably alter the analytical characteristics of an assay by lowering analyte immunoreactivity

3.4.4.5 Use of antibody fragment for tracer synthesis

To minimize interference from anti-Ig antibodies, it is also worth using antibody fragments (Fab' or F(ab')₂) in the synthesis of tracer or in the preparation of the solid phase. This abolishes interference due to recognition of the Fc fragment. In our hands, this approach has proved effective in IL1 assays and has reduced the frequency and amplitude of interference. The use of tracers with antibody fragments also improves assay sensitivity, in so far as it reduces nonspecific binding (47).

The use of antibody fragments does not, however, completely abolish interference, since we have shown (in our assays at least) that the interference is largely due to recognition of idiotopes carried by the assay antibodies.

3.4.4.6 'Two-step' assay procedures

As we have defined it, positive interference in two-site immunometric assays is due to the simultaneous binding of heterophilic antibodies to the capture antibody and the tracer antibody. This interference will be enhanced in a one-step assay, i.e. simultaneous addition of sample and tracer to the solid phase. It can, therefore, be expected that the frequency and amplitude of the interference may be reduced by means of a two-step protocol, in which the sample alone is first added to the solid phase, and the tracer is added in a second step after washing of the solid phase.

3.4.4.7 Summary

A multifaceted approach is probably necessary if one is to have a good chance of reducing to tolerable levels anti-Ig interference in all samples. Our IL1 assays were applied largely to samples from patients with rheumatoid disease and represent a good test case because such samples, practically by definition, contain anti-Ig antibodies. However, for almost *any* clinical assay some samples will be from such subjects. The final assay had a specially selected pair of antibodies (α185/α29), the tracer had an Fab' fragment, the assay buffer was supplemented with 50 μg/ml mouse IgG and contained 0.01 M dithiothreitol, and a two-step procedure was used (48).

4 Conclusions

Although immunoassays have become the technique of choice in clinical chemistry and in many research areas, the question of their reliability is still a matter of debate.

In the field of pharmacokinetic studies the role of immunoanalysis has become less important in recent years. This is because standard immunoanalytical techniques do not meet the high standards of robustness and specificity required for drug estimations in biological fluids, and physicochemical techniques such as the coupling of liquid chromatography and mass spectrometry are often preferred (49). Despite being expensive and requiring highly qualified personnel, these techniques could become more attractive than immunoanalysis in an increasing number of fields in the near future. Where the analytical specifications are rigorous, immunoassays will be able to compete successfully only if they exhibit maximum accuracy combined with a high level of sensitivity.

Maximum assay sensitivity is obtained by properly adjusting reagent concentrations. In addition, assay sensitivity is often limited by the specific activity and the nonspecific binding of the tracer, and it is likely that the next decade will see the introduction some of the new labels which have been recently proposed in order to improve immunoassay performance (50, 51).

Nevertheless, parallel to these technological advances, clinical, pharmacological and other researchers using immunoassays should continue to regard optimization and the identification and elimination of potential interference as top priorities when developing any immunoassay.

References

1. Rodbard, D. (1978). *Anal. Biochem.* **90,** 1.
2. Jackson, T. M. and Ekins, R. P. (1986). *J. Immunol. Methods* **87,** 13.
3. Ezan, E., Tiberghien, C., and Dray, F. (1991). *Clin. Chem.* **27,** 226.
4. O'Connor, T. and Gosling, J. P. (1997). *J. Immunol. Methods* **208,** 181.
5. Reiken, S. R., van Wie, B. J., Sutisna, H., Kurdikar, D. L., and Davis, W. C. (1994). *J. Immunol. Methods* **177,** 199.
6. Keane, P. M., Walker, W. H. C., Gauldie, J., and Abraham, G. E. (1976). *Clin. Chem.* **32,** 97.
7. Bilek, R., Hampl, R., Putz, Z., and Starka, K. (1987). *J. Steroid Biochem.* **28,** 723.
8. Wheeler, M. J., Shaikh, M., and Jennings, R. D. (1986). *Ann. Clin. Biochem.* **86,** 23.
9. Miller, J. J., Straub, R. W., and Valdes, R. (1994). *Clin. Chem.* **40,** 1898.
10. Laurie, D., Mason, A. J., Pigott, N. H., Rowell, F. J., Seviour, J., Strachan, D., and Tyson, J. D. (1996). *Analyst* **121,** 951.
11. Datta, P., Xu, L., Malik, S., Landicho, D., Ferreri, L., Halverson, K., Roby, P. V., Zebelman, A. M., and Kenny, M. A. (1996). *Clin. Chem.* **42,** 373.
12. Cheli, C. D., Marcus, M., Levine, J., Zhou, Z., Anderson, P. H., Bankson, D. D., Bock, J., Bodin, S., Eisen, C., Senior, M., Scwertz, M. K., Yeung, K. K., and Allerd, W. J. (1998). *Clin. Chem.* **44,** 1551.
13. Mire-Sluis, A. R., Das, R. G., and Thorpe, R. (1997). *J. Immunol. Methods* **200,** 1.
14. Seth, J., Hanning, I., Bacon, R. R.A., and Hunter, W. M. (1989). *Clin. Chim. Acta* **186,** 67.
15. Cassutt K. J. and Pincus S. H. (1998). *Biotechniques* **25,** 801.
16. Abraham, G. E. (1969). *J. Clin. Endocrinol. Metab.* **29,** 866.
17. Miller, J. J. and Valdes, R. (1992). *J. Clin. Immunoassay* **15,** 97.
18. Sinha, B., Semmler, J., Haen, E., Moeller, J., and Endres, S. (1995). *J. Pharmacol. Toxicol. Methods* **34,** 29.
19. Lee, J. W., Pedersen, J. E., Moravetz, T. L., Dzerk, A. M., Mundt, A. D., and Shepard, K. V. (1991). *J. Pharm. Sci.* **80,** 284.
20. Adamczyk, M., Fishpaugh, J. R., Harrington, C. A., Hartter, D. E., Hruska, R. E., and Vanderbilt, A. S. (1993). *Therap. Drug Monitor.* **15,** 4361.
21. Peinhardt, G. (1997). *Pharmazie* **52,** 12.
22. Riutta, A., Nurmi, E., Weber, C., Hansson, G., Vapatalo, H., and Mucha, I. (1994). *Anal. Biochem.* **220,** 351.
23. Oosterkamp, A. J., Irth, H., Heintz, L., Marko-Varga, G., Tjaden, U. R., and van der Greef, J. (1996). *Anal. Chem.* **68,** 4101.

24. Itoh, M., Misaki, A., and Kominami, G. (1983). *Anal. Lett.* **29** 1377.

25. Ezan, E., Morge, X., Lelievre, E., Créminon, C., Piraube, C., and Grognet, J-M. (1993). *Therap. Drug Monitor.* **15,** 488.

26. Wong, F. A., Juzwin, S. J., Tischio, N. S., and Flor, S. C. (1995). *J. Chromatog.* **1851,** 18.

27. Pellegati, M., Braggio, S., Sartori, S., Franceschetti, F., and Bolleli, G. F. (1992). *J. Chromatog.* **105,** 573.

28. Ueno, H., and Matsuo, S. (1991). *J. Chromatog.* **57,** 566.

29. Kramer, P. M., Quing, X. L., Bruce, D., and Hammock, C. (1994); *J. AOAC Int.* **77,** 1275.

30. Lewis, J. G. and Elder, P. A. (1988). *J. Steroid Biochem.* **29,** 191.

31. Earl, R., Sobeski, L, Timko, D., and Markin, R. (1991). *Clin. Chem.* **37,** 1774.

32. Boutten, B., Ezan E., Mamas, S., and Dray, F. (1991). *Clin. Chem.* **37,** 394.

33. Debberg, M., Houssa, P., Frank, B. H., Soddoyez-Goffaux, F., and Sodoyez, J-C. (1998). *Clin. Chem.* **44,** 1504.

34. Nelson, R. W., Krone, J. R., Bieber, A. L., and Williams, P. (1995). *Anal. Chem.;* **67** 1153.

35. Vinning, R. F., Compton, P., and MacGinley, R. (1981). *Clin. Chem.* **27,** 910.

36. Ezan, E., Mamas, S., Rougeot, C., and Dray, F. (1987). In *Handbook of Pharmacology* : (eds Patrono, C. and Beskar, P.), Vol. 82, pp. 143–179, Springer-Verlag, Berlin.

37. Ezan, E., Emmanuel, A., Valente, D., and Grognet, J-M. (1997). *Therap. Drug Monitor.* **19,** 212

38. Malvano, R. (1983). In *Radioimmunoassay of Steroids* (eds Odell, R. P. and Franchimont, P.), pp. 161–181. Lipincott, Philadelphia.

39. Ezan, E., Drieu, K., and Dray, F. (1989). *J. Immunol. Methods* **122,** 291.

40. Ballard, P., Malone, M. D. and Law, B. (1994). *J. Pharm. Biomed. Anal.* **12,** 47

41. Boscato, L. M. M. and Stuart, M. (1988). *Clin. Chem.* **34,** 27.

42. Levinson, S. (1992). *Clin. Biochem.* **25,** 77.

43. Reinsberg, J. and Gast, B. (1994). *Clin. Chem.* **40,** 951.

44. Grassi, J., Frobert, Y., Pradelles, Ph., Chercuite, F., Gruaz, D., Dayer, J-M., and Poubelle, P. (1989). *J. Immunol. Methods* **123,** 193.

45. Grassi, J., Roberge, C. J., Frobert, Y., Pradelles, Ph., and Poubelle P. (1991). *Immunol. Rev.* **119,** 125.

46. Primus, F. J., and Kelly, E. A., Hansen, H. J., and Goldenberg, D. M. (1988). *Clin. Chem.* **34,** 261.

47. Ishikawa, E., Imagawa, M., Hashida, S., Yoshitake, S., Hamaguchi, Y., and Ueno, T. (1983). *J. Immunoassay*, **4,** 209.

48. Grassi, J. (1994). *Immunoanal. Biol. Spéc.* **9,** 124.

49. Mehta, A. C. (1992). *J. Clin. Pharm. Therap.* **17,** 325.

50. Kricka, L. J. (1994). *Clin. Chem.* **40,** 347.

51. Joeger, R. D., Truby, T. M., Hendrickson, E. R., Young, R. M., and Ebersole, C. R. (1995). *Clin. Chem.* **41,** 1371.

Chapter 8
Validation

Peter O'Fegan

National Diagnostic Centre, National University of Ireland Galway, Galway, Ireland

1 Introduction

In the past three decades, RIA systems have diversified to give microtitre plate enzyme-immunoassays, time-resolved immunofluorimetric assays, automated random access immunoanalysers and single-step qualitative immunotests that are usable by members of the general public. To be acceptable to end users, all must be validated and these validation criteria are to a large extent independent of test format. Validation criteria revolve around the key concepts of precision and accuracy.

However, with respect to many important details, how assay validity may be demonstrated depends on the analyte in question and on its chemical nature. When the analyte is available in highly pure form and is chemically definable, a true reference method may be available and the validation procedure may be more rigorous and straight-forward in many respects. However the analyte may be a specific antibody, be biochemically poorly characterized, genetically variable, biologically or chemically glycosylated to various degrees or exist in different forms owing to partial denaturation and partial hydrolysis (e.g. peptide nicking). In many such cases, validation procedures may be peculiar to the kind of analyte in question but they all would adhere to the principles outlined in this chapter.

1.1 Validation in the development cycle

In developing any immunoassay, a broad range of aspects must be considered, such as the choice of antibody, the type of tracer and the type of solid phase, all of which have been discussed in previous chapters. The selection of the various components, the choice of format and the optimization and validation of the procedure all have to be considered each in relation to the others. There is a great deal of overlap and a certain amount of component substitution, re-optimization and re-validation can be expected before a satisfactorily validated assay is achieved. It must be emphasized that for an assay to be officially approved for a commercial application, any change in components or procedure shown to be necessary during validation will usually necessitate complete re-validation of the entire test system.

Prior to commencing a validation study, it is essential to ensure that all equipment to be used is calibrated and that excess supplies of standardized materials are available and stored in single-use quantities. These materials should include real samples, dilution matrix, tracer conjugate, pure standard material, and pure crossreactant materials. All the reagents should be stable on storage and if any are unstable in wet solution, liquid or frozen, they should be freeze-dried. Repeated freezing and thawing of any reagent should be avoided. Strict standards of 'Good Laboratory Practice' should be adhered to throughout (1).

1.2 Validation criteria and analytical goals

Once the desired assay system has been optimized (Chapter 7) the validation study can commence. First, the assay developer must decide how stringent the validation criteria that are to be met must be. The required stringency will be based on the end use of the assay and on the consequent necessity, or not, of meeting criteria set by an established scientific body such as the National Committee for Clinical Laboratory Standards (2–7). In this chapter, we discuss generally applicable validation methods relevant to research applications but, hopefully, the reader will find sufficient guidance to enable as thorough a validation as may be necessary.

The need for objective analytical goals for immunoassays is well recognized and has been reviewed by Fraser (8) with respect to human clinical applications. He concluded that the analytical goal for lack of 'trueness' (bias) should be zero, meaning that the assay should be accurately calibrated and resistant to all potential crossreactants and interferants. Therefore, according to Fraser, the goal for total analytical uncertainty should be based on that for total analytical imprecision. The view that for clinical assays the analytical goal for imprecision should be based on within-individual biological variation is now widely held and the following definition of what is desirable is generally recommended.

$$CV_{analytical} \leq 0.5 \times CV_{individual}$$

Ricos and Arbos (9) calculated analytical goals for a range of hormones on this basis, or, in practice, on half the normal intra-individual coefficient of variation found in samples taken from a cohort of 15 healthy subjects. For example, their goal for serum cortisol is 7.6%, which is realistic according to the imprecision results derived from external quality assessment schemes. Therefore, for many analytes and for whatever the application, a robust method operated by an effective user should contribute only about 10% or less to overall uncertainty.

2 Specificity

A test system with absolute specificity would measure its target analyte and only that compound. No other enantiomer, isomer, metabolite, precursor or any chemically different compound would crossreact or interfere in such an assay. In practice, an assay system may be acceptably specific if it can be demonstrated that no other compound that may occur in the analyte matrix (that is in the samples to be analysed) crossreacts sufficiently to produce a response of a magnitude relevant to the concentrations of analyte being measured. Frequently, an assay is expected to measure any molecule or molecular complex with one or more common attributes, for example all hCG molecules whatever their degree of glycosylation, all antibodies against an antigen whatever their subclass or idiotype, or all strains of a specific pathogen. Therefore, in relation to the validation of an assay, specificity must be assessed in the context of the nature of the analyte, the concentrations to be measured, the samples to be analysed and the purposes of such measurements.

While the most powerful and specific analytical systems have a separation step and a highly selective detection method (e.g. ID–GCMS), the specificity of most immunoassays depends only on the discriminatory power of one or two antibody-binding sites. Although preliminary chromatographic purification or even simple solvent extraction steps can very effectively improve the specificity of some immunoassays, they are no longer feasible in many laboratories, particularly when large numbers of samples must be analysed. However, assay specificity is never exactly equivalent to antibody specificity (Chapter 3). No crossreactivity study for the purpose of validation is analytically valid unless the procedure being validated is carried out with all its preliminary and ancillary steps under conditions that are effectively identical to those to be used for its routine operation.

2.1 Crossreactivity studies

2.1.1 Role and limitations

When a good panel of relevant potential crossreactants is available, a formal survey of specificity is very important to the validation process. It allows comparisons to be made with other assay methods and may give invaluable pointers as to necessary adjustments in the assay procedure or the necessity for replacing the antibody or antibodies used.

However it is important to be aware of the limitations of crossreactivity studies.

1. Precursors and metabolites of the analyte that may occur in normal samples and/or in samples from individuals with a disease or taking medication may be unknown or unavailable in pure form.

2. Small and large molecular mass compounds that are structurally unrelated to the analyte and occur in a greater or lesser number of samples and may crossreact in the procedure are not, and cannot normally be, tested in crossreactivity studies.

3. If the calibration curves for analyte and the crossreactant are not parallel then no single figure or percentage can adequately represent the crossreactivity.

Therefore, probably no panel of potential crossreactants is ever adequate. Even in the case of assays for common steroids for which many close relatives are available to be tested, when interference is encountered, it can rarely if ever be ascribed totally to known crossreactants. Therefore, most of the standard validation tests, other than the formal crossreactivity study, also have essential roles in the evaluation of specificity. For example, if during biological validation higher than normal baseline levels are consistently measured this may be taken to indicate reliably a susceptibility to endogenous crossreactants.

2.1.2 Planning

Of immediate relevance in planning a crossreactivity study is the number and variety of structurally related molecules that are available in pure form. With respect to assays for therapeutic drugs, a range of related variants may be available, and for some steroids the richness of the range of chemical relatives that may be purchased may appear to be quite close to ideal. For some protein analytes such as the glycoprotein hormones (hCG, LH, FSH and TSH), members of the growth hormone family (growth hormone, prolactin, placental lactogen and the insulin-like growth factors), the variety and availability of structurally-related potential crossreactants may also be good.

However, in addition to structural relatedness, other criteria should be applied when making up the list of compounds to be tested. The practical importance of any potential crossreactant is greatly dependent on its maximum concentration relative to the lowest analyte concentrations in the samples to be analysed. For example, a compound crossreacting at only 0.1% relative to analyte but present in a sample at a 1000-fold excess over analyte will contribute equally to the apparent quantity measured. Therefore, all related compounds known to occur in routine samples at high concentrations and available in pure form should also be considered for inclusion. Very low levels of crossreactivity against such structurally unrelated compounds that would not be acceptable may be quite feasible in assays with very short incubation times.

It is impossible to generalize as to what would constitute an adequate number of compounds to be tested. The simplest situation would be if the sample matrix were consistent and highly defined, as in the quantitative analysis of a pharmaceutical in an 'in-process' liquid, because testing the matrix constituents individually or even collectively would be sufficient. For assays of poorly defined analytes such as cancer markers, the best list may include only a few crude preparations of chemically related, alternative cancer markers and some important serum constituents, including haemoglobin, lipids and bilirubin. When, as with many steroids, the ideal list could be long enough to threaten to swallow the entire project budget, guidance may be sought in previously published validations of assays for the same or related compounds. However, comparisons of such studies indicate that the lists used are sometimes haphazard and often err by significant omissions.

Finally, the reliability of estimates of crossreactivity also depends on the purity of the compounds tested and on the accuracy of their concentrations in solution. In any study designed to lead to formal certification, both of these should be ensured by certification and by the use of rigorous operating procedures.

2.1.3 Execution

Crossreactivity may be measured in two ways. Most commonly, while operating the assay procedure as usual, each compound to be tested is substituted for the analyte to give an alternative standard curve over a concentration range that often includes much higher levels than usual. Absence of crossreactivity (0%) is indicated by a reading equivalent to zero standard over the whole range tested. If a test compound gives a curve that is superimposable on the normal standard curve, it has a crossreactivity of 100%. This corresponds to the most common methods for calculating crossreactions and is based on that of Abraham (10). Briefly, the percentage crossreactivity is the concentration of analyte causing a chosen reading in the mid-range of the standard curve divided by the concentration of crossreactant causing exactly the same reading, multiplied by 100 (see also step 4 of *Protocol 1*). When the curves given by analyte and cross-reactant are parallel, the estimate of crossreactivity will be independent of the chosen reading over a wide range of readings.

After selecting the potential crossreactants to be tested, and having decided on the range of concentrations of each to be tested following the general 'Abraham method', the crossreactivity study is carried out as in *Protocol 1*.

Protocol 1

Performing a crossreactivity study on a competitive immunoassay

Preliminary investigations are essential to establish a range of concentrations for each potential crossreactant to be tested. For less strongly reacting compounds of sufficient solubility the highest concentrations tested may be two, three or even four orders of magnitude greater than the normal top standard concentration.

Equipment and reagents

- A panel of potential crossreacting compounds, each dissolved in the matrix solution normally used for the assay standards and each at a suitable range of concentrations that are sufficiently closely spaced to allow accurate curve fitting and interpolation

- Equipment and reagents required for normal operation of the assay under validation

Method

1. Use the same volumes and manipulations for each set of crossreactant concentrations as for the standard curve.

2. When many compounds are to be tested, sort into batches and include a standard curve with each batch.

3. Run each batch per established method and plot data.

Protocol 1 continued

4. For each batch, compare the crossreactant curves with the standard curve and estimate the crossreactivity of each one as follows:

$$\% \text{ Cross reactivity} = \frac{ED_{50} \text{ of standard curve}}{ED_{50} \text{ of cross reactant curve}}$$

5. Tabulate data as per *Table 1*.

Table 1. Tabulation of results from a crossreactivity study on an immunoassay for cortisol

Substance	Crossreactivity (%)	Concentration[a] (nM)	Apparent cortisol concentration (nM)
Cortisol	100	140[b]	140
11-Deoxycortisol	19	1000[c]	190
Deoxycorticosterone	4.8	0.303[d]	0.14
Progesterone	<0.1	660[e]	<0.7
Prednisolone	12.8	1700[f]	218

[a] The concentrations shown are maximum concentrations of the substance in question that may be encountered in patient samples, except for cortisol where the concentration cited is a low concentration that may be commonly encountered.

[b] The low end of the normal AM range (see text).

[c] A concentration that may be encountered during the metyrapone test. The top end of the 0.95-reference interval in healthy persons is 7.25 nM; this may be greatly increased in certain circumstances such as congenital adrenal hyperplasia or stimulation testing.

[d] The top end of the 0.95-reference interval in healthy persons; a greatly increased concentration is found in certain circumstances such as congenital adrenal hyperplasia or stimulation testing.

[e] Maximum concentrations as found during late pregnancy. Maximum concentrations during the luteal phase of the menstrual cycle are 89.4 nM.

[f] In patients being treated with prednisolone.

However, the ability of an antibody to bind a crossreactant relative to the analyte is not just dependent on their relative affinity constants. Frequently in studies involving many compounds, not all of the curves for the crossreactants are parallel to the standard curve. In competitive assays, crossreactivity may also depend on the fraction of the labelled analyte bound, with the effect of a crossreactant being least when the fraction of label bound is high and greatest when most of the label is free (11). Apparent crossreactivity can vary with the concentration of the analyte, the binding affinity and concentration of the crossreactant, and with the binding affinities and concentrations of all other crossreacting substances present. Nevertheless, the Abraham method is generally used for estimating the potential of compounds to crossreact in immunoassays, and the complex studies necessary to evaluate combined crossreactant effects are rarely carried out (12).

While crossreactivity is analysed graphically, it is always reported in tabular form with columns of compound names and percentage crossreactivities. However, Krouwer (13) pointed out that the simple reporting of percentage cross-reactivities for potential crossreactants deviates from many guidelines on crossreactivity testing and suggested that such data be tabulated as is shown in *Table 1*. Here, in addition to each percentage crossreactivity, the expected maximum concentration of the crossreactant and the estimated consequent increase in the apparent analyte concentration are shown. Crossreactivity data presented in this way emphasize the potential consequences of the presence of such substances on apparent analyte concentrations. Such a table should normally be accompanied by adequate footnotes to explain how the maximum concentrations of the crossreactants were estimated and when they may occur. It will clarify whether any of the low-reacting compounds tested may pose problems, or if the crossreactant is known to be present in the samples at low concentration relative to the analyte, it may indicate that a significant degree of crossreactivity would be acceptable. Alternatively, it may be clear from the corresponding footnote that an apparently significant crossreactant (e.g. a drug or a pregnancy hormone) will not be elevated in the sample matrix at any time when samples are likely to be taken.

Another general method for measuring crossreactivity is to test the effect of the presence of a fixed concentration of each potentially interfering substance on the standard curve obtained with the analyte, and to repeat this at a limited number of concentrations (12). This method should be seen as complementary rather than alternative to the Abraham method and should be applied when more detailed investigations are justified or when the results of other validation experiments indicate possible interference from a particular compound, which appeared to crossreact minimally.

3 Precision

The precision of a measurement is the degree of agreement that would be obtained if the measurement were repeated many times in exactly the same way and the replicate measurements compared. The SD and CV of the replicate results represent lack of precision (imprecision). Preliminary evaluations of precision should be carried out early in the development of a test system and, if necessary, measures taken to improve it as imprecision can mask many other serious faults. As stated above (Section 1.2), the general goal for total analytical imprecision (CV) may be as low as about 10% or less.

Data points that are apparently spurious, 'wild', or just 'further away from the mean than usual' (outliers) are of direct relevance at all stages of assay development, but are particularly relevant to discussions of precision. There is a tendency to ignore outliers but, especially if they recur, they merit thorough investigation in order to ascertain why they appear. Often, their incidence can be greatly reduced by giving greater attention to instrument calibration or maintenance, procedural detail or operator performance.

3.1 Materials

It is critical that an excess of stable sample material is obtained, stored in single-use quantities, and is readily available for use throughout the precision study.

Real physiological samples are preferable to lyophilized materials. The concentrations of analyte present should reflect the entire range of the standard curve and commonly this is achieved with just three large-volume samples with high, medium and low concentrations. Provided that the concentrations found in samples and the analytical range of the assay match well, these concentrations should give readings that span most of the standard curve or, in the case of a competitive assay, correspond approximately to B/B0 ratios of 0.2, 0.5 and 0.8. In the case of a qualitative assay, the samples should be grouped around the clinical positive/negative cut-off point of the assay as this is where maximum precision is required. When single samples of sufficient volume are not available, samples may be pooled (and mixed thoroughly) to give the desired sample concentrations.

3.2 Levels of precision

An assay procedure involves many component steps (e.g. weighing, pipetting, separation of bound fraction, absorbance measurement etc.) and, accordingly, total assay imprecision is the sum of the imprecision of all of these steps (a, b, c, etc.), or more exactly:

$$SD_{total} = \sqrt{SD_a^2 + SD_b^2 + SD_c^2 + \ldots}$$

Therefore the precision of each and every step should be maximized by all means available to reduce total imprecision.

Total imprecision may also be regarded as being constituted of three main levels of imprecision, namely: between sample, within-batch precision; within-sample, within-batch precision; and within-sample, between-batch precision. In broader studies, within-sample, between-operator or within-sample, between-laboratory precision may also be of interest and can be estimated separately to evaluate the importance of operator skill and/or durability during transport.

3.2.1 Between-sample, within batch precision

As early as possible in the development process, it is advisable to check full-batch or full-plate variation as a method for estimating positional effects, across-plate drift, 'edge effects' and also for checking the total inherent variability of all the assay steps (*Protocol 2*). The precision of antibody coating separate from some other steps may be checked with the use of a labelled anti-capture antibody.

The causes of assay drift and other positional effects include the sub-optimization of reactions and reagent concentrations, inefficient mixing after reagent additions, temperature variations across racks or plates, and incomplete Ab–Ag reactions owing to too short incubation times or too low incubation temperature. The timing of reagent addition may also be critical and must be consistent throughout the assay run for each assay step, up to and including the addition of stopping reagent (for EIA) and the endpoint reading step. With EIA, the final enzyme assay reaction should be completely inhibited before endpoint determination, and the readings should be stable for a reasonable length of time afterwards (see also Section 3.2 of Chapter 7).

Protocol 2

Estimating within-sample, within-batch precision and assay drift

Equipment and reagents

- Equipment and reagents as required for normal operation of the assay under validation
- Zero standard or high standard

Method

1. Run a full batch (or plate) of zero standards (competitive assay) or of a single high standard (reagent excess assay) following the established procedure. (There is no need for a standard curve.)

2. Plot the readings obtained against the order in which the tubes or wells were processed.[a]

3. Calculate the SD and CV of the readings across the whole batch.[b]

[a] Drift may be quite accurately assessed by eye and, if present, all aspects of the assay procedure must be reviewed, and testing continued until drift is abolished.

[b] If, even in the absence of drift, the CV is unacceptably high ($> 4\%$), all pipetting and dispensing equipment should be tested, the assay procedure reviewed, and testing continued until the level of precision is satisfactory.

For an assay under formal validation, drift can be estimated by repeat determinations of patient or quality control samples at intervals within the batch. It is often not linear and must be eliminated.

3.2.2 Within-sample, within-batch precision

To the end user, this is the most fundamental level of precision and, formally, it is most simply assessed by assaying, all in one batch, 10–20 replicates of the high, medium and low concentration samples just as if they were routine samples. After calculating the mean, SD and CV for each set of replicates, the results may be tabulated, perhaps along with data representing other levels of precision. Performing calculations of the means of duplicate measurements improves, in itself, within-sample, within-batch precision by a factor of $\sqrt{2}$ or 1.414 and, if this is done, it should be made clear.

However, the degree to which precision is dose-dependent is best assessed by constructing precision profiles. Greatest precision is usually observed around the centre point of the standard curve, where, for many assays, it should be no greater than 5–7%. A poor precision profile is convincing proof that all is not well with an assay. Within-sample, within-batch precision profiles are easily generated as per *Protocol 3* or *4* (see also Section 4).

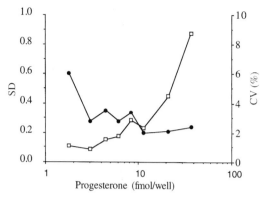

Figure 1. Precision profiles (SD, □ and CV, ●) for an enzyme immunoassay for oestradiol derived from data from routine duplicate determinations of 396 saliva samples. Each point represents data from about 50 samples and the eight concentration ranges covered are 0.8–2.3, 2.3–3.6, 3.6–5.4, 5.4–7.1, 7.1–9.7, 9.7–13.7, 13.7–32.4 and 33.5–40.1 fmol/well.

Protocol 3

Construction of a within-sample, within-batch precision profile by the measurement of selected samples

Equipment and reagents

- A sufficient number of routine samples or sample pools of sufficient volume that have been checked in a preliminary assay run to ensure that the concentrations and their spacing are suitable, and that they reflect the entire range of the standard curve

- Equipment and reagents required for normal operation of the assay under validation

Method

1. Run each sample in the assay at least 20 times, following exactly the established procedure.
2. Calculate the within-sample SD and CV for each individual sample or pool.
3. Plot CV and SD against concentration of analyte. Although the data in *Figure 1* was obtained with *Protocol 4*, the statistics are plotted in the same way.
4. A line drawn parallel to the *x*-axis at a CV judged as being acceptable, e.g. at a value of 7% may help establish the working measurement interval of the assay (see Section 3).

Alternatively, duplicate data from accumulated patient sample results may be used, thus saving reagent and labour costs and reflecting more closely actual routine precision (14).

Table 2. Form of spreadsheet or table used in the construction of a precision profile from accumulated duplicate data

A	B	C	D	E	F	G	H	I
Duplicate 1	Duplicate 2	Mean	Difference (d)	SD	Variance	Averages for duplicate sets		
x_1	x_2	$(x_1 + x_2)/2$	$x_1 - x_2$	$d/\sqrt{2}$	SD^2	'Mean'	'SD'	CV
2.5[a]	1.5	2.0	1.0	0.707	0.50			
3.6	3.0	3.3	0.6	0.424	0.18			
5.0	5.8	5.4	0.8	0.566	0.32			
7.8	7.2	7.6	0.4	0.283	0.08			
8.5	9.5	9.0	1.0	0.707	0.50			

[a] Dummy duplicate data (columns A and B) in order of increasing mean. With a spreadsheet, the data can be entered in any order, the formulae for the calculations on rows C–F entered and all the rows then sorted with reference to the figures in column C.

Protocol 4

Construction of a within-sample, within-batch precision profile from accumulated routine sample results

Requirements

- Individual duplicate results collected at random and without any omissions from routine data sets that were within the normal quality control limits for the assay[a]

- A standard spreadsheet program such as Excel® (Microsoft), or specialized software

Method

1. Select at least a few-hundred pairs of duplicate patient data at random and enter them columns, e.g. in columns A and B of *Table 2*.

2. In the columns C–F enter the calculated duplicate means, duplicate differences (d), SDs (d/$\sqrt{2}$) and variances (SD^2) and sort the six-column data set in order of increasing mean (column C).

3. After surveying the range and distribution of the means, select 5–10 subranges with an adequate ($\approx$ 50 or more) number (N) of data in each set. This may be done on the basis of fixed analyte concentration intervals (e.g. 0.31–0.50, 0.51–0.70 units/l. etc.) but then the number of data per interval may vary widely. Alternatively, fixed numbers of data points can be included in each set, with the interval limits varying in consequence.

4. For each interval set, count the number of points and calculate the average duplicate mean, average duplicate SD and average duplicate CV, where:

$$\text{Mean} = \frac{\Sigma \text{ duplicate mean}}{N},$$

Protocol 4 continued

$$SD = \sqrt{\frac{\Sigma \text{ duplicate variance}}{N - 1}} \text{ and}$$

$$CV = \frac{SD}{\text{mean}} \times 100,$$

and insert the results (opposite the last data points of each set) into columns G–I.

5. For all sets, plot average duplicate CV against average duplicate mean, as in *Figure 1*. Evaluate as in *Protocol 3*.

[a] To obtain reliable statistics for concentration ranges into which few measured levels fall, very large amounts of data will have to be collected and analysed.

3.2.3 Within-sample, between-batch precision

This statistic is normally estimated with internal quality control pools that are placed in each batch to be analysed. The SD and CV for each pool is calculated from the results collected over the required number of batches, each result being the average of duplicate determinations if patient samples are assayed in duplicate. There should normally be three such pools, with concentrations representing low, medium and high, spanning all diagnostically relevant levels.

Protocol 5

Estimation of a within-sample, between-batch precision by analysis of control samples

Equipment and reagents

- Equipment and reagents required for normal operation of assay under validation
- Three samples or sample pools of sufficient volume that are spaced over the range of the standard curve

Method

1. Run each sample in duplicate in the assay at least 10 times, following the established procedure.
2. Calculate the within-sample CV for each individual sample (pool).
3. Calculate the between-batch CV for each individual sample (pool).
4. Record and tabulate results.

4 Sensitivity

The working measurement interval of an assay may be defined as the range of analyte concentrations over which the within-sample, within-batch CV is less than a specified value, and the lowest concentration in this range may be regarded as the functional sensitivity of the assay. Davies (12) advocates the use of functional sensitivity as a true measure of sensitivity in an assay system.

However, no clear convention exists defining a degree of within-batch imprecision for this purpose, but a CV of 5–7% may be reasonably realistic for many assays and is consistent with a goal of about 10% for total assay imprecision. However, higher levels (up to 15 or even 20%) of imprecision are sometimes used to define the working interval. Two methods for the construction of such imprecision profiles are described above (*Protocols 2* and *3*). Because higher level samples are often quite rare, precision profiles do not always extend to high enough concentrations of analyte to allow estimation of an upper limit of detection. This may not be relevant, but some applications may require a wide and defined measurement interval, in which case the construction of a broader profile (perhaps with samples spiked with analyte) and/or re-optimization of the assay may be required. A more detailed discussion of the generation and use of precision profiles is given by Ekins (15) and Davies (12).

Apart from the lower working limit determined in this way, the ability of a procedure to quantify low concentrations of analyte is often characterized by the LLD (or lower limit of detection), which is primarily determined by the precision of the zero dose estimate (15). This defines the LLD as the lowest dose of analyte that can be distinguished from a sample containing no analyte. For a competitive assay, this would be:

$$\text{LLD} = B_0 - x \times \text{SD}_{B0}.$$

For reagent excess assays, the error component is not subtracted but added to the zero reading before interpolation of the LLD. Many authors quote as the lower detection limit a value calculated with $x = 2$, but $x = 3$ should be universally adopted. At least 10 replicates of the zero calibrator should be determined when calculating the LLD of an assay.

Protocol 6

Estimating a lower limit of detection

Equipment and reagents
- Equipment and reagents required for normal operation of assay under validation

Method
1. Run the standard curve in duplicate or triplicate following exactly the established procedure, but with at least 10 zero calibrant wells or tubes, .
2. Plot the standard curve as usual.
3. Calculate the standard deviation for the total number of zero readings (SD_{B0}).
4. Where B_0 is the average zero reading, interpolate from the standard curve the dose equivalent to:
   (a) $B_0 - 3 \times \text{SD}_{B0}$ in a competitive assay, or
   (b) $B_0 + 3 \times \text{SD}_{B0}$ in a reagent excess assay.

When defined as LLD, highest sensitivity is attained where an assay system exhibits a high degree of precision as it nears zero. In competitive assays where the tracer and antibody are both optimized at high dilutions, lack of precision is the main concern when considering sensitivity. In reagent excess assays, non-specific binding, causing loss of accuracy, is the main concern when considering sensitivity.

However, whatever the definition of sensitivity, the detection limit of a procedure depends on the volume of sample analysed, and this can only be estimated after the sample volumes to be routinely determined have been fixed. Larger sample volumes can be used with a procedure that is more resistant to matrix effects, thus decreasing its effective detection limit. If the normal serum sample volume is 100 μl and the LLD (or lowest point on the measurement range) is 10 pmol per tube, 100 nmol/l serum can be detected. See also Section 2 of Chapter 7.

5 Accuracy

The accuracy of a test system is dependent on the ability of the system to detect all of the specific analyte present and only that specific analyte. However, in addition to being specific, an accurate assay must also be precise and correctly calibrated. Accuracy is, therefore, the ability of the test system to measure the true concentrations of the analyte in the samples being tested. When a proper reference test method is available, accuracy can be readily assessed by running calibrated reference materials that reflect the range of the standard curve in the immunoassay test system and then determining whether the immunoassay results agree with the reference method results (Section 5.3). However, the thorough validation of a quantitative immunoassay requires a range of validation procedures.

5.1 Recovery of added standard

Analytical recovery is estimated by analysing samples into which known amounts of standard analyte have been added. Demonstration that added standard is determined as efficiently as endogenous analyte indicates both correct calibration and resistance to interference. Aliquots of a reasonably large number (about 10–25) of varied samples are spiked with one or more concentrations of standard, assayed with and without spiking, the concentration differences calculated and the percentages of added standard calculated.

Somewhat more complex, N × M experimental designs are sometimes useful because they may be designed to test the procedure over the full range of its standard curve. However, they are more complex and, consequently, must involve a smaller number of samples. For example, each of three (N) serum samples or pools containing low, medium or high concentrations of endogenous analyte may be spiked with a low, medium or high concentration of standard (M = 3). The concentrations are chosen to give a spread of endogenous and endogenous-plus-standard concentrations, which are evenly spaced and all on the standard curve. Again, the recoveries of added standard are calculated and tabulated (16). A procedure for a study of analytical recovery is outlined in *Protocol 7*.

Protocol 7

Estimating the recovery of added standard according to a 1 × 3 design

Equipment and reagents

- Equipment and reagents required for normal operation of the assay under validation
- Positive displacement pipettes, (e.g. Eppendorf)
- Samples or sample pools with a range of analyte concentrations

Method

1. Choose at least three analyte concentrations such that, when added to the concentrations in the samples, the sums (mostly) fall within the range of the standard curve.

2. Make up a highly concentrated stock solution of the analyte such that the addition of aliquots to portions of the sample pool will not cause significant dilution or other effects. This should *not* be the same stock from which the standard solutions were prepared, but it should be prepared with the same care.

3. Add calculated small volumes of analyte stock solution to three portions of each sample, add extra solvent to equalize the volumes added, and allow the mixtures to equilibrate.

4. Prepare at the same time, and in exactly the same way a fourth portion of each sample with zero analyte. (If the stock was prepared in organic solvent, prepare an extra 'solventless control' to ensure that this has no effect.)

5. Assay all four (zero + 3) samples by the established procedure.

6. Calculate the percentage recovery (%R) for each sample, for each of the three standard concentrations as follows:

$$\% \text{ Recovery} = \frac{\text{quantity measured}}{\text{quantity expected}} \times 100$$

7. Record final results as in *Table 3*.

Table 3. Sample set of results showing recoveries of analyte from four plasma samples (A, B, C, D) spiked with three analyte concentrations

Analyte added (ng/ml)	Concentration measured in ng/ml (recovered %)			
	A	B	C	D
0	5.0	6.3	6.8	3.2
5.0	13.75 (137%)	16.3 (144%)	14.5 (123%)	8.6 (105%)
10.0	17.6 (117%)	17.3 (106%)	18.7 (113%)	15.9 (120%)
15.0	19 (95%)	21.3 (100%)	22.7 (104%)	22.2 (120%)

225

When the percentage recovery for added standard has been calculated, one has to decide whether or not the recovery estimates are acceptable; they should be about 100% on average and be in the range 90–110% for readings involving the central portion of the standard curve. The actual criteria for the acceptability of recovery estimates are assay- and analyte-dependent. It is of paramount importance to consider diagnostic sensitivity and specificity (Section 7.2.2) when accepting recovery estimates as these criteria will dictate whether or not you can allow a larger variance in recovery.

5.2 Independence of volume

When a range of volumes of any sample are analysed, a valid immunoassay will measure amounts of analyte that are directly proportional to each other. Therefore, after correction for the volume analysed, the same concentration of analyte will always be found, i.e. it will be independent of the volume analysed. Owing to the different methods used to plot the results, the words parallelism and linearity are also applied to such studies. In practice, samples are generally diluted to different degrees with calibrator matrix solution and fixed volumes added to the assay mixture. The dilution matrix used in clinical situations may be serum that has been chemically or biochemically stripped of all analyte. Use of an unsuitable matrix solution may contribute to a lack of independence-of-volume.

Pronounced lack of independence is found in procedures prone to interference as interfering substances often act in a nonparallel, concentration-dependent fashion relative to analyte. However, the utility of any such studies carried out has often been very limited because the data has been presented in a way that would not always have indicated 'dependence-on-volume' when it was present and because of the limited variety and number of samples tested (17).

Preferably, the data may be analysed to give plots like those shown in *Figure 2*. Here the mass of analyte in each sample volume was interpolated from the standard curve, the concentration corrected for the volume assayed and the concentrations plotted against the actual volumes of serum assayed. Such plots should be parallel with the *x*-axis but, for example, in the presence of a factor that is less efficiently detected than the analyte, the apparent concentration will decrease markedly as the volume is increased. Another valid way of displaying the results is to plot the measured amounts (not concentrations) versus the volumes assayed, giving lines that should be straight with zero intercepts.

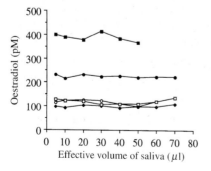

Figure 2. Results of a test of independence of volume for an oestradiol enzyme immunoassay. Plots of the concentration of oestradiol measured against the effective volume of saliva assayed for five saliva samples given by five different persons are shown.

The dilutions used should be arithmetically spaced to give an even distribution of points along the lines plotted. Ranges of volumes or dilutions that include volumes greater, or dilutions lower, than normally measured should always be used, if only to allow evaluation of the incidence and severity of crossreactivity or interference which could become relevant should the measurement procedure be changed.

The samples employed may be easy or demanding. Charcoal-stripped, standard-spiked sera are the easiest (and should never be used in formal validation studies), good quality sera from healthy, fasting, resting adults are the next best, while lipaemic or haemolysed samples may pose common problems of general interference. More demanding samples may also be available of types that have posed difficulties with previous assays and that the assay under development is intended to overcome .

If an assay displays dependence-on-volume with a high proportion of samples, the assay matrix solution may have to be reformulated, the volumes to be assayed reduced, or the principal reagents reassessed and the assay re-optimized to lower the LLD, or a combination of these.

Protocol 8

Establishing independence of volume

Equipment and reagents

- Equipment and reagents required for normal operation of assay under validation.

- Positive displacement pipettes (e.g. Eppendorf)

- Samples with a range of analyte concentrations

Method

1. With the same solution used to make up the standards, make at least five different dilutions of each sample. These dilutions should be spaced more or less arithmetically (e.g. 9/10, 7/10, 3/5, 1/2, 2/5, 3/10, 1/10) and *not* logarithmically (1/2, 1/4, 1/8, 1/16).

2. Calculate the effective volume of sample for each dilution. For example, since effective volume = sample volume $\times$ dilution factor, at a sample volume of 100 μl and a dilution of 3/10 the effective volume is 30 μl.

3. Assay in duplicate equal volumes (e.g. 100 μl) of all dilutions of all samples following exactly the established procedure and calculate the concentration of analyte while correcting for dilution

4. Plot the results as mean concentration (*y*-axis) against effective volume (*x*-axis) as in *Figure 2*.

The NCCLS guideline on linearity evaluation (3) states that data from valid-ation procedures equivalent to *Protocol 6* are acceptable, if by visual inspection the linear relationship and precision are appropriate to the requirements of the application. The guideline also suggests that the linearity relationship may be assessed by means of a statistical test for lack of fit.

5.3 Comparison with a reference method

Correlation studies with reliable reference methods are powerful validation tools. Briefly, samples reflecting the range of concentrations that will be en-countered by the new test are analysed by a reference method and by the assay under validation and the results compared (18, 19). The most important con-siderations when planning a correlation study are the number and variety of samples and the distribution of the values. For human clinical assays, the number of samples analysed should be sufficiently large (usually at least 120) to allow the inclusion of sufficient samples from both sexes, different age and racial groups and patients with relevant conditions or on relevant treatments.

If there already exists a gold standard reference method such as ID-GCMS, then a direct comparison of results will provide a reliable measure of the accuracy of the new method. However, proper reference methods are not available for many of the analytes measured by immunoassays, particularly protein analytes. In these cases, an established method, a more biological method or a market-leading kit is often used. For the purposes of the comparison, the formal assumption is made that the reference method is devoid of error but, if on the analysis of data, poor agreement is found there may be an argument for re-assessing the accuracy and precision of the reference method before con-demning the new method.

There is a divergence between how the results of correlation studies are generally analysed and how they should be analysed (18, 19). However, all agree that the first step should be the construction of a scatter graph with identical concentration scales on each axis. The insertion of a 'line of agreement' at 45° to each axis helps in the judgement of the degree of agreement between the two assays, and in the identification of deviations from linearity, homogeneity of variance and concentration-dependent relative bias (*Figure 3*).

In the literature, the data are usually analysed by means of the simple, un-weighted least-squares method with calculation of the Pearson product–moment correlation coefficient (r), and the intercept and slope of the fitted line. The correlation index (r^2) (20) is much more sensitive to deviations from a perfect correlation than the coefficient itself. Many computer software packages also give the errors for the intercept and slope, and these can be used to test whether the intercept is significantly different from zero and whether the slope is significantly different from 1.0. This method of analysis may be regarded as statistically reliable provided that the results from the more precise method are plotted on the *x*-axis; at least 10 points are included in the comparison and the points cover the concentration range in a roughly equidistant fashion.

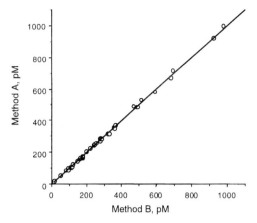

Figure 3. Scatter graph of the results of a correlation study in which method A is being tested against a 'reference' method (method B). Analyte was measured in 38 samples by the two methods. The included line of perfect agreement is at 45°.

However, Bland and Altman (18) convincingly argue against the use of correlation coefficients for assessing the agreement between two methods of measurement. They make two very important points.

1. The statistic r measures the strength of a relationship *not* agreement. There is perfect agreement only if the points lie on the line of equality, but there is perfect correlation if they lie on any straight line that is not horizontal. Therefore, the significance of the correlation is irrelevant to the question of agreement, and data that are in poor agreement can have a high correlation coefficient.

2. Correlation depends on the range of the true quantities of analyte in samples. If this is wide, the correlation will be greater than if it is narrow. If the two methods are compared over the whole range of analyte concentrations normally present in patient samples, a reasonably high correlation is almost inevitable.

Consequently, Bland and Altman (18) suggest an alternative method of analysis that is simple and graphical. In addition to the scatter graph described above, they propose highlighting any disagreements by plotting the difference between the results obtained for the same samples by the two methods against their means (*Figure 4*). This also allows identification of concentration-dependent measurement differences. The two simple statistics, mean difference (d) (or bias) and the standard deviation (SD) of the differences summarize any lack of agreement. Provided that the measurement error is reasonably equally distributed, the analytical or clinical significance of the lack of agreement is assessed with respect to the limits $d \pm 2SD$, referred to as the limits of agreement. Aspects of deficiencies of agreement that are clear when data are analysed in this way may not be immediately apparent from the equivalent scatter graph with fitted line (19). In fact, the fitted line is often a distraction and much less useful is assessing the degree of agreement than the line of perfect agreement (*Figure 3*).

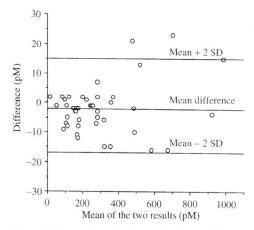

Figure 4. The graphical method of Bland and Altman (18) for the evaluation of a correlation study with two analytical methods, A and B. The difference in the measurements for each sample (Method A result minus Method B) is plotted against the mean for the two methods. The horizontal lines indicate the mean difference (2.07 pM), the mean plus twice the SD of the differences (15.04 pM) and the mean minus twice the SD (−19.18 pM).

Less formal and smaller-scale correlation studies may also be used to advantage at earlier stages of procedure validation. During analytical validation they may be used to test the effects of important procedural changes. They may also be used to evaluate the effect of an extraction or preliminary purification procedure, by testing such an assay without a preliminary extraction step versus the same procedure with a preliminary step or steps (21, 22).

6 Biological validation

Successful analytical validation of an assay builds confidence in its ability to deliver true analytical results, but an assay is not fully validated until it has been successfully applied to real biological samples obtained under circumstances associated with known concentrations, or well-understood changes in analyte concentration. Generally, biological or clinical validation is concerned with demonstrating that a procedure returns results that are biologically, physiologically and, if appropriate, diagnostically relevant.

It follows that the biological validation of the first assay for a completely new analyte is initially impossible, and that the extent and detail of biological validation must vary considerably with respect to the analyte and application in question.

6.1 Concentrations and changes in concentration

Concentrations of the analyte under standard conditions and under conditions known to be associated with higher or lower concentrations should be measured. For example with a clinical assay, levels should be measured in normal persons and in persons previously diagnosed as having particular relevant conditions or diseases. Longitudinal studies with repetitive sampling to establish endogenous pulsatile, diurnal or other cyclic patterns, to monitor analyte concentrations before and after environmental or activity changes, or after the administration of treatments should also demonstrate expected concentrations and patterns of change. With assays that detect antibodies against pathogens (or the pathogens themselves), the analysis of a set of samples taken at regular intervals after the time of infection (a seroconversion panel) also allows the biological evaluation of assay sensitivity. In summary, new test systems should be evaluated against the full range and, as far as possible, the full diversity of real samples likely to be found in the broad sample population base.

The range and variety of experiments that can be carried out as part of a biological validation generally increases as more becomes known about the biological roles of the analyte. With an assay for the reproductive glycoprotein hormone LH in an experimental animal species a full and thorough biological validation (16) could include the following (ethical approval may be needed for at least some of these):

- Basal levels in males and in females at about three stages of the oestrous cycle not including the time around ovulation,
- Serial measurement in females at short intervals over the period when ovulation is expected (pre-ovulatory peak),
- Serial measurement in females at very short intervals over 24-h periods at one or more stages of the oestrous cycle (pulsatile pattern of release),
- Serial measurements at short intervals before and after the administration of gonadotrophin releasing hormone (GnRH),
- Serial measurements before and after gonadectomy (removal of feedback inhibition of release).

6.2 Normal ranges and diagnostic cut-off levels

As described above, with a new assay for a well-characterized analyte, measurements on ranges of predefined samples are often done to establish that the assay under validation gives expected distributions of concentrations. However, when an analyte is not well characterized, the same exercise may be carried out to establish normal ranges of concentrations to be used to define diagnostic cut-off levels. The establishment of reference values is beyond the scope of this chapter and it is discussed by Sloberg in depth elsewhere (23).

In effect, the empirical result from any diagnostic test sample is translated into a diagnosis which is positive or negative, or into a prognosis which is good or poor, etc., and such translations are based on comparisons with one or more reference values. It follows that the both the accuracy of the measurement and the accuracy of the cut-off level are important and that, if different assays were used to do each, the results of both assays *must* be comparable. This is the concern of assay standardization which is impossible without accurate calibration, thorough validation and constant quality control (Chapter 10).

Diagnostic efficiency and its assessment are discussed further below (Section 7.2.2)

7 Qualitative and semiquantitative tests

True qualitative tests indicate the presence or absence of an analyte. Semi-quantitative tests also give some indication of the concentration present, which may be scaled relative to one or more significant cut-off values. Qualitative and semiquantitative tests require validation to ensure accuracy, precision, sensitivity and specificity, but the criteria for validation and the methods of validation may be more test-specific than for quantitative assays.

True qualitative assays, as used for the detection of hCG in pregnancy tests, of drugs of abuse, or of antibodies against HIV or hepatitis viruses, give positive results at the lowest level of analyte detectable. For some applications quali-tative assays may be optimized to read negative at concentrations lower than a certain level. Whether or not they also indicate that any analyte present is there at a 'low' or 'high' concentration may not be relevant or even desirable.

Semiquantitative assays may give only a little or quite a lot of quantitative information and there are no clear lines of division with either qualitative or quantitative tests. Basically, semiquantitative tests provide information such as 'undetectable', 'low', 'medium' and 'high' and this information is relevant to the applications of the tests.

Like quantitative assays, good choices of antibodies, antigens, conjugates, solid phases and other materials are essential to the successful validation of qualitative tests. In addition, efficient general optimization will ensure that most problems related to sensitivity and interference will have been overcome before the commencement of formal validation. However, with qualitative tests the often hazy distinction between optimization and validation procedures may be largely absent.

Finally, qualitative immunoassay systems are of great commercial import-ance and most are now carried out with the aid of disposable integrated devices. Therefore, much of the information on the fundamental technologies and their applications to specific tests is not readily available or is protected by patents.

7.1 Specificity

Consistent accuracy depends on good specificity and this must be formally assessed in so far as it is feasible. Basically, real negative samples are spiked with potential crossreactants at the highest concentration of each that may be found in routine operation. The choice of crossreactants is made judiciously, as mentioned previously in Section 2.1.2. In addition, since potential cross-reactants may be found in combination, a realistic range of likely double and multiple combinations should also be tested.

However, formal assessments of specificity may not be feasible with many analytes, particularly specific antibodies. In such cases, demonstrations of specificity may depend exclusively on the testing of panels of positive and negative samples of kinds that will be commonly encountered or that have previously been shown to cause problems in similar tests.

7.2 Validation criteria

The references in qualitative assays are positive and negative controls and the emphasis in test validation is on precision, sensitivity, accuracy at the test cut-off point. In clinical applications the cut-off point may determine a diagnosis and, therefore, during validation diagnostic specificity and sensitivity are major foci of attention.

Most analytes measured by qualitative assays fall into one of two groups that may be characterized as follows. In the first group accurate quantitative esti-mates of analyte concentrations at cut-off points are available (e.g. hCG, myo-globin) and in the second such estimates are not available (or feasible), and 'positive' and 'negative' are effectively defined with reference to panels of well-characterized samples (e.g. HIV-specific antibodies).

7.2.1 The grey zone

For analytes that can be quantified, the most important element in the validation of a qualitative or semiquantitative test is the analytical and bio-logical (diagnostic) reliability of the cut-off concentration. Given a reliable cut-off concentration, the zone around the cut-off in which there is ambiguity in the diagnosis or conclusion drawn must be defined. This zone is referred to as the 'grey zone'. A major objective in the optimization and validation of such a test is to ensure that the grey zone is as narrow as possible.

When determining the grey zone of a qualitative/semiquantitative test, it is of great benefit to have at hand a reliable quantitative reference method for the same analyte so that test results on panels of real samples may be compared, otherwise it will be necessary to use commercially available control materials of known analyte content that may differ significantly from the samples to be routinely tested.

To estimate the grey zone for a test, repeat the test 10–20 times on each of a range of real samples with analyte concentrations that fall around the cut-off concentration. In absolute terms the grey zone is the concentration range between which the results are 0% positive (100% negative) and 100% positive (*Figure 5*). The specifications for the test being validated may allow these criteria to be relaxed significantly (e.g. 5–95% positive) and the formal grey zone thereby made more narrow.

The width of the grey zone is a measure of the precision of the test and it should also be centered around the previously determined cut-off concen-tration. Should the zone be wider than acceptable, the test reagents and or conditions should be adjusted to improve precision and accuracy (re-optimization). The grey zone plot is not in any sense a standard curve and no dose–response relationship can be inferred.

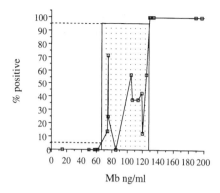

Figure 5. The results of a procedure to define the grey zone about the positive/negative cut-off of a qualitative test for myoglobin. The centre of the zone is the true cut-off point of the assay. (98 ng/ml in this instance). The grey zone is here defined as the range between the concentration above which 95% of the results are positive and the concentration below which 95% of the results are negative.

Protocol 9

Experiment to estimate the grey zone for a qualitative assay

Equipment and reagents

- A range of samples of known analyte concentration with concentrations evenly distributed around the cut-off concentration of the test

- Equipment and reagents required for normal operation of the test under validation

Method

1. Mix each sample and split into 10–20 aliquots.

2. Code and randomize the sample aliquots for all the samples to be tested and perform the tests below 'blind' to eliminate the possibility of subjective effects.

3. Test the samples in the assay as per established procedure.

4. Record the result for test as either positive or negative.

5. For each sample calculate the percentage of positive results obtained: (number of positive results/number of negative results) × 100.

6. Plot the frequency of positive results (%) against analyte concentration for all of the samples tested.

7. Insert a line on the graph parallel to the x-axis at, say, 5% positive.

8. Insert a line on the graph parallel to the x-axis at 95% positive.

9. Where the two horizontal lines intersect the plot, insert vertical lines. The concentration range between these two vertical lines defines the grey zone.

The analytical accuracy of qualitative and semiquantitative tests is also measured through method comparison with a panel of previously measured samples. The results obtained for all the samples with the new test are tabulated as 'negative' or 'positive', or (in the case of semiquantitative tests) as 'negative', 'low' and 'high', etc., and then compared with the known concentrations and the cut-off levels for 'positive', etc. Again, percentages are calculated to indicate the accuracy of the test with respect to each cut-off concentration.

7.2.2 Diagnostic sensitivity and specificity

The assessment of diagnostic accuracy or efficiency depends on the use of samples for which a confirmed diagnosis is already available. In principle, diagnostic accuracy is not necessarily the same as analytical accuracy, as the method(s) used to confirm the diagnoses may be completely different from the test being evaluated and numeric values for the concentrations of analyte present in the samples may be unattainable.

Diagnostic efficiency has two aspects, sensitivity and specificity, which have quite different definitions as compared with analytical sensitivity and specificity. Perfect diagnostic sensitivity means that a test will detect all cases with the property of interest (positives) and perfect diagnostic specificity means that it will correctly identify all cases without that property (negatives). Assessments of diagnostic efficiency must always be conducted as blind studies in order to avoid operator bias. The two statistics are calculated according to the following formulae:

$$\text{Diagnostic sensitivity} = \frac{\text{true positives}}{\text{true + false positves}} \times 100,$$

$$\text{Diagnostic specificity} = \frac{\text{true negatives}}{\text{true + false negatives}} \times 100.$$

Since 100% sensitivity and 100% specificity are rarely achievable together a test may be designed to give 100% for one and as high a figure as possible for the other, according to which is more significant, sensitivity or specificity. For example, since all patient samples testing positive for HIV on routine screening are automatically reanalysed with a confirmatory test, the sensitivity of the initial screening test is most important. In such a case, the test conditions and/or reagents should be adjusted to reduce any tendency to give false positive results even at the expense of a lower level of false negatives. The sensitivities of assays for antibodies to HIV are also routinely evaluated with seroconversion panels (see Section 6.1) and samples from persons infected with a variety of strains of the virus.

If the required levels of sensitivity and specificity are not achieved by re-optimization, alternate antibody and antigen reagents may have to be considered.

8 Evaluation of reagent stability

Even for assays that are intended for regular use within the laboratory in which they were developed, and not transported for use elsewhere, it is preferable that the reagents are highly stable. One obvious benefit is that inter-assay variation may be reduced by the use of a single batches or lots of reagents over longer periods of time.

On storage the biological components of immunoassays may be subject to many degradative influences, including proteases, oxidants, microorganisms and a broad range of other contaminant impurities. These degradative agents are often counteracted by the use of antiprotease cocktails (complete® Boehringer Roche), bacteriostatic agents (Thimerosal, Sigma), and by the use of bulking proteins such as BSA, HSA, fish skin gelatin, milk protein, etc.

Even with the use of protective/antidegradative agents there is often great variation in the shelf-lives of individual assay reagents. To establish good storage conditions and to estimate shelf-lives the stability of each component of the assay should be investigated. Reagent stability and full kit stability is normally accessed by subjecting them to accelerated decay at elevated temperatures (24–26), as outlined in *Protocol 10*.

Some preliminary work may be necessary to establish at what temperature and in what form the reagent being tested is most stable. Many reagent antibodies and some pure protein standards retain their activities at 4 °C in a simple stabilizing buffer (PBS/BSA) with a bacteriostatic agent. Some highly pure protein standards also retain their activities under similar conditions. Conversely, reagents involving cruder proteins may be highly unstable at 4 °C and require a complex cocktail of stabilizing agents and low storage temperatures (-20 °C or -70 °C) to ensure that they retain sufficient activity to remain active for reasonable periods.

Protocol 10

Investigating the stability of a reagent

A stability study should be designed to run over at least a 21-day period, with reagent testing at 3-day intervals and at about three temperatures. Here, the major test condition of interest is 37 °C and 4 °C represents (it is hoped) a stable storage condition. An intermediate condition (here 21 °C) may be included for purposes of comparison. For quantitative assays, the mean of duplicate endpoint readings for zero standard (competitive assays) or a high standard (reagent-excess assays) is usually taken as an indication of the activity of the test reagent.

Equipment and reagents

- Equipment required for normal operation of the assay
- A sufficient volume or quantity of the test reagent

- Reagents (other than reagent being tested) required for normal operation of the assay, in sufficient quantities for the whole test regimen and stored under optimal conditions

Method

1. Split the (freshly prepared) reagent being tested into a sufficient number of aliquots, e.g. 20. Store in containers as similar as possible to those the reagent will be stored

Protocol 10 continued

in permanently, as the nature of the container may be relevant. The volume of each aliquot should be enough for duplicate measurements with at least a 20% excess and should not be less than 200 μl. A study at three temperatures (e.g. 4, 21 and 37°C) with measurements on days 0, 3, 7, 10, 14, 17 and 21 requires 21 aliquots. However, always include at least an extra three aliquots.

2. Store the aliquots in refrigerators/incubators at the required temperatures and preferably in the dark.

3. At the same time (day 0) use the reagent in the assay as per the established method. At this time the aliquots 'stored' at different temperatures are identical and the extra replicates may be used to give a more precise zero time reading (baseline reading).

4. At approximately the same time on each of the designated days test the reagent for each storage condition.

5. For each aliquot tested, calculate the activity retained: (endpoint reading/baseline reading) × 100.[a]

6. At the end of the study, plot the activities retained at each temperature against day tested.

7. Repeat whole protocol for each of the principal assay reagents. Adjust storage conditions as necessary and continue until all the conditions to be routinely used have been shown to be satisfactory.

[a] For unknown reasons, reagents on accelerated stability at 37°C quite often show a retained activity of greater than 100% at one or more early time points.

Results may be interpreted as outlined by Kirkwood (25). As a rule of thumb, any reagent retaining more than 80% activity after 14 days at 37°C, can be given a 4°C shelf life of 1 year. Accelerated stability studies should always be supported by a real-time stability study on the reagent stored at its ambient storage temperature. Real-time stability testing often shows that the reagents retain more activity than previously indicated by accelerated stability studies.

References

1. Good Laboratory Practice. (1989). *UK Compliance Programme*. Department of Health, London, UK.

2. NCCLS. (1992). *Publication EP5-T2*, (2nd edn). National Committee for Clinical Laboratory Standards, Villanova, PA., USA.

3. NCCLS. (1986). *Publication EP6-P*. National Committee for Clinical Laboratory Standards, Villanova, PA., USA.

4. NCCLS. (1986). *Publication EP7-P*. National Committee for Clinical Laboratory Standards, Villanova, PA., USA.

5. NCCLS. (1995). *Publication EP9-A*. National Committee for Clinical Laboratory Standards, Villanova, PA., USA.

6. NCCLS. (1998). *Publication EP10-A*. National Committee for Clinical Laboratory Standards, Villanova, PA., USA.

7. NCCLS. (1998). *Publication EP14-P*. National Committee for Clinical Laboratory Standards, Villanova, PA., USA.

8. Fraser, C. G. (1991). *Ann. Inst. Super. Sanità*. **27**, 369.

9. Ricos, C. and Arbos, M. A. (1990). *Ann. Clin. Biochem.* **27**, 353.

10. Abraham, G. E. (1974). *J. Clin. Endo.* **27**, 966.

11. Ekins, R. P. (1974). *Br. Med. Bull.* **30**, 3.

12. Davies, C. (1994). In *The immunoassay handbook* (ed. Wilde, D.), p. 83. Stockton Press, New York.

13. Krouwer, J. S. (1986). *Clin. Chem.* **32**, 1980.

14. Seth, J. (1991). In *Principles and practice of immunoassay* (eds Price, C. P. and Newman D. J.), p. 154. Macmillan, London.

15. Ekins, R. P. (1976). In *Hormone assays and their clinical application* (eds J. A. Loraine and E. T. Bell) p. 1. Churchill Livingston, Edinburgh.

16. Abdul-Ahad, W. G. and Gosling, J. P. (1987). *J. Reprod Fert.* **80**, 653.

17. Power, M. J. and Fottrell, P. F. (1991). *Crit. Rev. Clin. Lab. Sci.* **28**, 287.

18. Bland, J. M. and Altman, D. G. (1986). *Lancet*, **8 Feb.** 307.

19. Pollock, M. A. Jefferson, S. G. Kane, J. W. Lomax, K. MacKinnon, G., and Winnard, C. B. (1992). *Ann. Clin. Biochem.* **29**, 556.

20. Zar, J. H. (1974). *Biostatistical analysis*, 2nd edn. Prentice–Hall, Englewood Cliffs.

21. Tunn, S. Pappert, G. Willnow, P., and Krieg, M. (1990). *J. Clin. Chem. Clin. Biochem.* **28**, 929.

22. Lantto, O, Lindback B. Aakvaag, A. Damkjaer, M. Pomoells, U.-M., and Björkhem, I. (1983). *Scand J. Clin. Invest.* **43**, 433.

23. Sloberg, E. S. (1999). *Teitz textbook of clinical chemistry* (eds Burtis, C. A. and Ashwood R. A.), 3rd edn, p. 336. W. B. Saunders, Philadelphia.

24. Jerne, M. D. and Perry W. L. M. (1956). *Bull. WHO* **14**, 167.

25. Kirkwood, T. B. L. (1977). *Biometrics* **33**, 736.

26. Rhodes, C. T. (1984). *Drug Devel. Ind. Pharm.* **10**, 1163.

Chapter 9
Data processing

Barry Nix* and David Wild[†]

*School of Mathematics, Cardiff University, Senghennydd Road, PO BOX 926, Cardiff CF2 4YH, UK, and [†]Ortho-Clinical Diagnostics, Forest Farm, Whitchurch, Cardiff CF4 7YT, UK

1 Introduction

Immunoassay developers need to be aware of the concepts involved in calibration curve-fitting and data interpolation, if only because of the ever-present risk of inaccurate results caused by the computational procedure itself. Although the computerized curve-fitting algorithms used are often highly sophisticated and have improved in recent years, they are still not universally applicable or totally reliable and can introduce bias or poor precision to assay data. Researchers may need to become involved in curve-fitting in a number of situations, such as:

1. Assay development in an open format (with the need to choose a suitable curve-fit method)
2. Assay development for an existing system (where curve-fit method is already decided).
3. Investigations of problems with assays.
4. The development of curve-fit programs themselves.

We will concentrate on (1) above but in all cases it is important that curve-fit weaknesses do not unduly affect assay results. In (2) there is the additional complication that the assay may have to be modified to work within the limitations of the curve-fitting algorithm. In all four situations the keys to success are to:

- Understand the underlying limitations of the type of curve-fit method employed, and
- Recognize the tell-tale signs of curve-fit error in assay results.

The purpose of this chapter is to raise awareness of the whole area of curve-fitting and data interpolation as it applies to immunoassays. In particular, we wish to discuss the capabilities and limitations of computerized calibration curve-fitting methods and to dispel the myth that they can only be understood by mathematicians.

2 Fitting calibration curves

In quantitative assays a 'calibration curve' is used to determine the analyte concentrations in samples from the levels of signal measured. Curve-fitting provides an interpolatory device so that a limited number of standards (or 'calibrators') can be used to determine the relationship between concentration and signal (the 'dose response') over the whole concentration range of the assay. Historically, dose–response curves were drawn by hand, by means of a sheet of graph paper, a pencil, and a ruler or flexicurve. This manual technique is often referred to as the 'gold' standard but it has drawbacks, as do all methods. The two main disadvantages of hand-drawn curves with manual interpolation are their subjectivity and the considerable time required, and these are the main reasons why computer/mathematical models have become almost essential. However, it would be wrong to conclude that the power of computers and mathematical algorithms necessarily always leads to better interpolations for the unknowns. The user should constantly be aware of the potential for odd-looking calibration curves to be produced by computer-based approaches, and as a result should always be in a position to inspect the curve produced.

> ## Tip
>
> Use a curve-fit package that provides a high-quality graphics output and always inspect the degree of agreement between the fitted line and the standard points.

2.1 Definitions

2.1.1 Dose–response metameters

The two fundamental variables involved in curve-fitting are analyte concentration (known as dose) and signal level (or response). Instead of plotting signal against concentration it often proves necessary to transform the variables first, e.g. by plotting signal against the logarithm of concentration. If such transformations are used, we refer to the quantities that are plotted as the response metameter and dose metameter to distinguish them from the original variables.

2.1.2 Response–error relationship

Precision usually varies according to the concentration of analyte present. The mathematical form that describes the way this precision varies (whether that be the variance, standard deviation or coefficient of variation) with signal level is called the response–error relationship.

2.1.3. Homoscedasticity and heteroscedasticity

A response variable is said to be homoscedastic if its variability (standard deviation) is constant for all signal levels, otherwise it is heteroscedastic.

2.1.4 Linearizing transformations

Effort is often expended trying to transform the response variable in such a way that the relationship between the transformed variables (or metameters) is linear. Such transformations are called linearizing transformations.

2.2 Manual and computer methods

This is a very broad topic, particularly given the way routine technology in the clinical laboratory is moving towards the use of 'master' calibration curves encoded with kits (e.g. on a bar code or magnetic card), and the reliance on perhaps two 'adjusters', that rescale the master curve for each assay. We will concentrate on the principles behind a number of the more popular curve-fit routines. There are three types of curve-fit: manual, empirical and theoretical.

2.2.1 Manual methods

Before attempting to create a manual plot one should be clear on exactly what one is trying to achieve. Replicate scatter is caused by imprecision of the method and makes manual plotting more difficult. The means of the replicate responses are less variable and will usually take the correct value, assuming outlier values are not present. Thus, it makes sense to fit to mean values. However, the information contained in the scatter within replicates should not be ignored since it enables the user to decide how much latitude they have when trying to connect the mean values in a smooth way. If there is little scatter every effort should be made to pass the curve through, or very close to, the corresponding mean values, whereas if the scatter is large the shape of the curve should be influenced by neighbouring points that are more precise.

> **Tip**
>
> Ensure that the plot of the calibration curve includes both the individual replicate values and, with a different symbol, their mean values. Then remove any *clear* outliers.

Another aspect is that one has to decide whether to plot the raw responses or to use dose and response metameters. This is a difficult area to give advice on as there is an element of subjectivity in such choices and many people have their own preferred metameters. However, the subjectivity of manual plots can be reduced and accuracy improved if the points are evenly spaced and curvature is minimized.

Manual plots have one significant virtue: they do not suffer from inherent systematic bias of the kind that can occur with computer curve-fitting techniques, due to unsuitability of the method or the constraints imposed by a mathematical model. Carefully drawn curves can produce surprisingly consistent results, the precision of which can be checked from the control values over a series of assays. (See *Protocol 1* and the associated text for further information relevant to manual methods.)

Table 1. Standards data set from an RIA[a]

Standard dose (pg/ml)	c.p.m.				Mean	Fraction bound	SD (c.p.m.)	Reps
0	1627	1567	1720	1660				
0	1704	1689	1759	1722	1681		30.183	8
0.625	1182	1291	1294	1312	1269.75	0.750	59.230	4
1.25	1029	1112	986	1074	1050.25	0.616	54.640	4
2.5	702	784	733	777	749	0.433	38.618	4
5	486	485	501	460	483	0.271	16.990	4
10	307	277	285	275	286	0.151	14.652	4
20	196	204	193	182	193.75	0.095	9.106	4
NSB	25	39	51	38	38.25		10.626	4

[a] Note that for the zero dose there are two rows corresponding to a replication order of eight. The SD column contains the standard deviations of the replicate responses.

To illustrate the above points we will consider the data shown in *Table 1*, which is from a RIA for oestradiol. The plots of the individual points, together with the means, are shown in *Figure 1* for the raw data and different metameter combinations. It is quite possible to fit a line to the untransformed dose–response curve (*Figure 1A*) with a flexi-curve. However, it can be difficult to make judgements about potentially biased points for competitive assays because of the very strong curvature at low concentrations. This is especially difficult where duplicate points are some distance apart. Immunometric assays (not shown) have a more linear response, so a plot of untransformed data may be satisfactory, provided that sensitivity is not an important requirement and the assay does not have a wide working range.

A plot of the raw response against the natural log of dose (*Figure 1B*) can provide considerable linearization of competitive assay curves. However, departures from linearity usually occur at the ends of the curve. Like all transformations that involve plotting log dose, this approach has the disadvantage that the zero concentration calibration point cannot be used (log zero is undefined). Therefore, it is essential to include a calibrator with a value near zero if values are to be determined in this part of the assay range. Log dose plots expand the lower part of the assay curve, so that the data for low concentration samples can be read with greater ease. They also produce evenly spaced values when the concentrations follow a power pattern (i.e. doubling dilutions), and easily cover a very wide range of concentrations (as appropriate for immunometric assays).

Graphing and comparisons between different assays are facilitated if the raw response data are treated by subtracting the mean NSB from each and expressing them as decimal fractions of the mean count at zero standard. If the NSB is not known, assume it has a value of zero. This is not a transformation. Response data treated in this way are sometimes represented as 'B/B$_0$', or as here, and in Section 2.3.2 below, as r.

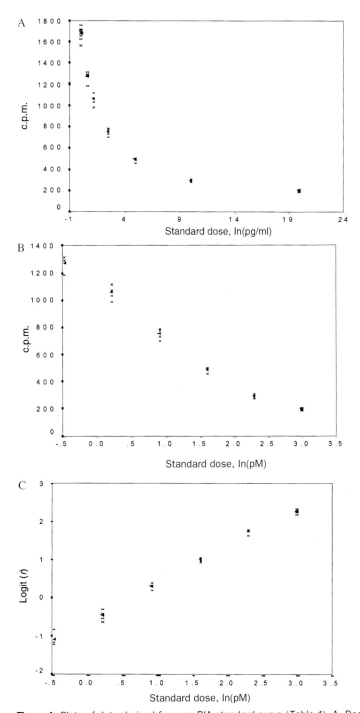

Figure 1. Plots of data derived from an RIA standard curve (*Table 1*). A. Dose response, showing individual and mean c.p.m. against dose. B. Dose response, showing individual and mean c.p.m. against natural log of dose. C. Dose response, showing individual and mean logit of the standardized variable (*r*) against natural log of dose.

A plot of logit (*r*) against the natural log of dose (*Table 2* below and *Figure 1C*) where

$$\text{logit}(r) = \ln \frac{1 - r}{r}$$

converts the calibration curves of many assays into an approximate straight line, making it much easier to detect any bias caused by individual calibrators. Even if this plot exhibits a small degree of nonlinearity, once a few curves have been plotted with the aid of a flexicurve, the user becomes familiar with the curve shape of that particular assay. Some prefer to use $\log_{10}$ for the dose metameter in both situations above and this makes no difference.

Manual plotting methods with appropriate dose and response metameters can be very effectively computer assisted. The ubiquitous spreadsheet program gives great versatility and can provide instant columns of means, logs, 'B/B$_0$' or *r* values and logits, and can subsequently be used to correct interpolated values for dilution, extraction efficiency, and units.

In summary, the logit-log approach gives linear, or near-linear plots, for most competitive (*Figure 1C*) and immunometric assays and we would recommend it when doing manual plots. However, plotting the raw response against log dose may be equally acceptable for competitive assays (as in this case), and involves less preliminary calculation. For immunometric assays, plotting log response versus log dose may give the most linear presentation of the calibration curve, while expanding the scale for low concentrations (see also *Protocol 1*).

2.2.2 Empirical methods

The use of empirical methods assumes that the function connecting the points is continuous and smooth, but does not assume any overall functional form for the dose–response relationship. Examples of this approach are simple linear interpolation, where straight line sections are drawn between the mean responses for neighbouring calibrators, and cubic splines, where a cubic polynomial is fitted. Both methods are limited in that they place far too much emphasis on the accuracy of the response variable. Both linear and spline methods should be avoided if the response has any tendency to be nonmonotonic or irregular, a not unfamiliar situation for calibration curves with asymptotes (*Figure 2*). For such a calibration curve, accurate interpolation would not be possible. This is a weakness of the curve-fit method used and is not necessarily due to poor assay performance.

2.2.3 Theoretical methods

Theoretical methods fit a given functional form to the calibration data and so errors in data may be partly corrected for. This is because the mathematical form of the fitted curve greatly restricts the range of shapes it may assume. A drawback is that such models are based on simplified molecular and kinetic models of immunoassay and, as such, might not be completely appropriate for

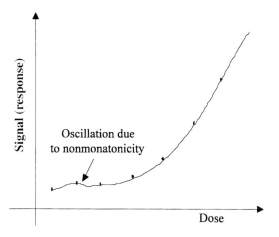

Figure 2. A simple cubic spline fit that shows oscillations when the data points are not monotonic.

any particular assay. However, despite this limitation, these are the best available curve-fit algorithms for most applications.

> **Tip**
>
> When using a computer curve-fitting method, choose an approach based on a theoretical model, e.g. a four or five parameter log logistic model.

2.3 Computer methods in common use

The two most common calibration curve-fit methods are the four-parameter log logistic (4PL) and the logit-log, which both belong to the same family of models. These models are described and two examples are given that highlight many of the most important points.

2.3.1 Four-parameter log-logistic (4PL)

Let Y_T denote the true mean signal level and X the concentration. The mathematical form of the four parameter log logistic (4PL) model is:

$$Y_T = A + \frac{(B - A)}{(1 + Z)} \quad \text{where} \quad Z = e^{C + D \times \ln(X)} \qquad [1]$$

and where A, B, C and D are the four parameters that need to be estimated. For those assays for which there is a decreasing mean signal level with increasing concentration, $D > 0$. For such assays, as $X \to \infty$, $Z \to \infty$, and so $Y_T \to A$. Also as $X \to 0$, $Z \to 0$, and so $Y_T \to B$. Thus A and B are the two asymptotes, as shown in the representation of a full theoretical curve for a competitive assay in *Figure 3*. Interpretation of these parameters in terms of assay curve characteristics is now possible. Accordingly, in a competitive format assay, A is the mean signal level

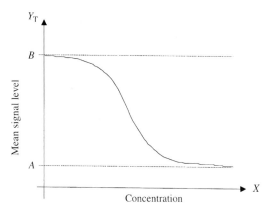

Figure 3. A plot showing the typical form of a competitive immunoassay calibration curve, which, as usual, is sigmoid in shape with two asymptotes and one point of inflection.

for 'infinite' dose, often referred to as the NSB, and B is the mean signal level for zero dose. The method works equally well with immunometric assays, which have ascending curves. However, although A still represents the NSB, which is the lower asymptote, it is now the response at zero dose. The parameter B still represents the upper asymptote, but in practice it is now normally well beyond the working range of the assay and not seen in the plot of the calibration curve. For all assays the 4PL curve-fit is obtained by using an appropriate nonlinear regression technique to estimate the four parameters A, B, C, and D, with the signal at zero and NSB being included in the fitting algorithm along with all the signal values associated with the other standard concentrations.

Nonlinear models such as the 4PL models (1–3) have been around for many years. They normally work very well with a wide variety of immunoassays; however, problems can still occur. One of us experienced first-hand a package specifically written to fit data with a 4PL model that kept producing a poor fit. At first appearance, the model appeared to be inappropriate, but it was found that the fitting algorithm in the program was inefficient and, therefore, unsuitable. Fitting nonlinear models requires powerful computational algorithms that are iterative in character. If the algorithm is not efficient, then after a preset number of iterations (normal practice) it may not have converged and the parameter values produced may give a very poor fit.

Most iterative algorithms require the iteration process to start with a set of values that are quite close to their optimal values, otherwise the numerical search may find the wrong solution. As in the case above, the use of an alternative curve-fitting program based on the same model may solve the problem. Care should always be exercised and expert help sought when the situation is unclear.

The five parameter log-logistic model is an elaboration of the 4PL model, with the extra parameter ('E') allowing some asymmetry of standard curves. However, as with all models, the greater the number of parameters to be fitted the more data are needed to give the same degree of confidence in the final fit.

For some applications the best solution is to use accumulated standard data to give a reliable estimate of 'E' and to keep 'E' constant rather than to estimate it each time.

2.3.2 Logit-log

The 4PL equation [1] can be rearranged to give:

$$r = \frac{(Y_T - A)}{(B - A)} = \frac{1}{(1 + Z)}$$

Now r (as above in Section 2.2.1) is the fraction of the signal that is bound and has values between 0 and 1. This equation can be further rearranged as:

$$ln\left(\frac{1 - r}{r}\right) = Ln(Z) = C + D \times \ln(X)$$

As we have seen, the function on the left-hand side of the above equation may be written as Logit(r), and so the equation reduces to:

$$\text{Logit}(r) = C + D \times \ln(X)$$

This is the so called logit-log model. As we have seen, it is just a rearrangement of the 4PL model and so is equivalent. The difference lies in the fitting of the curve. In the 4PL model the parameters A and B are estimated within the algorithm, whereas with the logit-log model A and B are assumed to be known and (in competitive assays) equated to the NSB and zero mean signal levels, respectively. This makes the model linear with the variable parameters C and D. Thus, in competitive assays, the two curve-fits will be equivalent when the fitted estimates of A and B derived from the 4PL model have the same values as the experimentally determined NSB and zero mean signal level, respectively. For immunometric assays, the same principle of equivalence applies, however parameter A, the NSB, is the same as the binding at zero dose, and parameter B is the upper asymptote, which in practice is difficult to ascertain experimentally (see also page 260).

2.4 Evaluating candidate methods

The curve-fitting and data interpolation method used is as much part of an immunoassay as sample preparation or liquid handling, and, if unsuitable, is just as capable of causing results to be spurious. Therefore, when the freedom to do so exists, choosing a curve-fitting method is a serious exercise and should be done systematically, perhaps according to *Protocol 1*.

If the data give a linear plot, or if the plot can be linearized by data transformation (*Protocols 1A and B*), a linear fitting procedure is allowable. If not, a nonlinear fitting procedure, preferably with a reliable theoretical model, is necessary (*Protocol 1D*). In either case, a weighted fitting procedure is desirable, and the dose–response error relationship must be known in order to calculate the weights (*Protocol 1C*).

Normally, immunoassays are not homoscedastic (i.e. they do not have a constant variance at different dose concentrations). Weighted least-squares fitting is a statistical technique that enables the fitting algorithm to pay more attention to those response values that are more precise. The weights are proportional to the reciprocals of the replicate variances (variance is SD^2) and so those points with highest precision, i.e. lowest variance, are given greatest weights. The relationship between dose and variance may be linear or quadratic. A suitable mathematical relationship is identified by plotting the observed variances against dose and testing the goodness of fit to candidate models with a statistical package (*Protocol 1C*).

However, there can be problems with weighted fits if a theoretical model is used that is not quite correct. The use of weights may produce a worse, and even unacceptable, fit. An example of this will be seen later.

Tip

Use a weighted curve-fit that takes account of the variation in error across the concentration range, but take care that the model used is appropriate.

There is a simple way to check the suitability of the curve-fit package. Most specialist curve-fit programs can automatically recalculate the concentration of each standard from the signal and the fitted curve-fit parameter values, as if they were unknowns. If the assay is run in triplicate with five standards, back calculation should produce 15 interpolated doses, five clusters of three, each cluster being centred on the 'true' standard value. Accumulating and analysing these data provides valuable information about the quality of the curve-fit, and a reliable estimate of curve-fit bias can be obtained. This is illustrated in *Figure 4*, where the distribution of interpolated doses is represented by the curve and the 'true' standard value by the solid vertical line. Such bias is represented by the distance between the 'centre' of the distribution and the target value. The

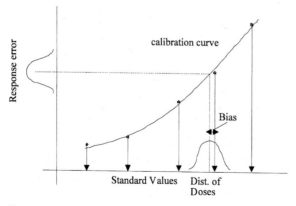

Figure 4. A plot showing the different forms of interpolation error.

variance of this distribution is affected by two sources of error: the response error of the standards and the variability associated with the fitting of the calibration curve, the latter also being a function of the curve-fit model selected. Knowledge of the bias profile for all standards should help to determine how to improve the curve-fit model being used and, if not, it will at least give an indication of the magnitude of bias. However, it is important to note that curve-fit bias can also occur because one or more calibrators have been miscalibrated.

Tip

Whether during assay development or during routine operation, checking the mean differences between the actual and fitted values of the calibrators over a series of assays is always worth doing. Consistent biases warn of either curve-fit or calibration error.

Protocol 1

Selecting a suitable curve-fit procedure

A and B describe testing whether a plot can be linearized by data transformation. C is concerned with determining the response–error relationship and choosing a suitable weighting function for line fitting, and D is about testing theoretical models for suitability.

Equipment and reagents

- Equipment and reagents for operation of immunoassay
- Graph paper, pencil, flexicurve
- Suitable computer and printer
- Curve-fit software
- Spreadsheet software
- Statistical software package (optional)

A. Can the curve be made linear by common data transformations?

1. Run at least three calibration curves for the assay in question with at least six calibrator concentrations in duplicate, or obtain historical calibration curve data.

2. Take the calibrator concentration and signal data sets from these assays, and for each set prepare a spreadsheet table with columns representing dose, signal and appropriate dose and response (signal) metameters for review.

3. Use the plotting function of the spreadsheet (e.g. Chart Wizard in EXCEL) to plot different combinations of dose and response metameters. Carefully inspect 'by eye' to identify those combinations that consistently linearize the data. Give preference to combinations where dose is linear or logarithmic.

4. If a particular method looks promising, continue checking with extra data sets. These should have been collected over a number of assays, encompassing a degree of variation in the assay protocol (time, temperature, etc.) and with more than one

Protocol 1 continued

set of reagents, to ensure that linearization is effective over as wide a range of conditions as will be encountered normally. Formally check linearity by performing a linear regression and comparing the residual sum of squares with that obtained from within replicates. This analysis may require the use of a special statistical package.

5. If the relationship is linear over most, but not all, of the range, consider the possibility of restricting the working range by omitting the highest or lowest calibrator concentration, depending on the application of the assay.

6. If linearization is unsuccessful, proceed to *Protocol 1B*.

7. If all the dose–response curves tested are linearized by the use of the same pair of response and dose metameters, you may routinely analyse your data manually or use the statistical or spreadsheet package to calculate the metameters *and* carry out the linear regression. An example of this approach, using a logit-log transformation was given earlier in the chapter. If you are using a curve-fitting package proceed to *Protocol 1C* to identify a weighting function and then to *Protocol 1D*, choosing the selected conditions from the appropriate menus.

B. Can the curve be made linear by a power transformation?

If common transformations to produce dose and response metameters do not succeed then an intelligent form of trial and error may work. Consider the family of power transforms proposed by Box and Cox (4):

$$\text{New Variable} = \frac{(\text{Old Variable})^\lambda - 1}{\lambda}$$

N.B. The logarithmic transformation is part of this family and can be obtained by letting λ tend to zero.

1. Initially, apply these transformations *only* to the response variable and plot against logarithmic or linear dose. First try the square root transformation ($\lambda = 0.5$).

    (a) If it improves the linearity then the power you require is between 0 and 0.5.

    (b) If it has reversed the curvature then the power required is between 0.5 and 1.0.

    (c) If it has made the plot even more nonlinear then the power required is greater than 1.0.

    A few trials will often give rise to a reasonable linearization.

2. In deciding on your final value of λ, give preference to common fractions of the form 0.5, 0.75 or 0.33.

3. As in *Protocol 1A*, check the selected transformation across a number of assays for consistency before applying it routinely.

C. Determining the dose–response error relationship

Ideally, investigate the dose–response errors with samples as well as standards. The relationships found should be similar.

Protocol 1 continued

With standards:

1. Run an assay standard curve with high-order replication at each standard value.

2. For each standard calculate the variance of the replicate endpoint readings, after transformation if necessary.

3. Plot variance against standard concentration with the scales to be used for the standard curve.

4. Examine the plot for any simple relationship between variance and concentration. Check the goodness of fit of candidate relationships (linear, quadratic etc.) with a statistical package.

With samples (unknowns):

1. Run a set of normal samples (selected to represent wide range of well-spaced analyte concentrations) with a high number of replicates for each.

2. For each sample determine the mean and variance of the replicate endpoint readings.

3. Since here the actual concentrations are unknown, plot variance against the mean endpoint response. (Alternatively, assay the samples and plot against concentration.) See also step 3 above.

4. Examine the plot for any simple relationship between variance and concentration. Check candidate relationships (linear, quadratic, etc.) with a statistical package.

D. Choosing a theoretical model

1. Select the model to be tested from the menu of the curve-fit program, and enter the weighting function as determined in *Protocol 1C*.

2. Fit at least three sets of assay standard data and examine carefully 'by eye' the agreement between the data points, their means and the fitted lines. Note also any statistics related to 'goodness of fit'.

3. Recalculate the concentration for each standard from the signal and the fitted curve-fit parameter values, as if they were unknowns.

4. If marked or consistent bias is evident, try adjusting weights as described below in Section 3.2, or select another model and start again at step 1.

5. If marginal bias is detected or if it is only occasionally found, examine all assay materials and procedure carefully for an explanation that can be tested. Always test a range of models.

6. If lines and points agree, no consistent or significant bias is seen on back-calculation and the results obtained agree closely with the results of manual plotting and interpolation, then continue checking with extra data sets to ensure that curve-fitting is robust. Check using a wide range of different conditions, within the allowed limits of the assay protocol.

Table 2. Spreadsheet layout for weighted logit-log fit, with data from an RIA that produce a good fit

Standard dose (pg/ml)	c.p.m.				Mean c.p.m.	Fraction bound	SD (c.p.m.)	Reps
0	1627	1567	1720	1660	1681		30.18278	8
	1704	1689	1759	1722				
0.625	1182	1291	1294	1312	1269.75	0.749658	59.23048	4
1.25	1029	1112	986	1074	1050.25	0.61604	54.64049	4
2.5	702	784	733	777	749	0.432659	38.61779	4
5	486	485	501	460	483	0.270735	16.99019	4
10	307	277	285	275	286	0.150814	14.65151	4
20	196	204	193	182	193.75	0.094658	9.10586	4
NSB	25	39	51	38	38.25		10.62623	4

Transformed data (logit-log)

Ln dose	Logit counts				Mean	SD
-0.47000363	-0.829	-1.167	-1.1771	-1.239	-1.1031	0.185179
0.22314355	-0.418	-0.635	-0.3102	-0.534	-0.4745	0.14083
0.91629073	0.3886	0.1847	0.3108	0.2019	0.271491	0.096007
1.60943791	0.9817	0.9847	0.93608	1.063	0.991375	0.052686
2.30258509	1.6317	1.7717	1.73299	1.7815	1.729463	0.068456
2.99573227	2.2422	2.1873	2.26338	2.3445	2.259325	0.065196

Weight[b] (wt)	M*wt[c]	M*D*wt[d]	D*wt[e]	D*D*wt[f]		
116.648056	-128.7	60.4775	-54.83	25.76795	Sum of wt[g] = 3987.936	
201.682432	-95.7	-21.354	45.004	10.04238	Sum ofM*wt = 4924.407	
433.968067	117.82	107.956	397.64	364.3547	Sum of M*D*wt = 12214.83	

1441.00964	1428.6	2299.21	2319.2	3732.633	Sum of D*wt = 7491.617
853.561507	1476.2	3399.08	1965.4	4525.496	Sum of D*D*wt = 17103.81
941.066498	2126.2	6369.45	2819.2	8445.518	

[h] Weighted estimator of slope for logit-log = 0.978121

[i] Weighted estimator of intercept for logit-log = −0.60264

[a] The top part of this table is identical to *Table 1* and is repeated here for convenience.

[b] Each weight is calculated as 'replication order/variance' where variance = SD^2, e.g. for a dose of 0.625 pg/ml the weight is $4/(0.185179)^2 = 116.648$, which is the first entry. Note that the standard deviation used is that for the logit values, since it is in this domain we are fitting the line.

[c] Each M*wt is 'mean logit × weight', e.g. for the lowest standard concentration $-1.1031 × 116.648 = -128.67$.

[d] Each M*D*wt is 'mean logit × Ln(Dose) × weight', e.g. for the lowest standard concentration $-1.1031 × -0.47000363 × 116.648 = 60.4775$.

[e] Similarly, D*wts = Ln(Dose) × weight = $-0.47000363 × 116.648 = -54.83$.

[f] Similarly, D*D*wt = $(Ln(Dose))^2 × weight = -0.47000363^2 × 116.648 = 25.768$.

[g] From the various column sums shown (X1 = Sum of Weights, X2 = Sum of M*wts, X3 = Sum of M*D*wts, X4 = Sum of D*wts, X5 = Sum of D*D*wts) (See footnote 'g' for definitions.)

[h] Slope = (X1*X3−X4*X2)/(X5*X1−X4*X4) (See footnote 'g' for definitions.)

[i] Intercept = (X2*X5−X4*X3)/(X5*X1−X4*X4)

3 More worked examples

3.1 A good logit-log fit

The first example involves the same set of standard data (from a competitive assay) that was used previously when explaining manual fitting methods (*Table 1*). The data, together with the necessary intermediate calculations for fitting a logit-log model are shown in *Table 2*, which is based on a printout of an EXCEL™ spreadsheet. The lower sections in *Table 2* contain the necessary intermediate calculations for fitting a weighted logit-log model. A plot of the SD of the signal counts against the natural log of the dose is shown in *Figure 5A*, and it is clear that the data demonstrate heteroscedasticity (non-constant SD). The mean signal for zero dose (B = 1681 c.p.m.) and the NSB (A = 38.25 c.p.m.) are used to obtain the fraction bound values (r) and, thereby the logits ($\ln([1 - r]/r)$). A plot of mean logit against log dose (corresponding exactly to the 'manual' plot of *Figure 1C*), but with a fitted line, is shown in *Figure 5B*.

A plot of the SD of the logit values against log dose is shown in *Figure 5C* and it is clear that the SD of the transformed values is not constant either, so a weighted fit should be considered. The weighting function can be obtained using a statistical package, as explained in *Protocol 1C*. (Normally the weighting function would be based on several sets of data.) However, here the calculated standard deviations rather than 'smoothed' values are used (*Table 2*). It can be seen that the weighted logit-log line is a good fit, without deviation from linearity (*Figure 5B*).

As mentioned in Section 2.3.2, when the logit-log fit is good, a similar fit will be obtained by the 4PL method. For example, when the two fixed (A and B) and two estimated (C and D) variables from the weighted logit-log fit (*Table 2* and *Figure 5B*) (A = 38.25, B = 1681, C = −0.60264 and D = 0.978121) are compared with the four estimated variables obtained by subjecting the same data set to a full nonlinear regression approach with the four-parameter method (A = 42.5, B = 1682.9, C = −0.60367 and D = 0.9876), the two sets of values are very close. This is not always the case, as the next example demonstrates.

3.2 Consequences of a poor logit-log fit

The second set of standard data, which is from a luminescence endpoint, EIA for oestradiol, illustrates what may happen when the standard 4PL and logit-log fits are poor, and what actions may be taken to improve the fit.

The raw data and calculations are shown in *Table 3*, which has the same layout as *Table 2*. The mean logit-log points with the weighted fitted line are shown in *Figure 6A* and it is clear that here the logit-log transformation has not successfully linearized the dose–response relationship. The slope and intercept for the weighted logit-log fit, as shown at the bottom of *Table 3*, are 0.87 and −5.4, respectively. For comparison, after an unweighted fit (all weights set at unity) the slope and intercept were 0.83 and −5.1, respectively (plot not shown). The lower slope in particular is a consequence of the removal of the weights,

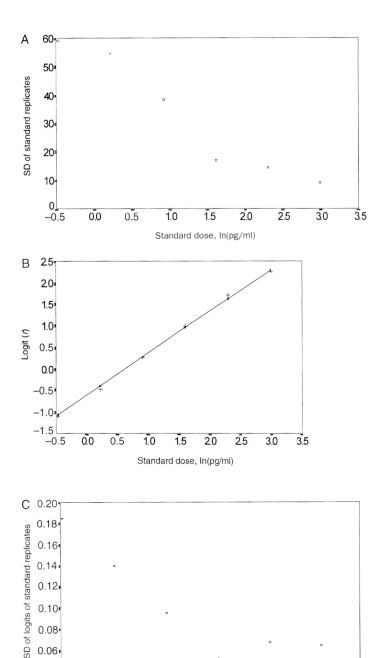

Figure 5. More plots of data derived from an RIA standard curve (*Tables 1* and *2*). A. Replicate SD (c.p.m.) plotted against the natural log of standard dose. B. Mean logit *r* plotted against log dose, with the weighted logit-log fitted line. (This employs the same data and is equivalent to *Figure 1C*.) C. Replicate SD of logit (*r*) against the natural log of dose.

Table 3. Spreadsheet layout for weighted logit-log fit (see *Table 2* for explanatory footnotes), with data from an RIA that produce a poor fit

Dose (pM)	Light units (LU)			Mean LU	Fraction bound	SD	Reps
0	2221.4	2397.8	2401.17	2326.134		88.50862	4
151	1539.4	1711.7	1713.87	1647.135	0.672627	83.21988	4
343	1299.7	1471.7	1453.03	1402.72	0.554785	77.80947	4
789	1098.8	1208.7	1189.45	1145.636	0.430835	62.41341	4
1653	815.25	917.61	906.503	866.4735	0.296239	53.0281	4
3404	585.19	651.1	624.07	610.753	0.172946	32.90352	4
7178	381.34	414.12	404.935	397.171	0.06997	15.02297	4
NSB	239.21	266.53	259.375	252.0478		13.02359	4

Transformed data (logit-log)

Ln dose	Logit-LU			Mean	SD
5.01727984	−0.492	−0.865	−0.8703	−0.669	−0.72423	0.1807
5.83773045	−0.021	−0.356	−0.3188	−0.188	−0.22087	0.151695
6.67076632	0.3712	0.1554	0.19275	0.3976	0.279228	0.122828
7.4103471	0.9868	0.7497	0.77435	0.9595	0.867578	0.122821
8.13270649	1.6536	1.4345	1.52064	1.6627	1.567867	0.110094
8.87877607	2.7108	2.4679	2.531	2.6549	2.591154	0.111362

Weight (wt)	M*wt	M*D*wt	D*wt	D*D*wt
122.502608	−88.72	−445.13	614.63	3083.77
173.827181	−38.39	−224.13	1014.8	5923.873
265.136009	74.033	493.859	1768.7	11798.32
265.162376	230.05	1704.74	1964.9	14560.93
330.014636	517.42	4208.02	2683.9	21827.47
322.541029	835.75	7420.47	2863.8	25426.77

Sum of wt = 1479.184

Sum of M*wt = 1530.141

Sum of M*D*wt = 13157.82

Sum of D*wt = 10910.67

Sum of D*D*wt = 82621.13

Weighted estimator of slope for logit-log = 0.87344

Weighted estimator of intercept for logit-log = −5.40817

because, since the weights are higher for larger doses, the weighted fit will tend to be closer to the data for such doses, which here produced a higher slope and hence greater bias for low doses. This effect can be much more dramatic than is seen here if the change in the values of the weights across the dose range is more than an order of magnitude.

This is shown very clearly in *Table 4*, in which the percentage bias figures (representing poorness of fit) are shown for the above weighted and unweighted fits, as well as for other fits that we will consider now. A four-parameter weighted fit ($A = 244$, $B = 2249$, $C = -5.7$ and $D = 0.91$), which can be expected to be more flexible than the simpler logit-log fit, did no better (*Table 4*) as the parameters are very similar to those for the logit-log fit. The reason that all of the models fail to provide a good fit is that the model is not completely correct, although the weightings adequately reflect the dose–error relationship. However, it would be wrong to consider that the situation hopeless, because, as explained previously, the weightings can be adjusted to compensate for some of the inadequacies of the model.

A feature of the four-parameter model is that, for some assays the model cannot 'bend' sharply enough to connect the zero and the first non-zero standard and, in attempting to do this, it produces a poor fit elsewhere, i.e. the model is not fully accurate. Some of the reasons for this are explained by Peterman (5). For example a competitive immunoassay may have a 'low dose hook' if the concentration of tracer is too low or the concentration of antibody is too high. The logit-log and 4PL models require symmetry in the dose–response curve, and may not respond adequately to this effect. However, if, as is normal, a good fit over the range of the non-zero standards is adequate, the fit can be improved by 'down-weighting' the zero and NSB, e.g. by arbitrarily increasing the standard deviations of these points by a factor of 10. StatLIA® (Brendan Scientific) effectively automates this process for the user (see Section 4).

If this is done, and the four-parameter model refitted (*Table 4* and *Figure 6B*), the agreement between the fitted curve and the data points improves greatly over the standard range. The parameter values become $A = 164$ (observed $= 252$), $B = 1804$ (2326), $C = -7.1$ and $D = 1.0$ (very different from the observed values and the first fit). The curved line in *Figure 6B* is a consequence of using the observed A and B values and *not* those derived from the 4PL fit. Had these fitted values ($A = 164$, $B = 2326$) been used to define the logits, points falling on a straight line would have been obtained.

What has happened is that the quality of fit near zero and above the top standard has been sacrificed to achieve a good fit throughout the range of the non-zero standards. From a user's point of view the model is now adequate. What has been described is not a 'fix' – it is recognition that the model being fitted is not exactly correct over the entire range, but is capable of a high degree of functional efficiency. If they are examined in sufficient detail it can be shown that, to a greater or lesser extent, all models suffer from such problems. However, it is essential that the resultant working range of the assay be limited to

Table 4 With the data set of *Table 3*, comparisons of actual vs. fitted standard concentrations using different curve-fit methods

Actual	Weighted logit-log		Unweighted logit-log		Weighted 4PL		Modified 4PL	
Std Conc. (pmol/l)	Fitted conc. (pmol/l)	% Bias[a]	Fitted conc. (pmol/l)	% Bias	Fitted conc. (pmol/l)	% Bias	Fitted conc. (pmol/l)	% Bias
151	214	42	191	26	219	45	127	−16
343	381	11	349	2	393	15	391	14
789	675	−14	635	−19	693	−12	810	3
1653	1325	−20	1288	−22	1334	−19	1615	−2
3404	2954	−13	2983	−12	2877	−15	3236	−5
7178	9534	33	10180	42	8606	20	7327	2

[a] Note that these figures for % bias are for only one assay run and include an elements of assay–assay error in addition to any systematic bias due to the curve-fit method. To estimate more accurately curve-fit bias, data from a number of assays should be analysed.

258

> **Tip**
>
> Selective adjustments of weightings, particularly of the zero and maximum dose data points, can improve the fit of a four-parameter model across most of the range.

that part of the dose–response curve that is adequately fitted. If this range is inadequate for the assay application, a better model is the only solution.

In this example we have shown the calculations for logit-log in detail. We have not shown the calculations for the 4PL fit because the fitting algorithms are highly computational. For research applications, logit-log is a useful tool and the process we have described may be used early on in the development of a new assay to provide a routine curve-fitting method. We have explained that

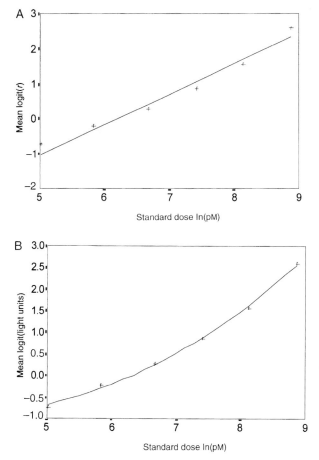

Figure 6. Plots of data derived from a standard curve for a luminescent EIA for oestradiol (*Table 3*). A. Mean logit *r* plotted against log dose, with the weighted logit-log fit. (This is equivalent to *Figure 5B*. B. Mean logit *r* plotted against log dose, with the weighted 4PL fit, using modified weights for the NSB (*A*) and zero (*B*) points.

weighting may have to be adjusted to compensate for model deficiencies, even with the excellent 4PL fit. If the cause of an inadequate fit is asymmetry, then use of a 5PL model will often, but not always, resolve curve-fitting bias.

The same process may be applied to immunometric assays. The main difference from a competitive immunoassay is that, instead of the NSB, an estimate of the signal level for the upper asymptote is required. This is normally well beyond the working range of the assay and, partly for this reason, logit-log is seldom used in practice. However, it is possible to experiment with a variety of values until a good fit is obtained. This is essentially what a 4PL curve-fit program does. In this way such programs usually provide good fits to immunometric assay standard curve data. Where asymmetry in the dose–response relationship causes curve-fit bias with the 4PL method (no matter what values are computed for the upper asymptote) the use of a good-quality 5PL fit will usually resolve the problem.

4 Calibration curve-fit software

Most immunoassay laboratories will have assay data processing software already available to them, but for those that do not, or wish to use another curve-fit method or have access to more features, the following commercial packages may be of interest.

StatLIA® by Brendan Scientific offers a range of curve-fit algorithms for immunoassays, including a weighted five-parameter log-logistic (5PL) program. It allows the back-fitting of data for standards and generates good-quality graphs of the fitted curves. In addition, it can accumulate information from up to 30 curves to define a reference curve for each assay, so that each new curve can be compared with the reference curve and any significant differences flagged. The program also attempts to identify the cause of any changes in curve shape from a list including pipetting, separation, tracer, antibody, buffer, incubation and standards. The package can be integrated with multiple workstations.

Another well-established assay data processing suite is MultiCalc™, from EG&G Wallac. This also includes a number of curve-fit algorithms, quality-control features and interface capability for multiple workstations.

References

1. Rodbard, D. and Hutt, D. M. (1974). In *Radioimmunoassay and related procedures in medicine*, Vol. 1, p. 165. IAEA, Vienna.
2. Faden, V. B. and Rodbard, D. (1975). *Radioimmunoassay data processing*, 3rd edn, (PB 246222–4). National Technical Information Service, Springfield.
3. Rodbard, D. and Feldman, Y. (1978). *Immunochemistry*, **15**, 71.
4. Box, G. E. P. and Cox, D. R. (1964). *Royal Stat. Soc. Ser. B* **26**, 211.
5. Peterman, J. H. (1991). In *Immunochemistry of solid-phase immunoassay* (ed. Butler, J. E.). CRC Press, Boca Raton.

Further reading

Box, F. E. P. and Hunter, W. G. (1962). A useful method for model-building. *Technometrics* **4**, 301–318.

Draper, N. R. and Smith, H. (1966). *Applied regression analysis.* Wiley, New York.

Dudley, R. A., Edwards, P., Ekins, R. P. *et al.* (1985).Guidelines for immunoassay data processing. *Clin. Chem.* **31**, 1264–1271.

Feldman, H. and Rodbard, D. (1971). In *Competitive protein binding assays* (eds Daughaday, W. H. and Odell, W. D.), pp. 158–203. Lippincott, Philadelphia.

Finney, D. J. (1978). *Statistical method in biological assay.* Charles Griffin, London.

Haven, M. C., Orsulak, P. J., Arnold, L. L., and Crowley, G. (1987). *Clin. Chem.* **33**, 1207–1210.

Healy, M. J. R. (1972). *Biochem. J.* **130**, 207–210.

Lynch, M. J. (1989). *J. Biolum. Chemilum.* **4**, 615–619.

Malan, P. G., Cox, M. G., Long, E. W. R. and Ekins, R. P. (1973). In *Radioimmunoassay and related procedures in medicine*, Vol I, pp. 425–455. IAEA Vienna.

Nisbet, J. A., Owen, J. A. and Ward, G. E. (1986). *Ann. Clin. Biochem.* **23**, 694–698.

Nix, B. Calibration curve-fitting. (1994). In *The Immunoassay handbook*, (ed. Wild, D. G.), pp. 117–123. Macmillan, London.

Peterman, J. H. (1991). In *Immunochemistry of solid-phase immunoassay*, (ed. Butler, J. E.), pp. 293–296. CRC Press, Boca Raton.

Raggatt, P. R. (1997). In *Principles and practice of immunoassay* (eds Pricen C. P. and Newman, D. J.), 2nd edn, pp. 269–297. Macmillan, London.

Rodbard, D. (1974). *Clin. Chem.* **20**, 1255–1270.

Rodbard, D. and Feldman, Y. (1978). *Immunochemistry* **15**, 71–76.

Rodbard, D. and Hutt, D. (1974). In *Radioimmunoassay and related procedures in medicine*, Vol. 1, 165–192. International Atomic Energy Agency, Vienna.

Chapter 10
Quality assurance

John Seth

Department of Clinical Biochemistry, Lothian University Hospitals NHS Trust,
The Royal Infirmary of Edinburgh, Lauriston Place, Edinburgh EH3 9YW, UK

1 Introduction

All analytical laboratories, whether in the field of health care, environmental monitoring or manufacturing industry must be able to demonstrate that their output meets defined quality standards. Basic research laboratories, which generally have operated independently of such controls and standards, are increasingly adopting them in response to the growing emphasis on 'evidence-based medicine', and/or as aspects of good management. An international guide to quality standards in analytical chemistry is available (1), and several general quality systems are in use, e.g. the ISO 9000 series from the International Organization for Standardization, and the European EN 45000 series, which evolved from earlier guides to 'good laboratory practice'. The practical implementation of these broad guidelines in the pathology laboratory and their role in laboratory accreditation has been described (2).

Quality assurance techniques in clinical biochemistry are well established (3), but immunoassays present some special requirements. In this chapter, the QA of immunoassays in laboratory medicine is described, with particular emphasis on their use in research and development. Good practices in some types of specialized laboratories in which immunoassays are used routinely may differ in detail, but the clinical laboratory provides a good general model and the general principles of QA are the same.

2 Quality assurance

2.1 Principles

Laboratory investigations comprise a sequence of complex steps that begin with specimen collection, and end with appropriate use of the assay data (*Figure 1*). QA describes all the measures taken to ensure that the entire sequence of events is carried out to a specified quality. QA procedures are systematic and ongoing, and include monitoring activities outside the laboratory. Internal quality control (IQC), which controls the analytical process, and external quality

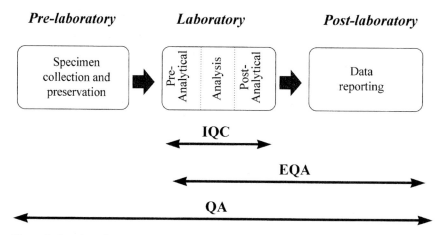

Figure 1. Overview of steps in laboratory measurements and the quality management tools used to monitor and control the laboratory output.

assessment (EQA) which assesses the performance of a laboratory in comparison with its peers, are parts of the QA process.

Figure 1 underlines the point that failure of any one of the steps of an investigation will undermine the value of the final measurements. Therefore, the laboratory worker, while requiring a sound practical knowledge of assay QC, must also be aware of the factors beyond the laboratory that can confound his/her best efforts. It can be surprising to find how little attention is given to events before the specimen reaches the laboratory, and after the results have been despatched, no doubt because these are often the most difficult to control and monitor. It is appropriate, therefore, briefly to review these aspects of QA first.

2.2 Specimen collection and preservation

The most diligent assay control may be worthless in ensuring quality data where specimens are not collected and stored under correct conditions. These concerns are especially relevant to immunoassay because of the wide range of analytes, many of which are subject to physiological variation and to instability. For example, in immunoassays for hormones, tumour markers and drugs, variables such as patient preparation (e.g. fasting, possible interfering medication, time since dose), time of collection (e.g. time of day or month) and stability (e.g. degradation during specimen transit) can markedly affect results. It is also vitally important to have a secure method of specimen identification at all stages from the point of collection and through the analysis, as specimen misidentification or transposition are potentially the most serious errors that can be made. Careful attention to procedures for specimen labelling and handling (e.g. minimizing transfers of specimens between racks and increased automation) may reduce these errors.

Although the above points may appear self-evident, their importance cannot be overstated, not least because poor specimen quality or misidentification will not be detected by IQC. The most appropriate practical advice for the laboratory worker is to anticipate such problems and, irrespective of whether specimens are collected as part of a routine service or research study, to ensure that there are written protocols for specimen collection, preservation and identification. It will usually be necessary, however, to monitor regularly that protocols are being adhered to.

2.3 Reporting results

From the perspective of the recipient of laboratory measurements, it is the return and format of results that defines their view of the laboratory, yet this is another area that is often neglected. Laboratory reports should be clear and informative, and arrive at the correct place without undue delay. The units of measurement should be clearly stated, a point which is especially relevant to immunoassay of peptide hormones, tumour markers and haptens, where different systems of units (e.g. international units per litre (U/l), mass/volume or molar), are in use. Peptide hormone and tumour marker results should be quoted in units of the current IS, especially when other standard preparations are in use that are not necessarily equivalent to the current IS. Where appropriate, therefore, care should be taken to give a full description of, and to quote the official WHO code number of, the standard preparation (e.g. Growth hormone, human, recombinant DNA derived, Code 88/624)

3 Internal quality control

3.1 Definitions

IQC describes the procedures undertaken by the staff within the laboratory to ensure that the analytical work is carried out to a specified quality. IQC procedures are systematic and ongoing, and include the formal monitoring of every assay run to decide whether the results are of suitable quality to be released.

The meaning of the terms commonly used in IQC are illustrated in *Figure 2* and are defined as follows.

Bias: difference between the true concentration of the analyte (X_t) and the mean concentration observed (X). Bias is also known as *systematic error*, and as *inaccuracy*. In immunoassay, the true concentration or value is often unknown, but may be approximated as the reference method value.

Precision: closeness of agreement between test results repeatedly and independently measured under stable conditions, expressed as sd_x or as the relative error (CV, coefficient of variation = $|sd_x \times 100|/X$). Precision is also known as *random error,* (cf. bias or systematic error above), and as *imprecision*.

Total error: The difference between an observed result, x_i, and the true value, X_t. It is the sum of errors due to imprecision and bias.

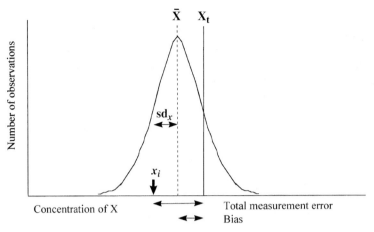

Figure 2. Fundamental concepts in quantitative measurement. X_t is the 'true' concentration of the analyte, and x_i is a single estimate of X_t. Replicated estimates are shown as a normal distribution with a mean of $\bar{X}$ and a scatter or standard deviation of sd_x.

Reference method: A method that, by means of exhaustive investigation, has been shown to have negligible bias in relation to its precision. (e.g. GCMS determination of steroids in biological fluids).

Run (analytical run): Set of measurements obtained under stable conditions, under which a minimum change in results would be expected to occur. A manual immunoassay in which a batch of tubes or plates is processed under identical conditions, or samples processed during 1 day on an automated analyser would be regarded as a run. Between runs, events may occur (e.g. recalibration) that may affect results.

The key features of IQC are summarized in *Table 1*, and their practical implementation described in the following sections. The division of the process into three phases, of preanalytical, analytical and postanalytical illustrates the often used saying that 'prevention is better than cure'. IQC begins long before the assay is set up, and only ends with the effective use of the IQC data in controlling the release of results from the laboratory.

3.2 Preanalytical quality control

3.2.1 Laboratory facilities and equipment

Adequate laboratory space, lighting and heating are prerequisites for analysts to perform skilled work. Equipment should be correctly specified for the task and be properly maintained, e.g. pipettes should be capable of the required accuracy and precision, and their performance periodically checked. For RIA, special attention to cleanliness and calibration of gamma counters is needed, including checks on detector equivalence of multidetector counters. Nonisotopic methods require special care to avoid environmental contaminants, e.g. dust, fluorophores

Table 1. Key features of IQC

Preanalytical quality control
- The laboratory facilities and equipment must be adequate for the assays to be performed
- The reagents and standards must be correctly prepared and be within their 'use-by date'
- The protocol for the method should be recorded, and adhered to
- The analyst should be appropriately experienced and trained

Analytical quality control
- The IQC specimens (e.g. serum pools) should have identical properties to the test specimens in the assay.
- Baseline assay performance (precision and bias) estimated under stable assay conditions (Section 3.3.2)
- The IQC specimens should be processed identically to test specimens through the entire assay procedure.
- The IQC results should be simply and clearly presented, e.g. on a control chart
- There should be defined criteria for run rejection, e.g. control rules
- The IQC plan should take account of the quality requirements.

Postanalytical quality control
- IQC failures should be explored in a constructive manner and remedial action taken.
- IQC and other data (eg EQA) should be reviewed regularly to search for trends in performance

---

or quenching agents. Where automated analysers are used careful adherence to analyser maintenance schedules is vitally important.

3.2.2 Calibrants and reagents

Working calibrants should be traceable to an analyte preparation of known purity. In the case of analytes that cannot be fully characterized by physico-chemical methods (e.g. many protein hormones and virological antigens) the appropriate WHO standard should be used. A catalogue of WHO biological standards and reference materials is available from the NIBSC (4). Calibrants and reagents should be prepared to written protocols, and the batch numbered and dated. In general, antibody and standard solutions should be stored frozen in aliquots sufficient for a single run to avoid repeated freezing and thawing, which can accelerate protein breakdown. Storage at $-30°C$ or colder is preferable to $-20°C$, as the set temperature will rarely be achieved in a freezer subject to frequent opening and closing. Experience will determine the shelf-life of standards and reagents but it is advisable to err on the side of caution.

3.2.3 Method design and protocols

Methods and reagents should be optimized so that minor changes in conditions have minimum effect on performance. The precision of any quantitative measurement is the square root of the sum of the variances of the component steps:

$$sd = \sqrt{sd_a^2 + sd_b^2 + sd_c^2 + \ldots}$$

where sd_a, sd_b sd_c, etc., are the standard deviations of steps a, b, c, etc. (e.g. pipetting, washing, absorbance measurement), and, therefore, attempts to improve assay precision must focus first on the steps that are least precise. There should be written 'standard operating procedures' (SOP) for the assay procedure and instrument operation, and, more importantly, these should be adhered to. The assay procedure should not be modified without formally verifying that performance is not adversely affected. Laboratory accreditation agencies will usually require documentary evidence of this.

3.2.4 Staff training

Manual immunoassays are among the more technically demanding of laboratory methods and can be vulnerable to changes in performance with changes in analyst. A compromise in staff rotation between the needs of training programmes and continuity of experience at the bench needs to be achieved. As a rough guide, staff changes should not be more frequent than 3-monthly. Immunoassay automation has the benefit of permitting greater flexibility in staff deployment, but does not obviate the need for adequate training in analyser operation and maintenance. Training should be the responsibility of a named person and not informally delegated to successive operators, which might risk undesirable changes from recommended practice-being introduced.

3.3 Quality control of the analysis

Figure 3 gives an overview of the design and implementation of an IQC plan for an immunoassay, and the overall process is described in detail in this section.

3.3.1 Choice of IQC material

The desirable properties of IQC specimens are summarized in *Table 2*, although for immunoassay, all the listed requirements are rarely met.

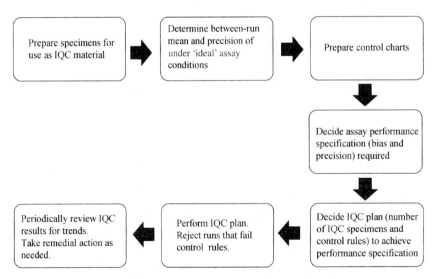

Figure 3. Overview of steps in planning and performing IQC of the analytical process.

Table 2. Desirable properties of IQC specimens

- Matrix identical to test specimens in assay
- Analyte concentrations close to decision levels of test
- Stable (before and after reconstitution if lyophilized)
- Free from infectious hazards (negative for hepatitis B, hepatitis C, and HIV antigens)
- Target value preassigned, or determined *in house*
- Large volume of single batch available

- Economical

Several types of control material may be used to assess precision and accuracy, and they are best regarded as complementary to each other rather than mutually exclusive alternatives.

3.3.1.1 Pooled material, prepared in-house

Possible sources of this pooled material are (a) pooled residues from test specimens routinely received at the laboratory, and (b) unwanted serum from blood donations or from therapeutic venesections. In some research applications it may be that (a) is the only available option, although the risk of introducing infected material into the IQC pools should be carefully considered. For tests on human serum, unwanted serum from blood donations that have been comprehensively screened for infectious hazards is generally preferable. *Protocol 1* is a generic procedure for preparation of pooled material for IQC.

Protocol 1

Preparation of liquid, pooled material for use in IQC

Equipment and reagents

- Supply of samples that have been tested by the methods for which the pool is to be used and stored under suitable conditions, and the results of the analyses
- Tests for infective hazards (hepatitis B and C, HIV, etc.) or the results of such tests

- Filtration apparatus or Sartorius Sartobran 300 capsules, 0.45/0.2 μm
- Tubes for storage

Method

1. Identify enough samples of the test material (e.g. serum, plasma) to provide sufficient volume for control samples for at least 50 assay runs. Screen the samples for infective hazards (e.g. hepatitis B and C, HIV). Depending on the sensitivity of the virological tests, reduce the number of screening tests by screening subpools. Discard infected samples by the locally approved procedure.

2. Group the samples according to analyte concentration to give a set of pools of different concentrations, preferably at levels representing cut-offs or other decision criteria. If necessary, store temporarily at −30 °C.

Protocol 1 continued

3. Pool each group of samples and mix gently. Stand at 4°C overnight. A protein precipitate may develop in some serum or plasma pools, which can be removed by filtration.

4. Check that the analyte concentration of each pool is suitable for IQC purposes by assay of an aliquot. If necessary, add a calculated amount of standard analyte in a very small volume of buffer or serum to increase the concentration.

5. Dispense suitable aliquots (usually 0.5 ml or more) into tubes for storage. Using smaller volumes may risk errors due to sample evaporation while frozen. Store at −30°C.

Because of the wide concentration ranges covered by many immunoassays, it is usual to use IQC specimens covering the low, medium and high concentration ranges and samples should be selected to achieve this. Where serum from blood donations is used, and analyte levels are normal, it may be possible to remove analyte by absorption on resin, charcoal, or immunoabsorbents, or to supplement the level by addition of analyte in the form of pure material, or a high-concentration specimen. However, these manipulations challenge the first of the requirements in *Table 2*. Liquid IQC sera should be stored at −30°C or colder to minimize degradation and not −20°C which, under working conditions, will give temperatures near the eutectic point of serum where protein breakdown may occur.

3.3.1.2 Lyophilized commercial IQC sera

These are convenient to use, can contain a wide range of analytes, and may have preassigned target values. However, they are relatively expensive and may not be suitable for many research applications. The use of lyophilized sera also introduces the potential for errors in reconstitution and they may not behave identically to patient sera, perhaps reflecting changes in the molecular forms of the analyte or in the serum protein matrix on lyophilization. It should be noted that the preassigned targets for immunoassay analytes cited by the supplier often vary according to the method used, and are of limited value in assessing accuracy. Therefore, it will usually be necessary to determine target values locally. Some suppliers of materials for IQC are listed in the Appendix.

3.3.1.3 Certified reference materials

A CRM is a material in which the analyte is certified to have a concentration within stated confidence limits, determined by a reference method, i.e. one that has been shown to have negligible inaccuracy in relation to its precision. The purpose of CRM is for the occasional assessment of accuracy, by providing traceability of results to an RMV. CRM for a limited range of analytes, e.g. serum proteins, α-fetoprotein, apolipoprotein, thyroglobulin, thyroxine, cortisol and progesterone are available through the European Commission (5).

3.3.1.4 Other types of specimen occasionally used in IQC

In view of the limited availability of CRM, other IQC materials are often used in the assessment of accuracy. *Recovery specimens* can be prepared by adding known quantities of the calibrant to analyte-free serum, taking care to use independently prepared solutions of the calibrant for assay calibration and preparation of the recovery specimens. *EQA scheme specimens* with a target assigned as the consensus mean may also provide an indication of accuracy, and are discussed more fully later in this chapter. *Blank specimens* may be helpful in assessing background interference as a cause of inaccuracy. They may be prepared by selection of appropriate samples, by pharmacological suppression in donor subjects (e.g. oral glucose for suppression of growth hormone levels), by specific removal with immunoabsorbents, or, if no better method is possible, by physicochemical removal of the analyte (e.g. charcoal absorption; see *Protocol 4* of Chapter 7).

3.3.2 Baseline assessment of assay performance

Having prepared and stored a new supply of IQC specimens (or obtained them otherwise), the next stage is to estimate the mean concentration and precision of the results for each pool in the set under stable or 'ideal' assay conditions. *Protocol 2* describes the steps involved.

Protocol 2

Determination of baseline assay performance with new IQC samples

Equipment and reagents
- All requirements for the performance of the relevant assay, which may be in routine operation with established controls

Method
1. Before each run, allow a set of frozen samples to thaw and to come to room temperature, mixing thoroughly by gentle inversion. If commercial lyophilized specimens are used, follow the manufacturer's directions. Include one specimen at each concentration in each run. If the assay is in routine operation, place randomly in the assay run among the unknowns.
2. Perform at least 15 assay runs under stable conditions, i.e. with reagents of proven reliability and with an experienced analyst.
3. Treat the IQC specimens identically to the unknowns, i.e. take the IQC specimens through all the steps, including any pretreatment (e.g. extraction, chromatography), and use the same number of replicates as is used for the unknowns.
4. For each IQC specimen calculate the between-run mean, standard deviation and coefficient of variation (see below). If sample results are calculated as the mean of duplicate determinations, then IQC specimen results are calculated in the same way, (i.e. not as two independent determinations)

If x_i is the control result in each of n runs, the between-run performance statistics are estimated using the formulae below. (Use the means, not the individual duplicate results for each sample when doing this.)

$$\text{Mean, } \bar{X} = \frac{\sum_{i=1}^{n} x_i}{n}$$

$$\text{Standard deviation, } SD = \sqrt{\frac{n\sum_{i=1}^{n} x_i^2 - \left(\sum_{i=1}^{n} x_i\right)^2}{n(n-1)}}$$

$$\text{Coefficient of variation, } CV = \frac{sd}{\bar{X}} \times 100$$

These statistics are easily calculated using a hand-held scientific calculator. They define the expected between-run mean and sd (or CV) for each IQC specimen in the assay, which, in turn, define the criteria for acceptance or rejection of future assay runs. Note that it would be incorrect to include more than one result per IQC specimen per run in the estimation of between-run performance statistics, as this would underestimate the between-run scatter.

3.3.3 Quality control charts

IQC data are intended to control the assay process in real time and their format and layout should be clear and straightforward. Recording the IQC results in tabular or spreadsheet form, together with details of assay run (date, reagent and calibrator batches, analyst name), is a basic minimum. However, significant

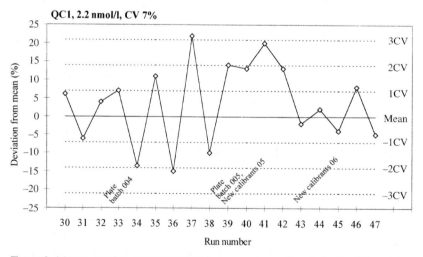

Figure 4. A Levey–Jennings chart for IQC of an immunoassay. Results for the IQC specimen are plotted as the relative error (per cent deviation form mean) and control lines are drawn at ± 1, ± 2, and ± 3CV for the QC specimen, corresponding to ± 1, ± 2, and ± 3 sd. The chart shows imprecision between runs 34 and 38, followed by positive bias from runs 39–42. Changes in reagents, calibrants, etc, can be marked to assist interpretation of events and trends.

trends may not be apparent without graphical presentation in the form of a Levey–Jennings chart (also known as Shewhart chart) (*Figure 4*). Details of the design and use of these charts have been described in standard texts (3) but for immunoassay some modification of the standard presentation is desirable. *Protocol 3* and *Figure 4* illustrate the preparation of a simple Levey-Jennings chart for the IQC of an immunoassay.

Protocol 3

Preparation of control chart

Equipment

- Graph paper, ruler, pencil, eraser

Method

1. Prepare the chart as shown in *Figure 4*, with 'Run number' along the x-axis, and IQC result as 'Deviation from mean (%)' on the y-axis. Scale the y-axis in units of relative error (a range of up to −25% to +25% will, hopefully, be adequate). This is preferable to scaling the axis in absolute error (concentration units) because in most immunoassays the sd increases with concentration, resulting in different y-scales for IQC specimens of different concentration. When, as is usual, there is more than one IQC in an assay, and the plot for each pool is stacked above a common x-axis on a single sheet of paper (e.g. *Figure 7*), a common y-axis facilitates interpretation.

2. Mark on the chart the identity of the IQC specimen, its mean and between-run CV, as previously estimated (e.g. according to *Protocol 2*).

3. Draw horizontal lines at ± 1CV, ± 2CV and ± 3CV around the zero line. (In the chart in *Figure 4* for an immunoassay with a between-run CV of 7%, the lines are drawn at ± 7%, ± 14% and ± 21%.)

4. Plot IQC specimen results on the chart the each assay run. It is helpful to subsequent reviews of assay performance to routinely note on the chart all changes in reagents and standards with the run number

Software packages for processing immunoassay data (Chapter 9) often provide facilities for plotting Levey–Jennings charts.

3.3.4 Interpretation of IQC results

The principle of interpretation is to detect significant changes in bias and precision while not rejecting in-control runs (false rejection). In a simple IQC procedure with one IQC specimen per run (*Figure 4*), basic statistical theory indicates that when the assay is in control, approximately 5% of IQC results will fall outside the ± 2CV limits, and that approximately 0.3% will fall outside the ± 3CV limits. Assay runs in which the IQC result is outside ± 3CV are unlikely to be in control and should, therefore, be rejected. Results outside the 2CV limits but not outside the 3CV limits might indicate a change in performance, but are not necessarily a signal for rejection. Intuitively, the assayist might await IQC results from subsequent assay runs and combine data across two or more runs to obtain a more complete assessment of trends.

Difficulties with the above simple approach are that the power of the rejection criteria to identify out of control runs is not objectively defined, and that when several IQC specimens are included in each run, and some are in control and others are out of control, the results are difficult to interpret.

These limitations can be overcome by a more formal approach based on the use of quality control rules.

3.3.5 Quality control rules

The approach developed by Westgard and coworkers (6,7) is based on computer simulation techniques to estimate the probability for detecting stated sizes of systematic error (bias), and random error (precision) with different numbers of control observations and different rejection criteria, or control rules. *Figure 5* shows power function graphs for the control rules listed in the right hand panels. The nomenclature of these, and other more complex 'multirule' rejection rules is shown in *Table 3*.

Figures 5 also demonstrates some important points about the power of IQC procedures to detect errors. For example, using a simple IQC procedure with one IQC specimen per run and the 1_{3s} rejection rule (*Figure 4*), the probability of detecting a systematic error of just 2sd (e.g. a 14% shift in bias in an assay with a between-run CV of 7%) would be only 0.15 (*Figure 5A*), and the probability of detecting a twofold increase in random error (e.g. CV worsening from 7 to 14%) would be only 0.1 (*Figure 5B*). Increasing the number of IQC specimens per run to three with the same 1_{3s} rejection rule improves the chance of detecting the same errors to (nearly) 0.4 and 0.3 respectively. This remains a very unsatisfactory control procedure since less than half the affected runs would be detected. Tightening the rejection criteria to 1_{2s} with three IQC specimens per run would improve the chance of detecting systematic and random errors to 0.8 and 0.6. However, the chance of rejecting in control runs is then 0.15, i.e. one of every

Table 3. Nomenclature of IQC rejection criteria or control rules

1_{3s}	Reject when one control measurement exceeds ± 3SD control limits
2 of 3_{2s}	Reject when any two of three consecutive control measurements exceed the same +2sd or – 2sd control limits
R_{4s}	Reject when one control measurement exceeds the +2sd control limit, and another exceeds the –2sd control limit.
3_{1s}	Reject when three consecutive control observations exceed the same +1sd or –1sd control limit.
6_x	Reject when six consecutive control measurements fall on the same side of the mean.
$1_{3s}/2of3_{2s}/R_{4s}/3_{1s})$	'Multirule' approach. Reject when any one of the rules specified in the combination is broken.

Note that the quality control rules express errors on an absolute scale, although they can be applied to relative errors by substituting CV for sd

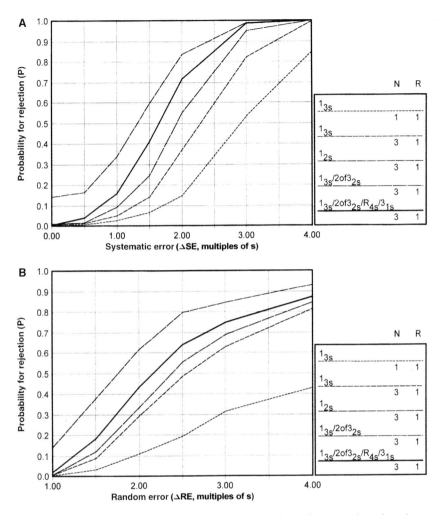

Figure 5. Power function graphs showing the probability of rejecting runs where there is a change in bias (A, systematic error) and in precision (B, random error), using alternative control rules. The changes are expressed in multiples of the assay precision (s). See *Table 3* for key to nomenclature of the control rules in the right panel. N= number of IQC results per run, R = number of runs. Graphs prepared using QC Validator software (8).

eight runs that are 'in-control' would be rejected. Combining results from multiple IQC specimens in a 'multirule' approach (e.g. $1_{3s}/2of3_{2s}/R_{4s}/3_{1s}$) reduces false rejections while providing probabilities of detecting the systematic and random errors of 0.7 and 0.45.

The conclusions from these simulated data are that:

- Increasing the number of IQC specimens per run, or tightening the rejection criteria, improves the probability of error detection, but also increases the probability of false rejection.
- A multirule approach, combining results from multiple IQC specimens can

maintain error detection without incurring a high probability of false rejection.

- For the majority of common control rules, changes in assay bias are more reliably detected than changes in precision.

3.3.6 Planning and implementing an IQC strategy to achieve quality goals

The above concepts provide a basis for planning a control strategy to achieve a level of performance appropriate to the intended use of the data. Thus, the routine clinical analyst might define performance in terms of clinical decision requirements, or the total error allowable in proficiency testing (EQA) schemes. The research analyst wishing to derive optimum value from a series of measurements might set a performance specification to maintain bias and precision as close to 'ideal' as practically possible, e.g. bias within ± 10% and CV not more than twice ideal. Both approaches can be easily followed using the 'QC Validator' software (8), which guides the user interactively through the IQC planning process. A simple illustration of the approach is given in *Protocol 4*.

Protocol 4

Planning and implementing an IQC strategy

The next section describes the application of this protocol to an example.

Equipment

- Graph paper, ruler, pencil, eraser, or QC Validator software (see Appendix) and suitable hardware

Method

1. Determine the quality requirement for the results in terms of the change in bias and precision that will cause run rejection.

2. Calculate the changes in bias and precision (critical errors) that cause run rejection in multiples of the between-run precision (CV), determined under ideal conditions (*Protocol 2*).

3. Using power function graphs (8), identify the control strategy (number of IQC results per run, rejection rules, number of runs) that will give probabilities of error detection and false rejection for 3sd errors of about 0.9 and 0.05, respectively. Between two and four IQC specimens will usually be adequate.

4. Place IQC specimens in each assay run as described in protocol.

5. Calculate the percentage error from the mean for each IQC specimen and plot the per cent deviation on the control chart.

6. Using the chosen control rules and the 1, 2 and 3 × CV limits on the control chart, determine whether the run can be accepted or rejected.

Protocol 4 continued

7. If the run is rejected, investigate the cause of the run failure, and take remedial action.

8. Review strategy, as required, in relation to changes in quality requirements and changes in method performance.

3.3.6.1 Example of IQC planning and operation

Assume that the assay in question is a manual immunoassay for serum testosterone with a between-run precision of 7% in the concentration range around which clinical decisions are made (3.0–10.0 nmol/l). The quality requirement is to detect and reject runs in which there is a shift in bias of 15%, or where the precision has worsened to 20%. Expressed in multiples of the assay CV, this corresponds to a shift in bias of $15/7 = 2.1$, and $20/7 = 2.8$ in precision.

Referring to the power function graphs for candidate IQC procedures (*Figure 6*) and interpolating these critical errors from the *x*-axes indicates that using three IQC specimens per run with the $1_{3s}/2$ of 3_{2s} /$R_{4s}/3_{1s}/6_x$ multirule as rejection criterion could be suitable. This combination would give probabilities of detecting systematic and random errors of about 0.95 and 0.7, with less than 0.05 chance of false rejection on the grounds of bias. Note that an alternative approach with four IQC specimens per run, and a simple $1_{2.5s}$ rejection rule would achieve slightly better detection of random error, with a small loss in detection of systematic error, and a small increase in false rejection.

The control charts for this testosterone assay in routine operation are shown in *Figure 7*. Using three control specimens and applying the multirule, the runs marked with arrows were rejected. Comments on the rejected runs are given in *Table 4*.

3.3.7 Benefits and limitations of IQC planning approach in immunoassay

3.3.7.1 Benefits

Benefits include:

1. The quality requirement is an explicit part of the IQC plan.

2. The probability of detection of significant errors is known approximately.

3. The size of the analytical errors in relation to quality requirements highlights those aspects of the process that most need attention. Where the critical error is large (allowable error large in relation to assay error) a minimum of IQC samples with a simple control rule and wide limits (e.g. 1_{3s}) might be adequate. When the critical error is small (allowable error small in relation to assay error), a more intensive IQC plan and efforts to reduce analytical errors are indicated.

4. Where IQC results fail control rule criteria, the rule that fails can indicate the type of error (bias or precision) occurring.

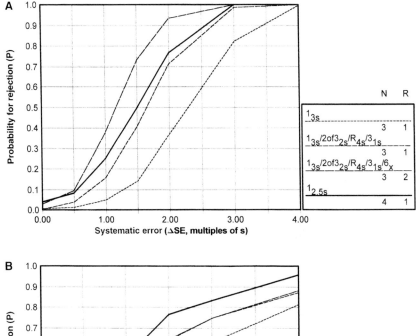

Figure 6. Power function graphs for alternative IQC strategies for a manual immunoassay for testosterone in serum (A, systematic error; B, random error). Graphs prepared using QC Validator software (8).

3.3.7.2 Limitations

Limitations include:

1. The approach of Westgard *et al.* (6) assumes constant measurement errors throughout the assay run. While this is appropriate for many biochemical analyses performed on automated equipment, it may not be applicable to some immunoassays. For example, because of the wide concentration of analyte measured in immunoassay, both systematic and random errors may vary with concentration. This is most likely to be the case in limited antibody (competitive) assays rather than in excess antibody (noncompetitive) assays, where the working range is greater.

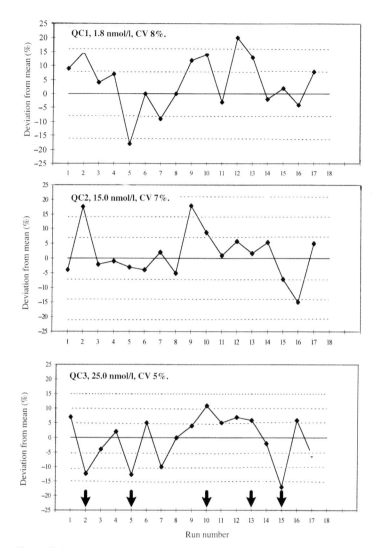

Figure 7. Levey–Jennings chart for the IQC of a manual immunoassay with three IQC specimens per run, and the $1_{3s}/2$ of $3_{2s}/R_{4s}/3_{1s}/6_x$ rejection rule. The broken lines show the ± 1, ± 2, and ± 3CV limits for each IQC specimen. The arrows show runs that fail the rejection rule; *Table 4* gives the details of the rules failed and possible causes.

Table 4. Application of the $1_{3s}/2$of$3_{2s}/R_4$s$/3_{1s}$ multirule to the testosterone RIA IQC data shown in *Figure 7*

Run No.	Rule failed	IQC specimen	Probable cause
2	R_{4s}	QC2, QC3	Imprecision
5	2of3_{2s}	QC1, QC3	Negative bias
10	3_{1s}	QC1, QC2, QC3	Positive bias
13	6_x	QC1, QC2, QC3 (Runs 12,13)	Positive bias
15	1_{3s}	QC3	Imprecision

2. Errors may vary across the immunoassay run, especially in manual assays due, for example, to nonuniformity of temperature or shaking conditions across microtitre plates or tube racks.

3. The multirule approach is more complex to apply than simple rejection criteria. Some automated analysers incorporate user-defined rules in their data-processing facilities.

3.3.8 Automated assays: particular considerations

Fully automated immunoassays present different operational features from manual batch assays and these should be taken into account in planning an IQC protocol.

1. Calibration is performed relatively infrequently, with sample results being calculated from stored calibration-curve parameters, in contrast to batch assays, where calibrators are included in every run. This economy of calibration is made possible by the stability of analytical process, but implies that errors of bias are most likely to occur after the instrument has been idle, or maintenance work has been done. Where IQC results fall outside limits at analyser start-up, a one- or two-point recalibration may be done to adjust the calibration-curve parameters. An IQC plan with high error detection at start-up is therefore advisable.

2. In many automated systems, tests are performed sequentially during the working day, whereas in batch analysis, tests (unknowns and IQC) are run simultaneously. Consequently, in batch analysis all IQC results are available at the time of reporting, maximizing the power of the QC rules. This is not practicable with automated sequential analysers unless IQC validation of results is delayed until the end of the working day. Unlike batch mode, run acceptance should be confirmed before the unknowns have been analysed. This again implies the need for an IQC plan with high error detection at start-up. From this point onwards, IQC specimens can be randomly placed throughout the day, culminating in one IQC specimen before close down at the end of the day.

3. The reagent and consumables costs of IQC on automated systems are relatively high, and the IQC plan must be carefully defined to balance effectiveness and economy. In order to comply with regulatory requirements, laboratories should, at minimum, follow manufacturers' recommended IQC protocols. However, the IQC planning approach of Westgard and coworkers (6, 7) provides a more objective approach. Application of this process to several immunoassays run on automated equipment (Abbott IMx®) led to the conclusion that proficiency testing performance criteria could be met by a two-stage IQC process. That is, with a 1_{3s} or $1_{2.5s}$ rule with $N = 6$ at weekly instrument start-up when measurement instability might be greatest, and $N = 2$–3 for daily monitoring.

The availability of analysers with on-board data processing facilities to store user-defined control rules and alert the operator to failures will simplify the routine application of this approach.

3.3.9 Other strategies in IQC

Other techniques in IQC may be used, although these are usually in addition to, rather than as an alternative to, the above use of stable control material.

3.3.9.1 Cumulative sum chart

CUSUM charts can be helpful in identifying trends in performance. The chart is prepared using IQC specimen results as in the Levey–Jennings chart. The run number is plotted on the x-axis, but the y-axis now shows the cumulated sum of the difference between the observed result and the target value of the IQC specimen, i.e. in *Figure 4* where the percentage deviations in runs 30–34 are 6, −6, 4, 7 and −13, the plotted CUSUM values would be 6, 0, 4, 11 and −2. A horizontal line is drawn at the mid-point of the y-axis at CUSUM = 0, and for an in-control assay, the CUSUM plot would follow, with minor positive and negative deviations, the zero line. IQC results falling persistently on one side of the mean will cause the CUSUM plot to slope away from the zero line. A persistent positive or negative CUSUM slope therefore indicates assay bias.

The problems with CUSUM charts are that the target value must be assigned with care to avoid a sloping plot under 'in-control' conditions, and determination of a significant change in slope can be somewhat subjective. A variant of this method, which may be more objective, is to scale the chart so that the distance between two consecutive runs on the x-axis equals twice the between-run sd on the y-axis. A 45° slope then represents a bias of 2sd.

3.3.9.2 Repeat analytical controls

Some of the limitations associated with pools can be overcome by the repeat analysis of from one to three selected patient specimens from each previous assay run. Repeat analytical controls (RAC) reflect performance on authentic patient specimens over a wide concentration range and can detect errors in specimen identification, while IQC pools reflect performance with specimens that have often been modified (addition or removal of analyte), and at a few concentrations that become well known to the analyst. RAC do not, however, provide an indication of long-term assay stability. Between-run precision can be estimated as:

$$sd = \sqrt{\frac{\Sigma d^2}{2N}}$$

where d = difference between repeat observations, and N = number of repeated specimens.

3.3.9.3 Patient data

The mean or median of results on patient specimens within an assay run, calculated after trimming to remove low and high values (e.g. by exclusion of values outside the range mean ± 3sd), has been used as an additional control parameter in general clinical biochemistry. The technique is not widely used because it cannot detect imprecision and has poor sensitivity to bias changes relative to the use of stable IQC material. However, it may have a value when large numbers of samples are being routinely screened. For example, in maternal serum screening programmes for Down's syndrome and neural tube defects, continuous monitoring of patient medians for serum α-fetoprotein, chorionic gonadotrophin and other analytes can provide information on assay stability and confirmation of the validity of the parameters used for risk calculation.

3.3.9.4 Assay parameters

IQC results on test material indicate the quality of the entire assay procedure, but it may be helpful to also record key parameters of assay performance. These include the background and maximum signals (absorbance, radioactivity, luminescence, etc.), the calibration curve parameters (slope, intercept) and the degree of scatter of the calibrator points about the calculated curve. Inspection of these parameters, together with records of reagent or kit batch number, can assist in determining the cause of trends and failures IQC results.

3.4 Postanalytical quality control

3.4.1 Review of QC data

It must be emphasized that IQC is a collaborative activity involving all staff and attempts to operate IQC as a 'policing' regime are not likely to be successful. Where a run fails to meet quality criteria, the reasons should be explored in a constructive, noncritical manner. Often, a lesson will be learned that benefits future practice. When a procedure is the responsibility of a single analyst it is beneficial to have a second person involved in assessing the daily QC results.

3.4.2 Troubleshooting

It is difficult to generalize causes of IQC failure, as these depend on the type of immunoassay. However, a summary guide to features of assays to examine in the event of IQC failure is given in *Table 5*.

3.5 Limitations of IQC

IQC ensures that assay runs conform to defined quality standards: it cannot ensure that errors do not occur with individual test specimens. *Table 6* summarizes some of the errors that might go undetected.

However, another aspect of the QA process can detect some of these errors, and this is discussed in the following sections.

4 External quality assessment

4.1 Principles

EQA describes the set of procedures operated by an external agency to compare objectively a laboratory's results with an agreed target. In contrast to IQC, EQA

Table 5. Some causes of errors in bias and precision in immunoassays

Assay stage	Bias	Precision
Set-up	Incorrect or degraded calibrant	Imprecise pipetting of samples and reagents
	Incorrect calibrant matrix	Reagents not mixed
	Delay between set-up of calibrants and test samples	Temperature gradients
Separation of free and bound label	Separation reagents not optimized	Inadequate washing
		Inadvertent loss of solid phase
Signal detection	High background signal	Nonequivalence of detectors (especially multihead gamma counters)
		Contaminants on reaction tubes or detectors.
		Environmental contaminants (esp. fluorescence, chemiluminescence)
Data processing	Incorrect curve fit model	
	Incorrect calibrant conversion factor (mass to IU)	

Table 6. Errors in immunoanalysis that may not be detected by IQC

Pre-analytical	Analytical	Post-analytical
Incorrect specimen identity	Insufficient sample due to pipette/probe blockage	Incorrect results transcription
Specimen degraded on storage	Incorrect reagent addition	
Incorrect type of specimen tube	Interference in test specimen, e.g. heterophilic antibodies, lipaemia	
	High-dose hook effect	
	Incorrect/missing dilution factor	

is not used to decide on the acceptability of results in real time, but provides a retrospective assessment of a laboratory's performance in relation to others.

The principles of EQA are shown in *Figure 8*. Identical aliquots of test material are distributed to participating laboratories from a designated laboratory or organizing centre. In each laboratory the aliquots are assayed and the result returned to the EQA centre, from which the statistics shown in *Figure 8* can be calculated. These statistics provide objective measures of overall (all-method) performance, individual method performance and laboratory performance.

4.2 Uses and availability of EQA schemes

From the above, it is evident that EQA has several important uses (*Table 7*). It provides a major information resource at several levels that, together, are a stimulus towards laboratory and method improvement.

EQA schemes operate in all major laboratory disciplines but vary in their approach. EQA schemes may be provided commercially, or on behalf of

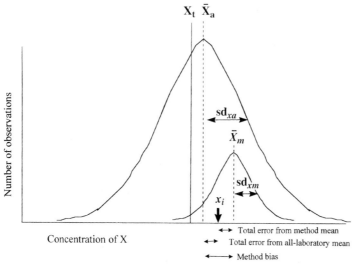

Figure 8. Principles of EQA, showing distribution of results on a single sample, assayed by different methods, in different laboratories. $\bar{X}_t$ is the 'true' value of analyte X. The statistics $\bar{X}_a$ and sd_{xa} are the mean and scatter of results for all laboratories, $\bar{X}_m$ and sd_{xm} are the corresponding statistics for laboratories using a single method. x_i is the result reported by a single laboratory. In the absence of a reliable estimate of X_t (e.g. a RMV) to set a target, laboratory performance is usually expressed as its deviation from the overall mean $[100(x_i - \bar{X}_a)/\bar{X}_a]$ or the method mean $[100(x_i - \bar{X}_m)/\bar{X}_m]$. The mean deviation over several samples issued over a period of time gives an estimate of the laboratory's bias relative to the target.

Table 7. Uses of EQA data

The laboratory
Provides information on a laboratory's performance in relation to peer laboratories
Complementary role to IQC in quality assurance:
Educational value towards best practice
Provides objective data to permit inter-laboratory comparison or combination of results in research
Provides objective data to assist laboratory accreditation
Diagnostics industry
Information on method performance in relation to peer methods
Guide and stimulus to method design and improvement
Professional associations, government departments
Information on overall quality of service, e.g. in healthcare and in environmental monitoring laboratories
Guide to activities requiring additional resources
Aid to public confidence in laboratory services

professional associations. Appendix 1 lists some of the providers of EQA schemes in pathology, which include analytes measured by immunoassay. The research analyst might, however, find that EQA is not available for a particular novel analyte and in such circumstances an exchange of samples among interested laboratories might be of value. Thereby, a new EQA scheme may become established.

4.3 Operation of EQA schemes for immunoassay

As noted above for IQC, the EQA of immunoassays presents some difficulties arising from the use of biological reagents to measure complex analytes. *Table 8* summarizes the key points that the laboratory should look for in the selection of an EQA scheme.

4.3.1 Sample material distributed

Identity of behaviour between EQA samples and those routinely received (e.g. patients' samples) can be difficult to ensure. The use of pooled sera can obscure differences in bias that might be revealed by use of serum from individual patients (9). In addition, serum specimens containing pure exogenous analyte can erroneously demonstrate closer agreement between laboratories than can be achieved with serum containing only endogenous analyte, owing to the greater heterogeneity of analyte structure in the latter.

Many EQA schemes use lyophilized samples, but this can induce changes in the matrix of serum samples and lead to differences in behaviour between the lyophilized EQA sera and the test sera. In addition, reconstitution errors may occur. Liquid specimens avoid some of these difficulties, but they can only be used where rapid specimen delivery (e.g. 48 h or less) can be guaranteed.

4.3.2 Definition of target values

The target value is the analyte concentration in the sample against which performance is assessed, and its validity (i.e. closeness to the 'true' value) is of central

Table 8. Key requirements of an EQA scheme for immunoassay

Scheme design

Frequent (e.g. monthly) sample distribution to provide practically relevant and statistically valid data
Rapid return of EQA reports to participants (e.g. within monthly cycle)
Accurate documentation of methods used
Common units for reporting results
EQA samples assayed by participants in exactly the same way as routine specimens
Reports clear and concise

Sample material distributed

Properties identical to patient samples in all assay systems
Analyte concentrations appropriate to use of test
Stable under conditions of sample distribution
Present no avoidable infectious hazard

Definition of target values

Accuracy and stability of targets (e.g. consensus means) can be demonstrated
Reference method values provided where possible

Assessment of performance

Appropriate statistics used, plus record of data reported to scheme
All-laboratory, method-group and individual laboratory performances estimated
Gross errors (outliers) highlighted
Other aspects of performance (e.g. test interference, interpretation) assessed where appropriate

---

importance to the credibility of the scheme. It may be defined on the basis of one of the following:

4.3.2.1 Reference method value

This is the preferred target if EQA is to promote the use of accurate methods, but in practice such targets have limited application in immunoassay owing to the lack of reference methods for other than a few analytes. They have been most widely used for steroid assays, where isotope-dilution mass-spectrometry methods are available. Replication of RMVs in more than one centre is essential and considerable financial and experimental resources are needed to sustain this approach.

4.3.2.2 All-laboratory consensus mean

The mean (or median) of results from all laboratories is applicable to a wide range of analytes, is easily calculated, and provided that there are sufficient participating laboratories (10 or more), is statistically reasonably robust. The stability of the estimates of mean and overall scatter can be improved by excluding 'outlier' values, which is best done by the trimming technique described by Healy (10). Although its relationship to the true value is rarely known for immunoassays and it is vulnerable to being overly influenced by the most commonly used methods (which may be inherently biased), its general applicability and simplicity ensures its use as the most widely used target for EQA schemes.

4.3.2.3 Method or grouped method means

This is analogous to the all-laboratory consensus mean but includes users of only a single method, or of a group of closely related methods. Method means should be used with caution: they might assist comparison of laboratory performance with that of its immediate peers, but unsatisfactory or changing performance of the method will remain undetected.

4.3.2.4 Value defined by preparative procedure

This can be used where an adequate supply of the pure analyte is available, and can be accurately weighed in to the specimen, for example in EQA of drug immunoassay. However, such specimens will not reflect the effect of metabolites in endogenous specimens and can seriously underestimate the scatter of results between methods and laboratories.

4.3.3 Assessment of performance

As outlined above, EQA schemes provide data describing all-laboratory, method-group and laboratory performance. The details of how this is done differ between schemes, e.g. choice of target, use of log-transformation, methods of outlier rejection, etc.

4.3.3.1 All-method (overall) performance

The all-laboratory mean ($\bar{X}_a$) and scatter (sd_{xa}) of results provide a measure of the 'state of the art' for measurement of the analyte (*Figure 8*). The closeness of the overall mean to an RMV, (where available), or to a recovery-validated target can indicate the accuracy of methods in use. The scatter (sd_a) of the overall distribution reflects the closeness of agreement between methods and laboratories. The limits of the overall distribution ($\bar{X}_a \pm 3sd_{xa}$) may be used to define the criteria for acceptable performance in some proficiency testing schemes.

Overall between-laboratory agreement for a wide range of immunoassays in the UK NEQAS is summarized in *Table 9*.

Several points are illustrated: agreement is relatively good for high concentration, structurally well-defined analytes (total thyroxine, α-fetoprotein), but is less good at low concentrations (e.g. female compared with male testosterone), and for unstable, technically demanding analytes (e.g. adrenocorticotrophin). Several EQA schemes show a modest trend towards improved overall agreement with time, in part reflecting increased automation of methods; however, differences between methods (in calibration and in specificity) are important factors limiting further improvements.

4.3.3.2 Method performance

EQA provides a powerful tool for assessing method performance. Provided that the method has a sufficient number of users (10 or more), and that the target value can be validated as above, the method bias $(X_m - X_t).100/X_t$ and the

Table 9. Overall between-laboratory agreement (geometric coefficient of variation, GCV %) in the UK NEQAS for a range of immunoassays for hormones and tumour markers in serum (1998)

Overall between-laboratory agreement	Analyte
Very good (GCV < 10 %)	α-fetoprotein
	Total thyroxine
Good (GCV 10 to 15%)	Cortisol
	FSH
	Progesterone
	Testosterone (male)
	TSH
	Total tri-iodothyronine
Moderate (GCV 16 to 20%)	Calcitonin
	Free thyroxine
	Growth hormone
	hCG (total and intact)
	Oestradiol
	Prolactin
	Parathyroid hormone
Poor (GCV 21 to 40)	Adrenocorticotrophin
	Carcinoembryonic antigen
	Free triiodothyronine
	LH
	Testosterone (female)

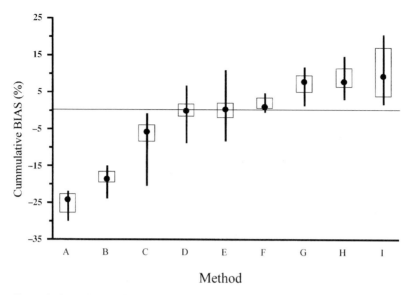

Figure 9. Bias of methods in the UK NEQAS for serum FSH. Bias is expressed as the percentage deviation from the all-laboratory mean and is based on 30 specimens distributed over a 6-month period. The box and whisker plot shows the median, interquartile range and extreme range of bias of laboratories using methods A to I.

within-method, between-laboratory scatter of results (sd_{xm}) may indicate, respectively, the security of method calibration and the stability of the analytical system.

Clear differences in performance of different immunoassay methods are a regular finding in EQA schemes. *Figure 9* shows that bias of immunoassays for serum FSH ranges from −25 to 7%. The causes of bias are complex, but calibration and specificity are important factors. The precision profiles (*Figure 10*) show that automated nonisotopic FSH methods give better between-laboratory agreement than manual RIA, but there are differences in precision among the automated methods, which might indicate differences in the robustness of assay reagents and/or instrumentation. Such comparative data from EQA schemes can be helpful to laboratories in their selection of new methods.

4.3.3.3 Laboratory performance

EQA is unique in providing the laboratory with objective assessments of its bias and precision, although the way in which these statistics are estimated differ between schemes. Bias is usually estimated as the mean percentage deviation of the laboratory results from the chosen target, either the all-laboratory consensus mean or the method mean. The estimation of precision depends on the sample distribution plan. Some schemes distribute duplicated sample aliquots over a period, precision being estimated directly from the sd of the duplicates. Other schemes distribute nonreplicated samples, and estimate precision as the scatter of relative total error [sd of $(x_i - \bar{X}_a).100/\bar{X}_a$, *Figure 8*]. Note that the latter

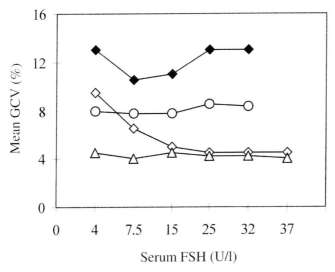

Figure 10. Between-laboratory precision profiles of four methods in the UK NEQAS for serum FSH. Solid symbols indicate laboratories using RIA methods and open symbols indicate automated nonisotopic immunometric assays. The data are based on 30 specimens distributed over a 6-month period.

estimate will also reflect concentration- and sample-dependent differences in bias. In order to provide sufficient data for performance estimates, schemes combine data over several months and an episode of poor performance may take some time to pass through the assessment 'window'. Nonanalytical errors (e.g. sample transposition) which cause incorrect results may be recorded separately to avoid distorting the record of assay performance.

Many schemes use scoring systems in order to simplify data presentation. These often combine bias and precision estimates (i.e. reflect the total error) and are intended to alert laboratories to a possible problem requiring more detailed investigation. Scoring systems may also be used with performance criteria, based on what is achievable and desirable, as a stimulus towards good practice. Figures 11 and 12 are extracts from an actual EQA report.

4.3.4 EQA and audit of laboratory practice

EQA provides an effective audit tool to assess laboratory practice. Clinical laboratories can be asked to interpret their results in the context of a given clinical presentation (11). Differences in normal ranges, even among laboratories using the same methods, can be shown, as can changes in methods used and test profiles offered (e.g. for thyroid function tests). Feedback of this information to participants through the EQA scheme is a valuable means of encouraging best laboratory practice.

4.4 Limitations of EQA

Although EQA is a powerful tool for improvement in quality of analysis it has limitations and can present some risks (*Table 10*).

UK NEQAS for AFP, CEA and hCG.

Laboratory

Distribution : 126   Date : 4-Aug-1998

Page 3 of 5

Analyte : C.E.A. (U/L IRP 73/601)

Your BIAS (%) is	−8.7
Your VAR (%) is	14.4
Your method is	Method D

Spec.	Pool	Pool description / Treatments / Additions
391	T446	Base pool of sera obtained at therapeutic venesection.
392	T447	Colorectal cancer patient serum (B) in base pool T446.
393	T431	Colorectal cancer patient serum (A) in base pool T429.
394	T448	Colorectal cancer patient serum (B) in base pool T446.
395	T449	Colorectal cancer patient serum (B) in base pool T446.

☐ All methods
▨ Method D

Specimen : 391

	n	Mean	GCV
All methods	159	29	18.0
Method A	49	27	14.9
Method B	8	28	1.0
Method C	5	35	16.4
Method D	25	30	9.9
Method E	16	26	5.6
Method F	9	30	5.3
Method G	9	26	13.2
Method H	22	35	7.6

no. of laboratories

Your result	29
Your target (ALTM)	29
Your deviation (%)	−0.6

Specimen : 392

	n	Mean	GCV
All methods	162	78	15.3
Method A	49	71	9.4
Method B	8	72	17.4
Method C	5	91	14.4
Method D	26	78	9.9
Method E	16	79	6.1
Method F	9	75	6.2
Method G	9	75	8.9
Method H	23	97	4.3

no. of laboratories

Your result	75
Your target (ALTM)	78
Your deviation (%)	−3.9

Figure 11. Extract from a monthly report in the UK NEQAS for serum carcinoembryonic antigen (CEA), showing overall, method and individual laboratory performance.

Figure 12. Extract from a monthly report in the UK NEQAS for serum carcinoembryonic antigen (CEA), showing a cumulative performance table for a single laboratory. Pool identifiers are listed down the left column, in order of increasing concentration. The laboratory result, all-laboratory mean target value, and the difference between these are listed in columns, for five specimens issued each month. BIAS and VAR are the bias and scatter of the bias for the 6 months to date. See text for further details.

Pool (exclusion) [Type]	Distribution 121 10-Mar-1998 result	target	% bias	Distribution 122 7-Apr-1998 result	target	% bias	Distribution 123 12-May-1998 result	target	% bias	Distribution 124 9-Jun-1998 result	target	% bias	Distribution 125 7-Jul-1998 result	target	% bias	Distribution 126 4-Aug-1998 result	target	% bias
(T433) [B]																		
(T446) [B]				(<29)	19											(29)	29	(-0.6)
(T429)	(39)	38	(+2.3)							29	38	-23.7						
T440																		
(T432) [N]				(54)	41	(+30.6)												
T444 [B]																		
T419	75	75	+0.7				59	59	+0.1				36	42	-15.1	75	76	-0.9
T431				87.6	88	0.0	75	75	-0.4				64	75	-14.7	75	78	-3.9
T447 [N]																		
T434	121	121	-0.4															
T427 [N]							121	121	-0.1	10	121	-91.7	102	120	-14.9	103	146	-29.5
T441										146	154	-4.9						
T448 [N]																		
T435 [N]				146	155	-5.7	182	182	-0.1									
T439 [N]																		
T407				140	184	-23.8	230	230	-0.2									
T438 [N]													265	310	-14.4			
T405	301	305	-1.3							467	484	-3.5	530	623	-15.0	250	387	-35.5
T430	380	377	+0.9															
T449										657	715	-8.2						
T442																		
T445 [N]																		
T443																		
method	Method D		+0.0	Method D		-9.8	Method D		-0.1	Method D		-26.4	Method D		-14.8	Method D		-17.5
mean bias BIAS	+1.0			+0.1			+0.2			-3.6			-5.7			-8.7		
VAR	10.6			9.3			7.2			11.5			10.8			14.4		

291

Table 10. Limitations and risks in EQA

• Consensus mean target value not accurate
• May inhibit development of improved methods giving numerically different results
• EQA scheme samples do not behave identically to patient samples in assay method
• EQA scheme samples not processed in laboratory identically to patient samples
• Laboratory performance may differ in different EQA schemes

The major limitation of EQA is that the target value, unless defined by a reference method, may be inaccurate. Consensus means reflect the performance of the most commonly used method(s), which may be incorrectly calibrated, or exhibit changes in performance with reagent reformulations. A combined approach to targeting EQA samples has been proposed (12), based on regular use of method targets to assess laboratory performance, with occasional distribution of material with an RMV to assess method bias, and establish traceability of results.

Other limitations of EQA are those that arise in any audit or survey using artificially introduced material (i.e. nonstandard treatment of EQA samples and results).

Finally, the validity of EQA data on method and laboratory performance may be challenged because performance data in different schemes do not agree. This may be due to differences in sample material (e.g. lyophilized or liquid), differences in methods mix or differences in the performance indices used. Laboratories should evaluate carefully EQA schemes against the principles set out in *Table 8*.

4.5 Making use of EQA and IQC data

EQA data should be reviewed and interpreted in relation to IQC performance, taking particular account of the nature of the specimens on which the data are based. Gradual shifts in bias and or precision may be identified. Such reviews are best undertaken at regular (e.g. monthly) meetings of all staff involved. Audit of pre-and post-analytical errors can also be reviewed at such meetings, providing a forum for continuous and comprehensive audit of the laboratory service.

References

1. CITAC (1995). *CITAC Guide 1, International Guide to Quality in Analytical Chemistry. An aid to accreditation*. Laboratory of the Government Chemist, Teddington, Middlesex, UK.
2. Burnett, D. (1996). *Understanding accreditation in laboratory medicine*. ACB Venture Publications, London.
3. Westgard, J. O. (1994). In *Tietz Textbook of Clinical Chemistry* (eds Burtis, C. A. and Ashwood, E. R.), 2nd edn, p. 548. W. B. Saunders, Philadelphia.
4. National Institute for Biological Standards and Control (1999). *Biological reference materials 1999*. NIBSC, South Mimms.

5. Joint Research Centre, Institute for Reference Materials and Measurements (IRMM) (1999). *BCR Reference materials, catalogue 1999*. IRMM, Geel. http://www.irmm.jrc.be/mrm.html

6. Westgard, J. O., Barry, P. L., Hunt, M. R., and Groth, T. (1981). *Clin. Chem.* **27**, 493.

7. Mugan, K, Carlson, I. H., and Westgard, J. O. (1994). *J. Clin. Immunoassay* **17**, 216.

8. Westgard, J. O. and Stein, B. (1997). *Clin. Chem.* **43**, 400.

9. Bacon, R. R.A., Hunter, W. M., and McKenzie, I. (1983). In *Immunoassays for clinical chemistry* (eds Hunter, W. M. and Corrie, J. E. T.), p. 669. Churchill Livingstone, Edinburgh.

10. Healy, M. J.R. (1979). *Clin Chem.* **25**, 675.

11. Sturgeon, C. M., Seth, J., Ellis, A. R. (1996). *Proceedings of the UK NEQAS participants meeting,* **2**, p. 110. Association of Clinical Biochemists, London.

12. Thienpoint, L. M. and Stockl, D. (1995). *Proceedings of the UK NEQAS Participants Meeting, 1994,* **1**, pp. 44–47. Association of Clinical Biochemists, London.

Appendix 1
Suitable reagents and other requisites

Core list of suppliers is available on-line at
http://www4.oup.co.uk/biochemistry/pas/supplier

Antibodies

Linscotts Directory:
www.antibodyresource.com; www.wenet.net/~sjdanko/solidusbiotech.html
www.researchd.com
Sigma
Immunotech SA
Pierce Chemical Co
Roche Diagnostics

Cell lines

American Type Culture Collection, VA, USA
Imperial Laboratories Ltd., Hampshire, UK

Immunogens

Electrophoresis and chromatography equipment

Amersham Pharmacia Biotech UK Ltd, Little Chalfont, UK
Bio-Rad Laboratories Ltd

Polysacchamine

Bionostics Limited, Bedfordshire, UK.

Reagents for peptide synthesis and protein modification

Calbiochem-Novabiochem (UK) Ltd, Nottingham, UK
Pierce Chemical Company, Rockford, USA
Prochem Inc., Rockford, USA

OligoPrep and other media for gel electrophoresis

National Diagnostics (UK) Ltd, East Yorkshire, UK

Immunoassay kits

This a list of the largest manufacturers of immunoassay kits, mostly for human
clinical applications:

Abbot Laboratories
Bayer AG
Behringwerke AG
BioMerieux sa
Bio-Rad laboratories
Boehringer Mannheim Gmbh
Byk-Sangtec Diagnostica
Ciba corning Diagnostics Corp
Dako Corporation
E. Merck
Immunodiagnostic Systems Ltd
Incstar Corporation
Johnson & Johnson Clinical Diagnostics Inc.
Pharmacia Diagnostics AB
Randox Laboratories
Sanofi Diagnostics Pasteur
Syva Company
Walloc Oy

Labels

Chemical reagents from Sigma Aldrich
Heterobifunctional reagents from Pierce, Calbiochem and Sigma
Gel filtration from Amersham Pharmacia Biotech, BioRad and BioSepra
Enzyme substrate, from Sigma Aldrich, Calbiochem, Biosynth AG and
Boehringer-Mannheim
Steroids derivatives from Steraloids
Concentration and ultrafiltration, Millipore

Quality assurance requisites

QC Sera

Ciba Corning Diagnostics
Biorad Diagnostics Group
Nycomed Pharma AS
Sartorius Ltd

EQA scheme providers

CNR EQA Immunocheck, Pisa, Italy
College of American Pathologists, Northfield, USA
D Gesellschaft f Klin Chemie, (Dr Rolf Kruse), Bonn, Germany
Labquality, Helsinki, Finland
New York Department of Health, Albany, NY, USA
LWBA, Afd Experimentele en Chemische Endocrinologie, Nijmegen, The
Netherlands
Murex Biotech Limited, Kent, UK

Ontario Laboratory Proficiency Testing Program, Ontario, Canada
Randox Laboratories Ltd, Northern Ireland
RCPA–AACB Program, St Leonards, Australia
Welsh External Quality Assessment Schemes (WEQAS), Cardiff, UK
UK National Quality Assessment Schemes (UK NEQAS), Sheffield, S5 7YZ, UK

Useful contacts

National Institute for Biological Standards and Control (NIBSC), Potters Bar, Hertfordshire, UK
Joint Research Centre, Institute for Reference Materials and Measurements (IRMM), GEEL, Belgium
NCCLS, Wayne, PA, USA
Westgard Quality Corporation, Ogonquit, USA
Laboratory of the Government Chemist, Middlesex, UK

Solid-phase reagents

Microtitre plates

Passive Adsorption

Corning Costar: Ultra-low, Medium and High Binding
NUNC: PolySorp™ medium binding; MaxiSorp™ high binding
Pierce Chemical: ImmunoWare™ high binding
Dynex: Immulon® 1B (medium binding), 2 HB (high binding), 4 HBX (high binding extra)

Activated

Corning Costar: *N*-oxysuccindimide amine binding; hydrazide carbohydrate binding; maleimide sulfhydryl binding; universal covalent high binding (UV abstractable hydrogens)
NUNC: Covalink™ NH2 primary amine surface; Covalink™ NH Secondary amine surface
Pierce Chemical: Reacti-Bind™ maleic anhydride; Reacti-Bind™ streptavidin

Beads

Passive adsorption

Bangs Laboratories: polystyrene (PS); polymethymethacrylate (PMMA); styrene/divinylbenzene (DVB)
Interfacial Dynamics: PS, DVB
Seradyn: OptiBind™ PS
Polysciences: Polybead™ PS, PMMA, DVB

Activated

Bangs: aldehyde, amine, carboxylic acid, chloromethyl, epoxy, hydrazide, hydroxyl, sulfonate, *p*-toluene sulfonyl activated microsphere surfaces;

297

streptavidin; protein A; secondary antibody (e.g. goat anti-mouse) coated.
Interfacial: aldehyde, amine, carboxylic acid, chloromethyl surfaces
Seradyne: OptiLink™ carboxylate modified PS (CM)
Polysciences: Polybead™ amine, carboxyl, hydroxyl, melamine, zwitterionic, chloromethyl surfaces; covalently attached protein A, protein G, secondary antibodies

Magnetic

Bangs: carboxyl, amine, protein A, streptavidin, secondary antibody coated; encapsulated iron microspheres with surface chemistries
Dynal: Dynabeads® M-500 (5#micron diameter), M-450 (4.5 micron) and M-280 (2.8 micron) polystyrene shell; streptavidin coated; tosyl-activated.
Seradyne: Sera-Mag™ carboxylate modifed (MG-CM); covalently attached streptavidin (MG-SA)
Polysciences: PS, amino, carboxyl; protein A magnetite particles

Membranes

Passive adsorption

Pall: nylon 6,6 based products, Biodyne® A (amphoteric, amino/carboxyl surface groups), B (positively charged, quaternary amine surface groups), C (negatively charged, carboxyl surface groups); FluoroTrans® PVDF membranes
Schleicher & Schuell: nitrocellulose based products, Protran™, Optitran™; nylon 6,6 based products, Nytran™ and Nytran™ Plus; Westran™ PVDF membranes
Millipore: Immobilon™ -P (PVDF), -NC (nitrocellulose) -Ny (nylon) membranes

Activated

Pall: Immunodyne® ABC chemically activated, high binding hydrophilic membrane for the covalent immobilization of proteins
Millipore: Immobilon™-AV Affinity Membrane (covalent attachment of amino-ligands)

Filter bottom microplates

Millipore: MulitScreen™ Assay Systems with Immobilon™ membranes
Whatman Polyfiltronics: Unifilter® with Whatman filters; nitrocellulose; PVDF, nylon or custom membranes

Tubes

NUNC: MiniSorp™ low binding

Chemicals, other reagents and materials

Pierce Chemical: extensive selection of cross-linking reagents; protein modification reagents; blocking buffers
Sigma Aldrich: a variety of crosslinking reagents, protein modification reagents, blocking buffers, solvents and polymers
Polysciences: monomers and polymers for surface coating
KaPak Corp: KaPak™ polyester barrier film sealpaks

Index